IMPLANTS
in DENTISTRY

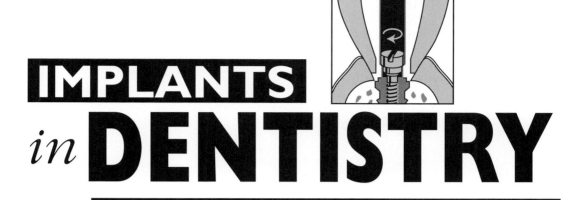

IMPLANTS *in* DENTISTRY

Essentials of Endosseous Implants for Maxillofacial Reconstruction

Michael S. Block, DMD
Professor
Department of Oral and Maxillofacial Surgery
Assistant Dean for Research
Louisiana State University
School of Dentistry
New Orleans, Louisiana

John N. Kent, DDS
Boyd Professor and Head
Department of Oral and Maxillofacial Surgery
Louisiana State University
School of Dentistry
New Orleans, Louisiana

Luis R. Guerra, DDS, MS
Professor
Department of Prosthodontics
Louisiana State University
School of Dentistry
New Orleans, Louisiana

W.B. SAUNDERS COMPANY
A Division of Harcourt Brace & Company
Philadelphia London Toronto Montreal Sydney Tokyo

W.B. SAUNDERS COMPANY

A Division of Harcourt Brace & Company

The Curtis Center
Independence Square West
Philadelphia, Pennsylvania 19106

Library of Congress Cataloging-in-Publication Data

Block, Michael S.

Implants in dentistry: essentials of endosseous implants for maxillofacial reconstruction / Michael S. Block, John N. Kent, Luis R. Guerra.

p.   cm.

ISBN 0–7216–2174–0

1. Implant dentures.   I. Kent, John N.   II. Guerra, Luis R.   III. Title.

[DNLM: 1. Dental Implantation.   WU 640 B651i   1997]

RK667.I45B57   1997   617.6′92—DC21

DNLM/DLC   96–50087

IMPLANTS IN DENTISTRY   ISBN 0–7216–2174–0

Printed in the United States of America.

Last digit is the print number: 9   8   7   6   5   4   3   2   1

To my wife, Colleen, and my daughters, Courtney and Celeste, for their support and love. In addition, I would like to dedicate this to all of my teachers, such as Drs. Kent and Guerra, for their dedication to teaching and for sharing their knowledge with me.

MICHAEL S. BLOCK

To my wife, Virginia, and children, John, Kelley, Jeff, Andrea, and Edwin, who are all, and will continue to be, students.

JOHN N. KENT

To my wife, Elizabeth, for her patience and understanding and to faculty everywhere whose efforts in education, service, and research ensure the future of the dental profession.

LUIS R. GUERRA

CONTRIBUTORS

Michael S. Block, D.M.D.
Professor, Department of Oral and Maxillofacial Surgery and Assistant Dean for Research, Louisiana State University School of Dentistry, New Orleans, Louisiana
Anesthesia, Incision Design, Surgical Principles, Exposure Techniques; Placement of Implants into Extraction Sites; Maxillary Sinus Bone Grafting

Gene K. Brown
Staff, Ozarks Medical Center, West Plains, Missouri
Team Management of Atrophic Edentulism with Autogenous Inlay, Veneer, and Split Grafts with Endosseous Implants

John Brunski, Ph.D.
Professor, Department of Biomedical Engineering, Rensselaer Polytechnic Institute, Troy, New York
Biocompatibility, Biofunctionality, and Biomechanics of Dental Implants—Tissue Response to Implanted Materials

Harold S. Cardash, B.D.S., L.D.S., R.C.S. (Eng)
Department of Restorative Dentistry, Tel Aviv University, Tel Aviv, Israel
Hybrid Dentures

Richard F. Caudill, D.M.D.
Associate Professor (Previously), Department of Periodontics, Louisiana State University School of Dentistry, New Orleans, Louisiana; Research Director, Implant Innovations, West Palm Beach, Florida
Guided Bone Regeneration and Implants: History and Case Reports—Guided Bone Regeneration in Conjunction with Dental Endosseous Implants

Thomas A. Collins, D.D.S., M.S.
Director, Mid America Center for Osseointegration; Staff, St. John's Regional Health Center, Cox Medical Center, and Springfield Community Hospital, Springfield, Missouri
Team Management of Atrophic Edentulism with Autogenous Inlay, Veneer, and Split Grafts with Endosseous Implants

Stephen D. Cook, Ph.D.
Professor and Director of Orthopaedic Research, Department of Orthopaedic Surgery, Tulane University School of Medicine; Clinical Professor, Louisiana State University School of Dentistry, New Orleans, Louisiana
Biocompatibility, Biofunctionality, and Biomechanics of Dental Implants—Tissue Response to Implanted Materials

Arthur W. Curley, B.S., J.D.
Assistant Professor, University of the Pacific; Faculty Lecturer, University of California, San Francisco, San Francisco, California
Medical-Legal Ramifications of Dental Implants

Jeanette E. Dalton, M.E.
Biomedical Research Associate, Department of Orthopaedic Surgery, Tulane University School of Medicine, New Orleans, Louisiana
Biocompatibility, Biofunctionality, and Biomechanics of Dental Implants—Tissue Response to Implanted Materials

Thomas D. Driskell, B.S.
Former Director of Research and Development, Dental Implant Division, Stryker Corp., Kalamazoo, Michigan
Dental Implants: A Historical Perspective

Israel M. Finger, B.D.S., M.Sc., M.Ed., D.D.S.
Professor and Coordinator, Postgraduate Prosthodontics, Louisiana State University School of Dentistry; Consulting Staff, Ochsner Clinic and Charity Hospital, New Orleans, Louisiana
Principles of Implant Prosthodontics; Fixed Prosthodontics; Development of the Occlusal Scheme in Implant Prosthodontics

Luis R. Guerra, D.D.S., M.S.
Professor, Department of Prosthodontics, Louisiana State University School of Dentistry; Chief, Department of Dentistry, Charity Hospital of New Orleans, New Orleans, Louisiana

Principles of Implant Prosthodontics; Implant Overdentures; Hybrid Dentures; Fixed Prosthodontics; Development of the Occlusal Scheme in Implant Prosthodontics

†David R. Hoffman, D.D.S.
Implants and Orthodontics

Keith Hoffmann, D.D.S., PhD.
Associate Professor, Department of Oral and Maxillofacial Surgery, Loma Linda University School of Dentistry; Chief of Service, Oral and Maxillofacial Surgery, Loma Linda University Medical Center, Loma Linda; Riverside County Hospital, Riverside, California
Anatomic Considerations—Maxilla

Aydogan Huseyin, B.D.S., M.S.
Fellow, Postgraduate Implant Prosthodontics, Ohio State University School of Dentistry, Columbus, Ohio
Implant Screw Mechanics

Neale Johnson, D.D.S.
Associate Staff, Cedar County Memorial Hospital, Eldorado Springs, Missouri
Team Management of Atrophic Edentulism with Autogenous Inlay, Veneer, and Split Grafts with Endosseous Implants

Eugene E. Keller, D.D.S., M.S.D.
Professor, Oral and Maxillofacial Surgery, Mayo Medical School and Mayo Foundation; Consultant, Oral and Maxillofacial Surgery, Mayo Medical Center, Rochester, Minnesota
Composite Grafting

John N. Kent, D.D.S.
Boyd Professor and Head, Department of Oral and Maxillofacial Surgery, Louisiana State University School of Dentistry, New Orleans, Louisiana
Healing of Endosseous Implants—The Wound Response; Maxillary Sinus Bone Grafting; Maxillofacial Reconstruction in the Compromised Patient

Richard Kraut, D.D.S.
Associate Professor, Department of Dentistry, Albert Einstein College of Medicine of Yeshiva University; Director, Oral and Maxillofacial Surgery Residency Training Program, Montefiore Medical Center, Bronx, New York
Radiologic Planning for Dental Implants

———————
†Deceased 1996

Jay P. Malmquist, D.M.D., F.A.C.D.
Associate Professor, Department of Oral Pathology and Oral and Maxillofacial Surgery, Oregon Health Sciences University School of Medicine; Private Practice, Portland, Oregon
Guided Bone Regeneration and Transplants: History and Case Reports: Use of Membrane Technique to Regenerate Bone with Endosseous Dental Implants

Ronald Marks, D.D.S.
Clinical Associate Professor, Oral and Maxillofacial Surgery, Louisiana State University Medical Centers, Shreveport and New Orleans; Clinical Assistant Professor of Surgery, Tulane Medical Center, New Orleans; Private Practice, Alexandria, Louisiana
Medical-Legal Ramifications of Dental Implants

John A. Mayo, Ph.D.
Professor of Microbiology, and Clinical Professor of Periodontics, Louisiana State University School of Dentistry, New Orleans, Louisiana
Microbiology of Dental Implants

Edwin A. McGlumphy, D.D.S., M.S.
Associate Professor, Restorative and Prosthodontics Dentistry, Ohio State University School of Dentistry, Columbus, Ohio
Implant Screw Mechanics

Arturo J. Mendez, D.D.S., M.Sc.
Professor, Department of Removable Prosthodontics, Louisiana State University School of Dentistry; Visiting Staff, Charity Hospital, New Orleans, Louisiana
Implant Overdentures

Paul Mercier, D.D.S., F.R.C.D.(C.)
Director, Maxillary Atrophy Clinic, St. Mary's Hospital, Montreal, Quebec
Resorption Patterns of the Residual Ridge

Dale J. Misiek, D.M.D.
Professor, Department of Oral and Maxillofacial Surgery, and Coordinator, Advanced Education Program in Oral and Maxillofacial Surgery, Louisiana State University School of Dentistry, New Orleans, Louisiana
Maxillofacial Reconstruction in the Compromised Patient

John P. Neary, M.D., D.D.S.
Assistant Clinical Professor, Case Western Reserve University School of Medicine, Cleveland,

Ohio; Assistant Clinical Professor, Louisiana State University School of Medicine, New Orleans, Louisiana; Private Practice, Kent, Ohio
Medical Evaluation

Bill D. Nunn, D.D.S.

Board Member, Center for Osseointegration; Private Practice, Springfield, Missouri
Team Management of Atrophic Edentulism with Autogenous Inlay, Veneer, and Split Grafts with Endosseous Implants

James D. Ruskin, D.M.D., M.D.

Associate Professor, Director of Residency Education Program, Department of Oral and Maxillofacial Surgery, University of Florida College of Dentistry, Gainesville, Florida
Inferior Alveolar Nerve Repositioning Procedures for Placement of Dental Implants

Leonard B. Shulman, D.M.D., M.S.

Lecturer, Division of Implant Dentistry, Department of Oral and Maxillofacial Surgery, Harvard University School of Dental Medicine, Boston; Private Practice, Waltham, Massachusetts
Dental Implants: A Historical Perspective

John Stover, D.D.S., Ph.D.

Resident, Department of Oral and Maxillofacial Surgery, Louisiana State University School of Dentistry, New Orleans, Louisiana
Anatomic Considerations—Mandible

Raymond A. Yukna, D.M.D., M.S.

Professor, Department Head, and Coodinator of Postgraduate Periodontics, Louisiana State University School of Dentistry, New Orleans, Louisiana
Periodontal Considerations for Dental Implants; Diagnosis and Treatment of the Ailing/Failing Implant

Jozef Zoldos, D.D.S., M.D.

Former Chief Resident, Department of Oral and Maxillofacial Surgery, Louisiana State University School of Dentistry, New Orleans, Louisiana; currently Resident in Plastic and Maxillofacial Surgery, University of Pittsburgh, Pittsburgh, Pennsylvania
Healing of Endosseous Implants—The Wound Response

PREFACE

Endosseous implants are important for comprehensive treatment planning in patients who have missing teeth. Dental implants are now included in dental school and graduate program curricula and have gained widespread acceptance in dental practice. This book is a version of *Endosseous Implants for Maxillofacial Reconstruction,* designed to meet the needs of dental students and clinicians who have little experience with dental implants. It provides historical background and fundamental and basic concepts in wound healing, anatomy, radiology, treatment planning, surgery, and prosthetics for dental implants. The material is presented in a format that allows the clinician to utilize a variety of implant systems successfully by following the fundamentals as taught in 26 chapters.

Section 1 concerns *Pretreatment Considerations.* The history of dental implants is presented in the first chapter. The resorption pattern of mandibular and maxillary bone resulting in edentulous ridges with varying anatomy is presented in Chapter 2 to put into perspective the problems that clinicians face in treating the edentulous patient. Chapter 3 presents a review of the preoperative medical assessment of the dental implant patient, with a rationale for adjunctive therapy for patients with medical problems. The anatomy of the jaws is described in a two-part chapter dealing with the mandible and the maxilla. Radiographic preoperative assessment of the patient, including the use of computerized imaging, is presented in Chapter 6. The tissue response at the implant site is described, along with classic principles of soft and hard tissue wound healing, and the biocompatibility and biofunctionality of implantable materials.

Section 2 covers the *Restorative Considerations* for dental implants. The prosthetic chapters describe fundamental concepts that when followed result in mechanically sound prosthetic reconstruction. Treatment planning is discussed from the prosthetic aspect, with separate chapters dedicated to overdentures, hybrid dentures, and fixed prostheses. The principles of prosthetic reconstruction are detailed in such a manner that

the clinician can extrapolate these principles to the patient. A unique chapter on the mechanics involved in connecting the prostheses to the implants allows the reader an understanding of how to keep a restoration connected to an implant without mobility. Occlusion is discussed in a separate chapter.

Section 3 focuses on *Surgical Considerations.* The first chapter in this section describes anesthesia, incisions, and exposure techniques that can be universally applied to all implants. Chapter 15 includes surgical principles and specific recommendations on placing implants into fresh extraction sites, with examples of when to delay immediate placement and how to handle bone defects. A separate portion of that chapter deals with anterior maxillary aesthetic restorations. A comprehensive review of the use of implants for orthodontic anchors, including visions of the use of implants or onplants for facial orthopedics, is included in Chapter 16. Nerve repositioning for implant placement is discussed, as well as the treatment of sensory nerve complications following implant placement in the posterior mandible. The chapter on guided tissue regeneration (GTR) comprehensively covers the history and current methods of GTR with membranes, including clinical examples of the use of membranes for osteopromotion. The following chapters demonstrate the surgical reconstruction of bone defects and the use of implants for reconstruction of the compromised patient. Maxillary sinus grafting is reviewed historically and then demonstrated through case examples. The techniques for onlay grafting are discussed first as principles and then demonstrated by clinical examples. The team approach for management of these compromised patients emphasizes that the restoration drives the implant placement and the requirements for adjunctive grafting procedures. Reconstruction in patients with severe maxillary resorption resulting in extreme atrophy is described, including the use of interpositional and onlay techniques. The rehabilitation of the patient with full thickness maxillary and mandibular defects resulting from tumor ablation or trauma is covered with attention to fundamental tissue manipulation that results in soft and hard tissue replacement in otherwise compromised tissue beds.

Section 4 concerns *Soft Tissue and Microbiological Considerations*, including the reaction of the soft tissue to implants. The microbiological aspects are discussed by a microbiologist. The periodontal considerations are discussed in general with recommendations for maintenance. The next chapter deals with the problem of bone loss resulting from periodontal-like mechanisms. The rationale for treatment of the "ailing" implant is discussed in detail. The final chapter discusses the medical-legal aspects of dental implants, with specific reference to risk management principles and avoidance of legal problems in the event of complications.

This book contains basic information for the beginner in this field, as well as an introduction to meticulous and comprehensive procedures for the more experienced clinician challenged with complicated reconstructions. The foundation of knowledge presented in this book allows the reader an appreciation for why, and then how, to utilize basic wound healing principles for re-establishment of missing anatomy.

We hope this book will be useful for dental students, hygiene students, assistants, lab technicians, and clinicians who are looking for an introductory, generic reference on the use of endosseous implants for reconstruction of the dental arches. The use of dental implants is here to stay and has evolved historically into a definite treatment option. Rapid improvements in techniques will demand that readers keep up with the literature and also attend meetings dedicated to dental implants. Portions of this book may not change in time, but other sections will need to be revised and updated.

MICHAEL S. BLOCK, DMD
JOHN N. KENT, DDS
LUIS R. GUERRA, DDS, MS

ACKNOWLEDGMENT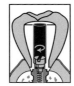

The editors would like to thank the efforts of the following Louisiana State University School of Dentistry staff members: Ms. Maureen Raymond in the word-processing center, Robert Raben in the photography studio, Kathy Martello in the art department, and Denise St. Clair, administrative assistant, Department of Oral and Maxillofacial Surgery.

CONTENTS

SECTION *1*

Pretreatment Considerations 1

CHAPTER *1*

Dental Implants: A Historical Perspective 2
Leonard B. Shulman
Thomas D. Driskell
Revised by Michael S. Block

CHAPTER *2*

Resorption Patterns of the Residual Ridge 10
Paul Mercier
Revised by Michael S. Block

CHAPTER *3*

Medical Evaluation 17
John P. Neary
Revised by Michael S. Block

CHAPTER *4*

Anatomic Considerations 21
a. Mandible 21
John Stover
Revised by Michael S. Block
b. Maxilla 27
Keith Hoffmann
Revised by Michael S. Block

CHAPTER *5*

Radiologic Planning for Dental Implants 33
Richard Kraut
Revised by Michael S. Block

CHAPTER *6*

Healing of Endosseous Implants—The Wound Response 45
Jozef Zoldos
John N. Kent
Revised by John N. Kent
and Michael S. Block

CHAPTER *7*

Biocompatibility, Biofunctionality, and Biomechanics of Dental Implants 54
Part 1. Tissue Response to Implanted Materials 54
Stephen D. Cook
Jeanette E. Dalton
Revised by Luis R. Guerra
Part 2. Biomechanics of Dental Implants 63
John Brunski
Revised by Michael S. Block
and Luis R. Guerra

SECTION *2*

Restorative Considerations 73

CHAPTER *8*

Principles of Implant Prosthodontics 74
Luis R. Guerra
Israel M. Finger
Revised by Luis R. Guerra

CHAPTER *9*

Implant Screw Mechanics 87
Edwin A. McGlumphy
Aydogan Huseyin
Revised by Luis R. Guerra

CHAPTER 10

Implant Overdentures 94
Arturo J. Mendez
Luis R. Guerra
Revised by Luis R. Guerra

CHAPTER 11

Hybrid Dentures 112
Luis R. Guerra
Harold S. Cardash
Revised by Luis R. Guerra

CHAPTER 12

Fixed Prosthodontics 122
Israel M. Finger
Luis R. Guerra
Neil Boner
Revised by Luis R. Guerra

CHAPTER 13

Development of the Occlusal
Scheme in Implant
Prosthodontics 138
Israel M. Finger
Luis R. Guerra
Revised by Luis R. Guerra

SECTION 3

Surgical
Considerations 149

CHAPTER 14

Anesthesia, Incision Design,
Surgical Principles, Exposure
Techniques 150
Michael S. Block

CHAPTER 15

Placement of Implants into
Extraction Sites 157
Michael S. Block

CHAPTER 16

Implants and Orthodontics .. 167
David R. Hoffman
Revised by Michael S. Block

CHAPTER 17

Inferior Alveolar Nerve
Repositioning Procedures
for Placement of Dental
Implants 175
James D. Ruskin
Revised by John N. Kent

CHAPTER 18

Guided Bone Regeneration
and Implants: History and
Case Reports 183
Part 1. Guided Bone
        Regeneration in
        Conjunction with
        Dental Endosseous
        Implants 183
Richard F. Caudill
Revised by Michael S. Block
Part 2. Use of Membrane
        Technique to Regenerate
        Bone with Endosseous
        Dental Implants 192
Jay P. Malmquist
Revised by Michael S. Block

CHAPTER 19

Maxillary Sinus Bone
Grafting 206
Michael S. Block
John N. Kent

CHAPTER 20

Team Management of
Atrophic Edentulism with
Autogenous Inlay, Veneer,
and Split Grafts with
Endosseous Implants 223
Thomas A. Collins
Gene K. Brown
Neale Johnson
Bill D. Nunn
Revised by Michael S. Block

CHAPTER *21*

**Composite Graft
Reconstruction of Advanced
Maxillary Resorption:
Autogenous Iliac Bone,
Titanium Endosseous
Implants** 232
*Eugene E. Keller
Revised by John N. Kent*

CHAPTER *22*

**Maxillofacial Reconstruction
in the Compromised
Patient** 242
*Dale J. Misiek
John N. Kent
Revised by Michael S. Block
and John N. Kent*

SECTION *4*

Soft Tissue and Microbiological Considerations 259

CHAPTER *23*

**Periodontal Considerations
for Dental Implants** 260
Raymond A. Yukna

CHAPTER *24*

**Oral Bacteria and Dental
Implants in Health
and Disease** 265
*John A. Mayo
Revised by Michael S. Block*

CHAPTER *25*

**Diagnosis and Treatment of
the Ailing/Failing Dental
Implant** 274
Raymond A. Yukna

CHAPTER *26*

**Medical-Legal Ramifications
of Dental Implants** 281
*Arthur W. Curley
Ronald Marks*

Index 289

SUGGESTED COURSE OUTLINE

This course outline is used by the Louisiana State University School of Dentistry for third-year dental students. The authors realize that all schools are different, and because of this the intended hours and number of sessions for dental students must be adapted for each school and course.

Implants in Dentistry

ATTENDEES: THIRD-YEAR DENTAL COURSE

1.0 Introduction

1.1 During the past several years great strides have been made in dental implants. The results obtained by using implants in a dental practice have proven reliable and predictable if they are used properly.

1.2 Information concerning dental implants has been made available from several departments in the dental school, each with its own perspective. There exists a need to bring all of this information together under one required course so that all students can benefit.

1.3. This course will allow students the opportunity to gain knowledge about implant design, the implant-bone interface, the implant–soft tissue interface, and prosthodontic considerations. All of these topics must be incorporated in the restoration to ensure long-term success. Well-known authorities in all these areas are presently on the faculty.

1.4. Total clock hours for this course are 38. Three laboratory sessions of 4 hours each are included in this number.

1.5 A multidisciplinary faculty will participate in this course from the Departments of Oral and Maxillofacial Surgery, Periodontics, and Prosthodontics. Guest speakers from other departments and outside sources will also be involved as appropriate.

2.0 Text and Materials

The recommended textbook is *Implants in Dentistry* by Block, Kent, and Guerra. Various reading assignments will be given during the course. Informational material from the manufacturers of various implant systems will be distributed at appropriate intervals.

3.0 Entry Level Skills or Prerequisites

Students entering this course will have successfully completed courses in the Departments of Prosthodontics, Oral and Maxillofacial Surgery, and Periodontics offered in the first and second year of the undergraduate dental school curriculum.

4.0 Instructional Objectives

Upon completion of this course the student will:

4.1 Understand the healing process that occurs around the implant and bone.

4.2 Understand the healing process that occurs around the implant–abutment head complex and the soft tissue.

4.3 Understand the dynamic effects on the surrounding bone of loading the implant.

4.4 Understand the effects on bone and soft tissue of the surgical procedures required to place the implant.

4.5 Be familiar with the surgical techniques required to place endosseous implants.

4.6 Be able to diagnose and plan treatment for implant prostheses.

4.7 Be able to design surgical treatment aids for use in specific prosthesis designs.

4.8 Be able to design prostheses to be supported by implants.

4.9 Understand the importance of occlusion on the loading of implants.

4.10 Be able to select appropriate attachments for use in specific prosthesis designs.

4.11 Understand the importance of selection of the proper impression material for use in implant prosthodontics.

4.12 Have had a hands-on experience in using the transfer mechanism available to ensure accuracy of the master cast.

4.13 Be able to determine the accuracy of the master cast as it relates to the relationship of the dentition to the implants and the implants to each other.

4.14 Understand the laboratory procedures required to ensure a well-fitting prosthesis over implants.

4.15 Recognize the features of a well-fabricated wax rim and its relationship to the final prosthesis.

4.16 Understand the needs for accurate jaw relation records.

4.17 Understand the importance of and relationship between the waxup and the final prosthesis.

4.18 Be able to design frameworks for various prosthetic applications.

4.19 Recognize the importance of the proper selection of materials when prescribing the fabrication of the various frameworks.

4.20 Be able to determine the need for overdentures in the edentulous patient.

4.21 Be able to determine the number of implants required for overdentures completely supported by implants.

4.22. Understand the use of implants in fixed prosthodontics.

4.23. Be familiar with the use of implants in complex restorations.

4.24. Be exposed to at least two different implant systems and be able to evaluate the commercial presentations of two manufacturers.

4.25. Understand the long-term maintenance required for successful implant therapy.

4.26. Be familiar with the salvaging procedures available for preventing implant loss.

4.27. Become aware of the more common problems associated with implants and the methods available to minimize these problems.

5.0 Course Sessions

Section 1: Pretreatment Considerations

Session 1: History of dental implants, morphology of the edentulous patient, and medical considerations for implant patients.

Reference:
Chapter 1. Dental Implants: A Historical Perspective

Chapter 2. Resorption Patterns of the Residual Ridge

Chapter 3. Medical Evaluation

Session 2: Anatomical considerations, radiographic planning, healing of implants, bioengineering principles of dental implants

Reference:
Chapter 4. Anatomic Considerations

Chapter 5. Radiologic Planning for Dental Implants

Chapter 6. Healing of Endosseous Implants

Chapter 7.

1. Biocompatibility and Biofunctionality—Materials

2. Biomechanics of Dental Implants

Section 2: Restorative Considerations

Session 3: Diagnosis and treatment planning

Reference:
Chapter 8. Principles of Implant Prosthodontics

Session 4: Overdentures

Reference:
Chapter 10. Overdentures

Session 5: Hybrid dentures

Reference:
Chapter 11. Hybrid Dentures

Session 6: Fixed prosthodontics

Reference:
Chapter 12. Fixed Prosthodontics

Session 7: Occlusal considerations and implant screw mechanics

Reference:

Chapter 13. Development of the Occlusal Scheme in Implant Prosthodontics

Chapter 9. Implant Screw Mechanics

Section 3: Surgical Considerations

Session 8: Surgical Considerations

Reference:

Chapter 14. Anesthesia, Incision Design, Surgical Principles, Exposure Techniques

Chapter 15. Placement of Implants into Extraction Sites

Chapter 17. Inferior Nerve Considerations

Session 9: Use of guided tissue regeneration in implant dentistry

Chapter 18.

　1. Guided Bone Regeneration

　2. Use of Membrane Technique to Regenerate Bone with Endosseous Dental Implants

Session 10: Advanced surgical procedures and applications

Reference:

Chapter 16. Implants and Orthodontics

Chapter 19. Maxillary Sinus Bone Grafting

Chapter 20. Team Management of Atrophic Edentulism with Autogenous Inlay, Veneer, and Split Grafts with Endosseous Implants

Chapter 21. Composite Grafting

Chapter 22. Reconstruction of the Compromised Patient

Section 4: Soft Tissue and Microbiological Considerations

Session 11: Soft tissue considerations for long-term success

Reference:

Chapter 23. Periodontal Considerations for Dental Implants

Chapter 24. Microbiology of Dental Implants

Chapter 25. Diagnosis and Treatment of the "Failing" Implant

Sessions 12, 13, and 14: Hands-on lab participation

Session 15: Review for final exam

SECTION 1

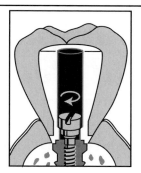

Pretreatment Considerations

CHAPTER 1

Dental Implants: A Historical Perspective

Leonard B. Shulman
Thomas D. Driskell
Revised by Michael S. Block

Historical Sequence of Events
Ancient Implants
Early Implants
Subperiosteal Implants
One-Stage Endosteal Pins, Screws, and
    Cylinders

Blade Implants
Transosteal Implants
Endosteal Root-Form Implants
References

HISTORICAL SEQUENCE OF EVENTS

The history of implant dentistry is best viewed in terms of critical periods and landmark events. The earliest dental implants were of stone and ivory, cited in archaeologic records of China and Egypt before the common era. Gold and ivory dental implants were used in the 16th and 17th centuries.[26]

Metal implant devices of gold, lead, iridium, tantalum, stainless steel, and cobalt alloy were developed in the early 20th century.[41] Cobalt-chromium-molybdenum subperiosteal and titanium blade implants were introduced in the 1940s[13, 31] and 1960s,[29, 37] respectively, and became the most popular and successful implant devices from 1950 through 1980. Exaggerated claims in the wake of long-term morbidity and unpredictability engendered disbelief and disinterest and even denial on the part of organized dentistry. These implants never really "caught on."[1, 6]

The first Dental Implant Consensus Conference, sponsored by the National Institutes of Health (NIH) and Harvard University in 1978 and cochaired by Schnitman and Shulman, was a landmark event; it was entitled *Dental Implants: Benefits and Risks*.[38] Retrospective data on implants were collected and analyzed using life-table methods (Figs. 1–1 and 1–2). The confer-ence established criteria and standards for implant dentistry and issued a mandate to organized dentistry for input and involvement in this new field.

Shortly thereafter, in 1982, at Toronto, Bråne-mark presented work begun 15 years before in Gothenberg, Sweden. In a seminal presentation by his basic and clinical research group, Brånemark's discovery and application of osseointegration were set forth.[50] Five- to 12-year data from clinical trials conducted in Sweden with the Brånemark two-stage titanium screw were presented. Such scientific documentation had never been gathered to this extent in implantology. The Toronto conference opened the door to prompt widespread recognition of the Brånemark implant, not heretofore granted to any implant by organized dentistry. The discovery of osseointegration has undoubtedly been one of the most significant scientific breakthroughs in dentistry over the past 10 to 20 years.

With osseointegration a clinical reality, the root-form implant once again became implantology's most dominant design. A multitude of solid- and hollow-screw and cylindrical forms developed with and without a titanium plasma spray or HA (hydroxylapatite) coating and are now successfully marketed.[22, 23, 39, 50] A flexible abutment to allow implant movement similar to natural teeth was a unique contribution of the plasma-spray press-fit IMZ implant.[23]

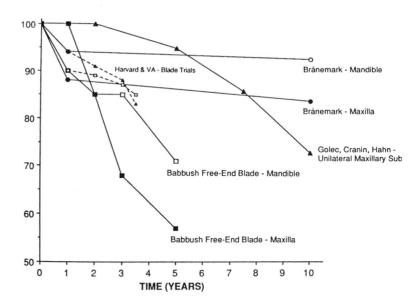

Figure 1–1. Comparative survival of encapsulated individual blade and unilateral subperiosteal implant and osseointegrated root-form implants. (From Shulman LB: Surgical considerations in implant dentistry. J Dent Educ 52:713, 1991.)

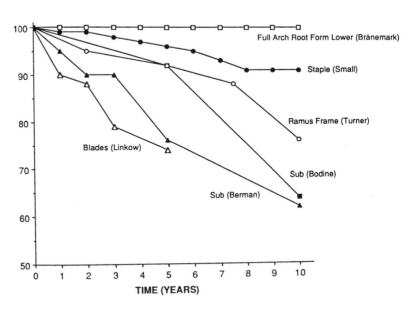

Figure 1–2. Comparison of continuously functioning complete arch restorations on osseointegrated and nonintegrated implants. (From Shulman LB: Surgical considerations in implant dentistry. J Dent Educ 52:713, 1991.)

ANCIENT IMPLANTS

Attempts to replace lost teeth with endosteal implants have been traced to ancient Egyptian and South American civilizations.[26] There is a skull from the pre-Columbian Era in the Peabody Museum of Harvard University in which an artificial tooth carved from dark stone replaced a lower left lateral incisor.[24] Curators of the museum now state that this implant was placed post mortem, a custom of South American Indians in that period.[11] Implanted animal and carved ivory teeth cited in ancient Egyptian writings are the oldest examples of primitive implantology. It is doubtful that any of these earliest attempts with crude materials and coarse methods enjoyed appreciable longevity.[24]

EARLY IMPLANTS

In 1809, Maggiolo placed a single-stage gold implant without a crown to heal passively in a fresh extraction site just above the gingiva. The crown was added after healing. The insertion of such teeth roots of gold was inevitably followed by intense pain and gingival inflammation.[14] Roughened lead roots held a platinum post and a porcelain crown[20]; tubes of gold and iridium were used.[6] Silver capsules were used[35] as was corrugated porcelain. Greenfield[19] used a two-piece hollow basket fabricated from 24-gauge iridium wire soldered with 24-carat gold in 1913 (Fig. 1–3); this was clearly the forerunner of today's hollow-basket design.

Adams[1] in 1937 patented a submergible

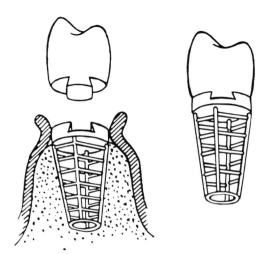

Figure I–3. Greenfield two-piece basket implant, 1913; precursor of hollow basket design.

threaded cylindrical implant with a round bottom, smooth gingival collar, and healing cap. A ball head screwed to the root was used to retain an overdenture in a manner similar to that done today. It is not clear whether or how much the Adams implant was used clinically, but it did portend many implants that were to come along 50 years later. Although the majority of these patented implant designs never succeeded, it is remarkable that modern implants appear to be variants or composites of some of the designs recorded in early implant literature.

Up to this point, success was marginal and measured in terms of a few years. It was left to Strock at Harvard to place the first *long-term* endosseous implant. In 1938, Strock placed into a fresh extraction socket a threaded Vitallium (cobalt-chrome-molybdenum) implant, custom-fashioned by Austenal, the predecessor of the Howmedica Corporation. This implant had a cone-shaped head for the cementation of a jacket crown. The socket filled in with bone around the implant, and it remained firm and asymptomatic until 1955, at which time the patient died in a car crash.

SUBPERIOSTEAL IMPLANTS

Because there is often not enough bone in which to place an endosteal implant, dentists turned to placing implants on and around bone rather than in it in the form of subperiosteal implants. In 1943, Dahl placed metal structures on the mandible and maxilla with four projecting posts.[26] Goldberg and Gershkoff[17] made an impression taken of the mucosa covering the edentulous ridge. On the model produced from this impression they generated a multifenestrated narrow cobalt-chrome-molybdenum casting with four abutments that had little bone coverage and a fit that was only reasonably accurate (Fig. 1–4).[10] The two-stage technique was refined by several clinicians.[4, 5, 21, 24, 27, 47] Subsequently a series of modifications were made in the implant design.[10]

A three-dimensional replica of the mandible can now be developed from CT images, making it no longer mandatory to carry out extensive surgical dissection for a direct bone impression.[18] CT-generated CAD-CAM models, however, are not as precise as those obtained from a direct bone impression,[3] and many surgeons still use the direct technique.

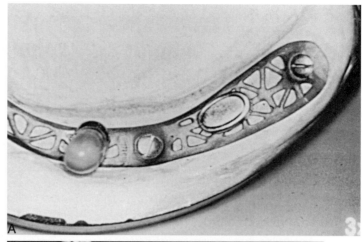

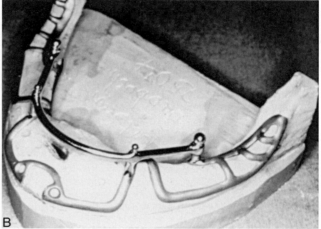

Figure 1–4. *A,* Original Gershkoff and Goldberg subperiosteal implant restricted by a closed impression. (From Goldberg NI, Gershkoff A: Implant lower denture. Dent Digest 55:490, 1949.) *B,* Subperiosteal design extended by direct impression techniques.

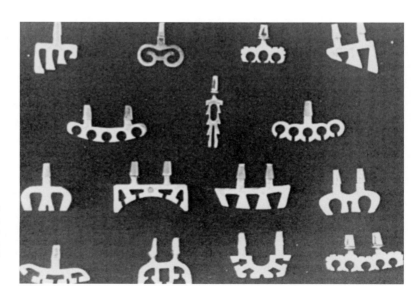

Figure 1–5. Early Linkow blade implant designs. (From Linkow L, Chercheve R: Theories and Techniques of Oral Implantology, St. Louis, Mosby–Yearbook, 1970, p 462.)

ONE-STAGE ENDOSTEAL PINS, SCREWS, AND CYLINDERS

Various implant designs emerged in the early 1960s.[25, 27, 30, 32, 34, 40, 46] The majority of these screw-shaped implants were one piece and were not submerged; they generally did not osseointegrate. Some workers theorized that the fibrous peri-implant membrane with its shock-absorbing feature was preferable to an implant fused to bone.[48] We now know that this is not the case.

BLADE IMPLANTS

In 1967, two variations of the blade implant were introduced independently by Linkow[29] and Roberts and Roberts.[37] Linkow[28] subsequently designed a myriad of configurations for the blade, making it suitable for broad applicability in the maxilla and mandible (Fig. 1–5), especially for placement in narrow ridges. It did require shared support with natural teeth and could not function on its own. The blade implant was restorable within a month of placement and soon became the most widely used device in implantology in the United States and abroad.

TRANSOSTEAL IMPLANTS

In 1975, Small[42–44] introduced the transosteal mandibular staple bone plate, a reconstructive device placed through a submental incision and attached to the mandible with multiple fixation and two transosteal screws to support a full arch prosthesis. Current application of this device has been limited to the mandible only. Other transosteal implants of historical and practical importance are the single transosteal implant of Cranin[9] and the transmandibular implant of Bosker.[7]

ENDOSTEAL ROOT-FORM IMPLANTS

A two-stage threaded titanium root-form implant was first presented in North America by Brånemark in 1978 at a conference in Toronto (Fig. 1–6).[36] Brånemark[8] had found in conjunction with vital microscopy studies that titanium oculars placed in the femurs of rabbits could not be removed from the bone after a

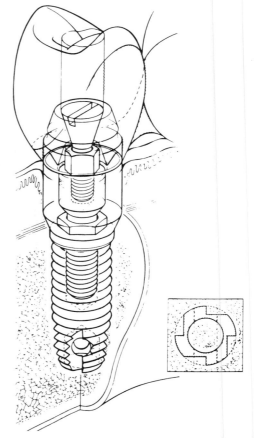

Figure 1–6. Two-stage threaded root-form (Brånemark).

period of healing. Brånemark developed and tested a two-stage dental implant system utilizing pure titanium screws, which he termed *fixtures.* The first fixtures were placed in patients in 1965, and intensive clinical studies have proceeded ever since. His well-documented, long-term prospective studies offered clear evidence of prolonged survival, freestanding function, bone maintenance, and significant improvement in the benefit-to-risk ratio over all previous dental implants.[2] Osseointegration undoubtedly represents the most significant breakthrough in dentistry in the past 20 years. It has revolutionized dental treatment planning. With the Brånemark implant came the concept of the premachined abutment and the fixed detachable prosthesis. Based on Brånemark's extensive and weighty documentation of implant efficacy and safety[2] and early replication by Zarb[49] and others, dental schools and dental specialties, which heretofore had avoided any involvement in this field, finally recognized and incorporated dental implants into their curricula and training programs.[12]

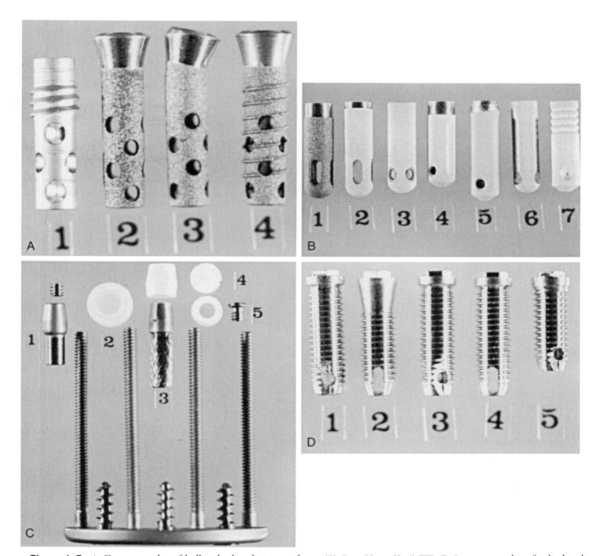

Figure 1–7. *A,* Four examples of hollow basket design implants: (1) Core-Vent; (2–4) ITI. *B,* Seven examples of cylindrical implants: (1) IMZ; (2) HA-coated IMZ; (3) Integral; (4,5) Steri-Oss; (6) Bio-Vent; (7) Sustain. *C,* Example of transosseous implant. Mandibular staple bone plate. *D,* Five examples of threaded, screw-shaped implants: (1,2) Brånemark; (3,4) Impla-Med; (5) Osseodent. (From English C: An overview of implant hardware. J Am Dent Assoc 121:360–370, 1990. Reprinted with permission.)

Subsequent to the Brånemark implant, many other root-forms have been introduced and enjoy widespread clinical use.[16] Some are traditional screws (ITI-plasma sprayed); others have platforms rather than threads (Stryker[15]); the IMZ implant is a press-fit stress broken titanium plasma-sprayed cylinder[23]; many are hollow cylinders (ITI,[39, 45] Core-Vent[33]); and some are HA coated (Integral, Calcitek, Inc.).[22] Plasma-sprayed or other induced surface roughness enhances bone deposition and maintenance as well as affording an increased surface area for stress transfer.[7] Figure 1–7 shows examples of a variety of endosteal and transosteal implants.

References

1. Adams PB: Anchoring means for false teeth. U.S. Patent No. 2, 112,007, March 22, 1938.
2. Adell R, Lekholm U, Rockler B, Brånemark PI: A 15 year study of osseointegrated implants in the treatment of the edentulous jaw. Int J Oral Surg 10:387, 1981.
3. Babbush CA: Personal communication, 1989.
4. Berman N: The physiologic and mechanical aspect of the implant technique and its application to practical cases. Dent Dig 8:342, 1952.
5. Bodine RL: Implant dentures: Follow-up after 7–10 years. J Am Dent Assoc 67:352–363, 1963.
6. Bonwell, First District Dental Society. In Greenfield EG: Implantation of Artificial Bridge Abutments. Dent Cosmos 55:364, 1913.
7. Bosker H, Van Dijk L: The transmandibular implant: A 12-year follow-up study. J Oral Maxillofac Surg 47:442–450, 1989.
8. Brånemark PI: Introduction to osseointegration. In Brånemark PI, et al (eds): Tissue Integrated Prostheses. Chicago, Quintessence Publishing Co, Inc, 1985, p 29.
9. Cranin AN, Dennison T: The anterior vertical transosseous implant. In Cranin AH (ed): Oral Implantology. Springfield, Ill, Charles C Thomas, 1970, pp 200–208.
10. Cranin AN, et al: Evolution of dental implants in the twentieth century. Alpha Omegan 80:25, 1987.
11. Curator, Peabody Museum, Harvard University: Personal communication, 1994.
12. Curriculum guidelines for predoctoral implant dentistry. J Dent Educ 55:751–753, 1991.
13. Dahl GSA: Om impjlighenten for implantetion i Keken au metaliskelett som has eller retention for fastoc eller avatagbara protesor. (Mandibular subperiosteal implants.) Odontol Tidskr 51:440, 1943.
14. Driskell TD: History of implants. J Calif Dent Assoc 15:17, 1987.
15. Driskell TD, O'Hara MJ, Greene GW: Surgical tooth implants, combat and field. Report No. 1, Contract No. DA DA17-69-C-9118. Supported by U.S. Army Medical Research and Development Command, 1971.
16. English C: An overview of implant hardware. J Am Dent Assoc 121:360–370, 1990.
17. Goldberg MI, Gershkoff A: The implant lower denture. Dent Dig 55:490, 1949.
18. Golec TS: CAD CAM multiplanar diagnostic imaging for subperiosteal implants. Dent Clin North Am 30:85, 1986.
19. Greenfield EJ: Implantation of artificial crown and bridge abutments. Dent Cosmos 55:364, 1913.
20. Harris SM: An artificial tooth. Quoted in Dent Cosmos 55:433, 1887.
21. Izikowitz L: Superplants. J Implant Dent 8:18–32, 1962.
22. Kent J, et al: Biointegrated hydroxylapatite coated dental implants: Five year clinical observations. J Am Dent Assoc 121:138–144, 1990.
23. Kirsch A, Mentag P: The IMZ endosseous two-phase system: A complete oral rehabilitation treatment concept. J Oral Impl 12, 1986.
24. Lee TC: History of dental implants. In Cranin AN (ed): Oral Implantology. Springfield, Ill, Charles C Thomas, 1970, pp 3–5.
25. Lehmans J: Contribution a l'etude des implants endosseus. Implant a arceau extensible. Rev Stomatolog 41:224, 1919.
26. Lemons J, Natiella J: Biomaterials, biocompatibility and peri-implant considerations. Dent Clin North Am 30:4, 1986.
27. Lew I: Progress in implant dentistry: An evaluation. J Am Dent Assoc 59:478–492, 1959.
28. Linkow LI: The endosseous blade vent—twenty years of clinical application. Alpha Omegan 80:36–40, 1987.
29. Linkow LI: The blade-vent—a new dimension in endosseous implants. Dent Conc 11:3, 1968.
30. Linkow LI: Intra-osseous implants utilized as fixed bridge abutments. J Oral Impl Transpl 10:17, 1964.
31. Marziani L: Radici artificidi come ancoraggio de protesi commplete mobili interiori. Clin Odont 2:244, 1947.
32. Muratori G: Personal system osseous implants with screw-in surfaces. [Italian.] Dent Cadm (Milano) 32:746, 1964.
33. Niznick GA: The Core-Vent implant system. Oral Implantol 10:379–418, 1982.
34. Pasqualini U: Anatomic-pathologic reports and clinico-surgical deductions from 91 alloplastic implants in 28 experimental animals. [Italian.] Riv Ital Stomat 18:3, 1963.
35. Payne RE: Implantation of teeth by silver capsule. Dent Cosmos 12:1401, 1901. [In Greenfield.]
36. Proceedings of the Toronto Conferences on Osseointegration in Clinical Dentistry. J Prosth Dent 49:50, 1983.
37. Roberts HD, Roberts RA: The ramus endosseous implant. J South Calif Dent Assoc 38:571, 1970.
38. Schnitman PA, Shulman LB: Dental implants: Benefits and risks. Proceedings of NIH-Harvard Consensus Conference, 1978.
39. Schroeder A, et al: Tissue reaction to a titanium hollow cylinder implant with titanium plasma sprayed layer surface. Schweiz Mschr Zahnleilk 86:713, 1976.
40. Scialom J: A new look at implants. A fortunate discovery: Needle implants. [French.] Inform Dent 44:737, 1962.
41. Shulman LB: Dental replantation and transplantation. In Laskin D (ed): Oral and Maxillofacial Surgery. Vol 2. St. Louis, CV Mosby, 1985, pp 132, 133, 136.
42. Small IA: Metal implants and the mandibular staple bone plate. J Oral Surg 36:604, 1978.
43. Small IA: Metal implants and the mandibular staple bone plate. J Oral Surg 33:571, 1975.
44. Small IA, Misiek DJ: A 16 year evaluation of the mandibular staple bone plate. J Oral Maxillofac Surg 42:421–428, 1984.
45. Suter F, et al: ITI hollow cylinder system: Principles and methodology. J Oral Implantol 11:168, 1983.
46. Tramonte S: A further report on intraosseous implants with improved drive screw. J Ora Impl Transpl Surg 11:35, 1965.
47. Weinberg L: An early unilateral subperiosteal implant. In Cranin AN (ed): Oral Implantology. Springfield, Ill, Charles C Thomas, 1970, p 19.

48. Weiss CM: Fibro-osteal and osteal integration: A comparative analysis of blade and fixture type dental implants supported by clinical trials. J Dent Educ 52:706–711, 1988.

49. Zarb G: Implants for complete denture therapy. J Dent Educ 52:721, 1991.

50. Zarb G: Proceedings. Toronto Conference on Osseointegration in Clinical Dentistry. St. Louis, CV Mosby, 1983.

Study Questions

1. How do different implant types (blades, subperiosteal, transosteal, Brånemark type) compare in regard to long-term survival?

2. What materials have been used for dental implants, and what are the current materials used?

3. Be able to discuss the importance of the 1982 Toronto conference.

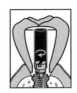

CHAPTER 2

Resorption Patterns of the Residual Ridge

Paul Mercier
Revised by Michael S. Block

Patterns of Resorption
General Changes
Maxillary Changes
Intermaxillary Relationship Changes

Soft Tissue Changes
Treatment Implications
    Prosthetic Considerations
References

Dental extraction is one of the most frequent injuries affecting the human skeleton. The alveolar bone reacts by remodeling its structures with bone removal at its outer surfaces and bone deposition in the empty sockets. This process of disuse atrophy is usually limited to the contouring of the alveolar bone surfaces, as it is commonly observed that people who have never worn dentures do not suffer from severe atrophy. The simple fact that maxillary ridges provided with larger denture-bearing surfaces are less affected by bone resorption than mandibular ones is a strong argument in favor of mechanical factors being primarily involved. Masticatory forces transmitted by dentures create a greater challenge to the integrity of the residual ridge than loss of teeth. On a long-term basis, this pressure-resorption phenomenon, associated with other factors, takes its toll to produce bone loss that may involve the whole basal-alveolar bone complex of the jaws.

The factors of resorption are divided into three categories: mechanical, biologic, and anatomic (Fig. 2–1). Their interrelations, along with the sex factor, are illustrated by four interconnecting rings. The larger central ring is one of the main factors of resorption, the mechanical ones among which the duration and type of compressive forces are those parameters that most influence the rate of resorption. People of either sex with multiple years of denture wear, associated with the harmful habit of wearing their dentures overnight, a history of bruxism, a closure of the bite, and an inadequate denture design are prime candidates for severe atrophy.

Women may be particularly disadvantaged in that they often have a longer period of denture compressive forces owing to earlier dental extractions than men, a decrease in bone density especially after menopause, and usually smaller bones than men and so less jaw volume to resorb. It is in this context of a combination of unfavorable mechanical, metabolic, and anatomic factors being present that the higher incidence of severe ridge atrophy for women must be considered. One should not assume, however, that men have a distinct advantage in treatment over women because usually there is more bone present to start with and normally more bone left after the same number of years of denture wear. Not only the volume of bone, but also its form and relationship with the opposing jaw, must be evaluated.

PATTERNS OF RESORPTION

Residual ridge morphology has been the object of multiple studies.[1–16] The general consensus is that variability constitutes the common rule of bone changes in edentulous ridges. Some patterns are specific to one jaw in particular. To get a clear understanding of the structural changes, one must not confine examination to one jaw but must include also the intermaxillary relationships and soft tissue changes that become more evident as the resorptive process proceeds to more advanced stages.

GENERAL CHANGES

The general changes in ridge shape following extractions include: a ridge broad enough at the

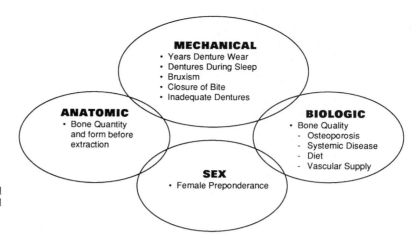

Figure 2–1. Multiple interrelated factors responsible for residual ridge resorption.

crest initially to accommodate the width of the recently extracted teeth to one that becomes pointed, then one flat to the level of the basal bone, and finally a concave ridge with resorption of the basal bone. These four stages of resorption correspond to the description and classification of residual ridges (Fig. 2–2).

The classifications of Kent et al[9] and Cawood and Howell[6] are descriptive variants of these four stages of ridge resorption described by Atwood in 1963.[2] Group IV atrophy is more often seen in the mandible than in the maxilla, which has little bone beyond the root apices in the posterior segments. This feature is in contrast with the large amount present between the apices of the lower teeth and the inferior border of the mandible.

The most obvious change for both jaws is a loss of ridge height that is associated with posterior and inward drift of the summit of the resid-

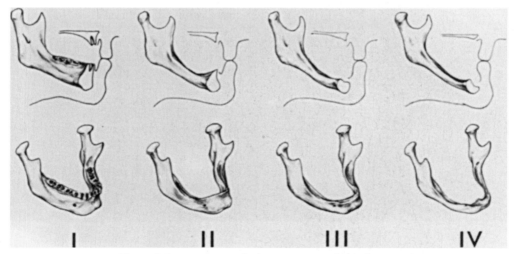

Figure 2–2. Four stages of ridge resorption and classification.

Group I	Minor ridge remodeling	Denture problems, if any, are more related to muscle interferences than to bone deficit.
Group II	Sharp atrophic residual ridge	Some alveolar bone is still present at different levels, from a high knife-edge ridge to a low residual crest.
Group III	Basal bone ridge	Resorption to the level of the basal bone.
Group IV	Resorption of basal bone	Resorption into basal bone with concavities present.

ual crest. The anterior vertical bone contour and external slope are more affected by this medial drift in the mandible than in the maxilla, where there is natural protrusion of the alveolar bone. Cawood and Howell[6] have illustrated these changes in a measurement study of 300 dry bone specimens (Fig. 2–3). The anterior maxilla is shown to maintain its anterior vertical slope, even at stage III of the resorption process.

To the contrary, one can observe rapid deterioration of the ridge form in the anterior region of the mandible. The profile is modified from a pear-shaped appearance at the time of dental extraction to a pointed one. Then the ridge loses its vertical slope, as it becomes flat and occasionally concave. The lingual plate in the genial tubercles region, however, seldom resorbs. The plate becomes palpable. Other structures, such as the mylohyoid crest or the external oblique line, behave in the same way.

MAXILLARY CHANGES

The external (labial) side of the maxilla is also resorptive as during growth the jaw expands by

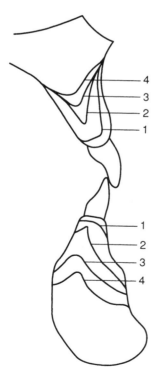

Figure 2–3. Four stages of resorption of anterior region superposed.

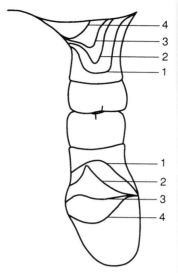

Figure 2–4. Four stages of resorption of posterior region superposed.

bone being added on the inside of the arch. In contrast to the mandible, however, there is less horizontal bone loss and posterior drift of the anterior crest owing to the normal protrusive characteristic of the anterior maxilla that holds central incisors at a 110 degree angulation with the palatal plane. The vertical anterior slope is better preserved (see Fig. 2–3). In the less protrusive posterior ridge segment, the inward drift of the crest is more pronounced. The width of the posterior maxilla is reduced. The maxilla becomes smaller as the mandible appears to widen (Fig. 2–4).

When the anterior maxillary bone disappears at a faster rate than the posterior part, it is related to a specific situation described by the term *combination syndrome*: excessive forces originating from natural mandibular incisors and inadequate posterior prosthetic support. Counterrotation of the mandible as the occlusal vertical dimension decreases and the dentures are not renewed accentuates the pressure-resorption phenomenon affecting severely the anterior residual ridge, whose level reaches the nasal spine.

INTERMAXILLARY RELATIONSHIP CHANGES

An inverse or crossbite ridge Class III ridges relationship is developed with advanced stages of ridge resorption (see Fig. 2–4). To get a better understanding of this resorption pattern, jaws must be represented in three dimensions. A pyramidal architecture is usually present with a mandibular base broader than the maxillary one. To respect this natural disproportion, teeth must be differently aligned: the lower molars inward to the lingual side and the upper ones outward to the buccal side (Fig. 2–5). As bone resorbs, the lower jaw becomes wider and the upper jaw narrower. The severely resorbed mandible appears to be wide because more of the external oblique line and buccal shelf and of the paralingual shelf have become integrated to the residual ridge form as the alveolar part of the bone had resorbed.

SOFT TISSUE CHANGES

Soft tissue changes also occur following tooth loss and denture wear. A crestal scar band is usually formed at the crest of the ridge. It represents remnants of the attached gingivae and in the mandible all of what is left in terms of keratinized mucosa. In the maxilla the situation is different. The delicate lining mucosa is confined to the vestibular side, whereas in the lower jaw it is present on both sides of the scar band. With increasing ridge resorption, more of the keratinized and thick mucosa of the palate migrates toward the crest (Fig. 2–6A).

As the residual ridge resorbs, the muscular attachments to the ridge interfere with the denture flange. The denture stability is adversely affected, most rapidly in the anterior region of the mandible, where the strong mentalis muscle is attached high on the ridge, at the limit of the mucogingival junction. In the upper jaw, the problem is lessened by muscle attachments placed at a higher level on the vestibular side. Interferences with the denture flange are mostly confined to the canine regions.

TREATMENT IMPLICATIONS

Prosthetic Considerations

The anatomic changes described in this chapter have important treatment implications. The changes must be well understood if one wishes to become fully aware of their adverse effects on denture wear and design. Solutions can then be applied more effectively. The main problem is one of bone loss leading to muscle attachment interferences with the denture base. The large interridge distance must be filled by a high acrylic base over which artificial teeth sit far from their center of gravity (Fig. 2–7A). One incorrect treatment alternative to improving denture stability without reconstructive surgery is to reduce the patient's vertical dimension but to risk temporomandibular joint problems or an aesthetic prejudice.

In the maxilla the situation is different for several reasons: a larger denture-bearing area owing to the presence of the palate, a more favorable residual ridge contour with fewer muscle interferences, and a residual scar band that is firmer and more useful for prosthetic support than the mandibular one. The quantity of bone

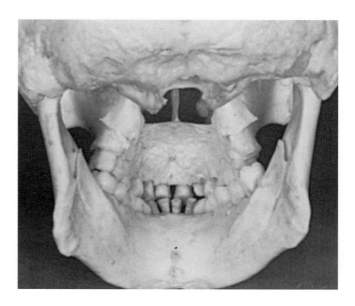

Figure 2–5. Pyramidal architecture of jaws with a broad mandibular base, a narrow maxillary base, and corresponding inclined axes of molars.

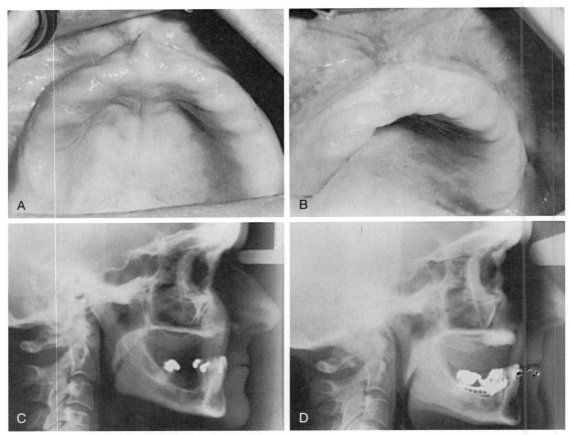

Figure 2–6. *A,* Keratinized crestal scar band with muscle interference in the canine region. *B,* Ridge reconstructed with HA augmentation on residual crest and over palatal side. *C,* Typical combination syndrome and anterior maxillary bone loss. *D,* Anterior vertical slope obtained with HA.

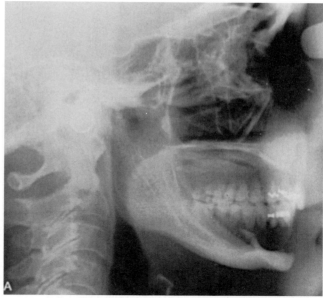

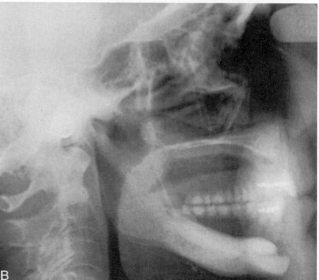

Figure 2–7. *A,* Typical resorption patterns: maxilla, persistence of the anterior slope, evenness of maxillary resorption; mandible, persistence of the genial tubercles, posterior mandibular concavities. *B,* Ridge relationship reestablished in all planes after reconstruction of the mandible.

left is less crucial to denture efficiency than the shape of the residual ridge and the quality of covering soft tissues. A small, firm ridge, free of muscle interferences, with a shallow but flat palate, favors surface tension and denture adherence. It is superior to a residual ridge with a narrow and deep inverted V-shaped palatal vault covered with thick mucosa. In the more severe atrophy case (situation A), the masticatory forces applied to the ridge and to the palate are distributed on a much wider surface at the base of the maxilla and counteract more efficiently the dislodging contracture of the lip and cheek.

There is often no need in these instances to apply surgical treatment.

References

1. Atwood DA: Reduction of residual ridges: A major oral disease entity. J Prosthet Dent 26:266–277, 1971.
2. Atwood DA: Post-extraction changes in the adult mandible as illustrated by microradiographs of mid-sagittal section and serial cephalometric roentgenograms. J Prosthet Dent 13:810–825, 1963.
3. Atwood DA, Coy WA: Clinical cephalometric and densi-

tometry study of reduction of residual ridges. J Prosthet Dent 26:280–295, 1971.

4. Bergman B, Carlsson GE: Clinical long term study of complete denture wearers. J Prosthet Dent 53:56–61, 1985.

5. Carlsson GE, Persson G: Morphological changes of the mandible after extraction and wearing of dentures: A longitudinal clinical and x-ray cephalometric study of 5 years. Odontol Rev 18:27–53, 1967.

6. Cawood JJ, Howell RA: A classification of the edentulous jaws. Int J Oral Maxillofac Surg 17:232–236, 1988.

7. Engstrom C, Hollender L, Lindquist S: Jaw morphology in edentulous individuals: A radiographic cephalometric study. J Oral Rehab 12:451–460, 1985.

8. Enlow DH, Bianco HJ, Eklund S: The remodeling of the edentulous mandible. J Prosthet Dent 34:685–693, 1976.

9. Kent JN, et al: Alveolar ridge augmentation using non-resorbable hydroxylapatite with or without autogenous cancellous bone. J Oral Maxillofac Surg 41:629–642, 1983.

10. Mercier P: Ridge reconstruction with hydroxylapatite: I.

11. Mercier P: Ridge reconstruction with hydroxylapatite: II. Ridge reconstruction based on residual anatomic structures. Oral Surg 65:641–652, 1988.

12. Mercier P, Lafontant R: Residual alveolar ridge atrophy: Classification and influence of facial morphology. J Prosthet Dent 31:120–132, 1979.

13. Pietrokowski J, Massler M: Alveolar ridge resorption following tooth extraction. J Prosthet Dent 17:21–29, 1967.

14. Tallgren A: The continuing reduction of the residual alveolar ridge in complete denture wearers: A mixed longitudinal study covering 25 years. J Prosthet Dent 31:120–132, 1972.

15. Tallgren A: Alveolar bone loss in denture wearers as related to facial morphology. Acta Odont Scand 28:251–270, 1970.

16. Tallgren A, Lang BA, Walker GF: Roentgen cephalometric analysis of ridge resorption and changes in jaw and occlusal relationship in immediate complete denture wearers. J Oral Rehab 7:74–94, 1980.

Anatomy of the residual ridge. Oral Surg 65:505–510, 1988.

Study Questions

1. Describe the pattern of resorption of the mandible and the maxilla.

2. As the result of the pattern of resorption of the mandible and maxilla, what is the resultant ridge relationship of the edentulous mandible to the edentulous maxilla?

3. To reconstruct the severely resorbed mandible and maxilla with implants, describe where to place and locate bone grafts to establish ideal implant placement in the original location of the patient's teeth.

CHAPTER 3

Medical Evaluation

John P. Neary
Revised by Michael S. Block

Evaluation
   Cardiovascular Assessment
Hypertension
Coronary Artery Disease
   Cigarette Smoking and Alcohol Abuse
Evaluation in the Healthy Patient
References

The medical evaluation in the implant patient should be no different than that a patient receives for any surgical procedure. The extent of the planned surgery, the type of anesthesia employed, and the general health of the patient are all factors in determining the magnitude of the preoperative evaluation. The preoperative evaluation may uncover facts that alter the planned surgery or anesthesia.

The practitioner must integrate his or her knowledge of the surgical procedure with the information provided by a medical consultant, when the patient's health status indicates consultation is appropriate. It is imperative that the consultant understand what procedure the patient is about to undergo, the type of anesthesia planned, and any special concerns the surgeon may have.

EVALUATION

Cardiovascular Assessment

Myocardial infarction is the most common cause of perioperative death in patients undergoing a surgical procedure. Other cardiovascular diseases, such as hypertension, congestive heart failure, valvular heart disease, and rhythm and conduction disturbances, are also commonly encountered. The question then becomes: How does the practitioner identify the patients at risk, and what type of workup do they require before implant surgery?

The Cardiac Risk Index developed by Goldman[3] identifies nine independent risk variables (Table 3–1) and assigns a point value to each. This results in four risk categories (I–IV) (Table

1	Past medical history	Illnesses, hospital admissions, immunizations
2	Past surgical history	What, why, any complications
3	Allergies	To what medications; describe the type of reaction
4	Medications	Names and dosages, including over the counter; why they are taken, and for how long
5	Family history	Major diseases of importance, problems with anesthesia
6	Social history	Cigarette smoking, alcohol and illicit drug use, risk factors for human immunodeficiency virus (HIV)
7	Review of systems	Questions should pertain to recent changes in well-being, weight changes, weakness, fatigue, or fever and specific items regarding each organ system: cardiac, pulmonary, endocrine, renal, hematologic, rheumatologic, and neurologic

Table 3–1. Computation of the Cardiac Risk Index

Criteria	Multivariate Discriminant Function Coefficient	Points
History	0.191	5
Age >70 years	0.384	10
Myocardial infarction in previous 6 months		
Physical examination	0.451	11
S_3 gallop or jugular venous distention	0.119	3
Important valvular aortic stenosis		
ECG	0.283	7
Rhythm other than sinus or premature atrial contractions on last preoperative ECG		
>5 premature ventricular contractions/min documented at any time before operation	0.278	7
General status	0.132	3
Po_2 <60 or Pco_2 >50 mm Hg		
K <3.0 or Hco_3 <20 mEq/L		
BUN >50 or creatinine >3.0 mg/dl, abnormal SGOT, signs of chronic liver disease or patient bedridden from noncardiac causes		
Operation		
Intraperitoneal, intrathoracic, or aortic operation	0.123	3
Emergency operation	0.167	4
Total possible		53

From Goldman L, et al: Multifactorial index of risk in noncardiac surgical procedures. N Engl J Med 297:845, 1977. Reprinted with permission of the Massachusetts Medical Society.

3–2), which correlate extremely well with cardiac risk. The significance of the index is that many of the risk variables can be evaluated in the surgeon's office without expensive laboratory tests. An understanding of this index is also important in communication with a consultant because many internal medicine physicians use this index to assess cardiac risk.

HYPERTENSION

Assessment of the patient with hypertension should focus on the detection of associated cardiac risk factors from the history and cursory examination. The history should focus on the duration of the patient's hypertension and specific treatment the patient is receiving and its effectiveness. The examination should include careful measurement of the blood pressure with a cuff of appropriate size.

It should be noted that perioperative hypertension occurs in about 25% of patients with hypertension regardless of preoperative control. With few exceptions, patients taking antihypertensive medications should be maintained on their medications, including the day of surgery. Patients with elevated diastolic pressures and patients with significant end-organ damage from hypertension require careful preoperative evaluation and possible consultation.[2] In patients with hypertension or myocardial disease, when local anesthetics are used that contain epinephrine, the minimum amount of epinephrine necessary to achieve good anesthesia is the rule. If 3% mepivacaine (Carbocaine) cannot achieve ade-

Table 3–2. Cardiac Risk Index

Class	Point Total	No or Only Minor Complications (N = 943)	Life-Threatening Complications (N = 943)	Cardiac Deaths (N = 19)
I (N = 537)	0–5	532 (99)	4 (0.7)	1 (0.2)
II (N = 316)	6–12	295 (93)	15 (5)	5 (2)
III (N = 130)	13–25	112 (86)	15 (11)	3 (2)
IV (N = 18)	>26	4 (22)	4 (22)	10 (56)

From Goldman L, et al: Multifactorial index of risk in noncardiac surgical procedures. N Engl J Med 297:845, 1977. Reprinted with permission from the Massachusetts Medical Society.

quate anesthesia, a local anesthetic containing 1:200,000 epinephrine should be used. The maximum recommended dose of epinephrine in patients with hypertension or cardiac disease is 0.04 mg. Inadequate anesthesia caused by poor local anesthesia owing to lack of a vasoconstrictor may cause more hypertension than the vasoconstrictor itself.

CORONARY ARTERY DISEASE

The preoperative evaluation of the patient with known or suspected coronary artery disease depends on the presence of residual myocardial ischemia, ventricular irritability, and overall ventricular function. For the most part, these variables can be translated into clinical practice based on history and electrocardiogram (ECG) testing. One of the most important factors is a history of a previous myocardial infarction. The risk of infarction is less than 1% in the general population in a perioperative setting. In patients undergoing surgery within 3 months of a myocardial infarction, the risk of reinfarction is 30%. In patients undergoing surgery 3 to 6 months following a myocardial infarction, the risk of reinfarction is approximately 15%. Delaying the surgery to at least 6 months after myocardial infarction reduces the risk to 5% to 6%, which then remains constant at that level of risk.[1]

The presence of angina is another finding that warrants further investigation. Stable angina alone is not associated with increased risk. When it is present after a myocardial infarction, however, its presence significantly increases the perioperative risk. If the patient experiences angina only during vigorous activity and responds readily to oral nitroglycerin, outpatient surgery can usually proceed without elaborate preoperative testing. Patients with unstable angina (defined as a change in their anginal pattern—increased frequency, duration, ease of provocation, or angina at rest) should receive thorough preoperative investigation before surgery proceeds.

Patients who have undergone coronary artery bypass grafting are generally considered to be low risk for perioperative cardiac ischemia and are statistically equal to patients without significant coronary artery disease.[1, 8]

The perioperative management of patients with coronary artery disease begins with appropriate preoperative evaluation. Implicit in the care of these patients is the need for intraoperative monitoring of vital signs and ECG monitoring. Patients prescribed medications should receive them up to and including the day of surgery. The surgeon should use all available preventive measures to reduce the possibility of an anginal episode during surgery. The increased oxygen demand during surgery is primarily due to patient anxiety. Therefore attention should be given to a good anxiety-reduction protocol. Supplemental oxygen should be delivered during the procedure. Preoperative nitroglycerin should be considered, and profound local anesthesia should be achieved before proceeding with the surgery.

Detailed discussions of congestive heart failure, cardiac rhythm disturbances, valvular heart disease, pulmonary problems, endocrine abnormalities, renal assessment, hematologic assessment, and other medical problems are included in *Endosseous Implants in Maxillofacial Reconstruction* by Block and Kent.

Cigarette Smoking and Alcohol Abuse

The effects of cigarette smoking on the respiratory and cardiovascular systems have been widely recognized as deleterious. Although the effects of cigarette smoking, and more specifically nicotine, on wound healing have not been widely studied, there is substantial evidence that cigarette smoking exerts a significant negative effect on wound healing.[4] Nicotine is a poisonous alkaloid that when inhaled or injected can produce significant vasoconstriction through the release of catecholamines and a direct effect. Nicotine has been demonstrated to impair wound healing in several animal models.[5] Cigarette smoking has also been shown to increase the incidence of skin necrosis in rhytidectomy patients (approximately 12.5 times the risk in a nonsmoker).[6] The speculation is that nicotine exerts its damaging effects on wound healing in several ways. Nicotine may cause direct damage to fibroblast precursors. The vasoconstrictive effects predispose to thrombotic microvascular occlusion, thus producing tissue ischemia. Nicotine may also inhibit epithelialization.

Consequently, consideration should be given to the effects of cigarette smoke on surgical healing as well as to its better-known effects on the human body. Although no conclusive evidence exists to guide in the length of abstinence from smoking, many surgeons empirically ask their patients to refrain from smoking for 10 days before surgery and for 3 weeks after surgery.

Alcohol abuse represents a significant problem

in our society, and it is common to see patients who abuse alcohol. Alcoholic patients range from being easily recognized to the high-functioning alcoholic who is most difficult to recognize. The importance of identifying patients with alcohol abuse problems lies in the underlying medical problems associated with alcohol abuse. The most notable problems for any proposed implant surgery include liver dysfunction, coagulopathies, abnormal white cell function, anemia, cardiac disorders, neurologic disorders, and alcohol withdrawal. The key to management is to obtain an accurate and thorough history from patients and to investigate any suspected alcohol abuse with laboratory studies so potential problems can be identified preoperatively.

EVALUATION IN THE HEALTHY PATIENT

Millions of people are operated on each year in the United States, and the majority of these patients are class I anesthetic risks or essentially healthy. How extensive should the evaluation be in these patients? Most studies indicate that the most efficacious is performance of an accurate history and physical examination, with pertinent findings directing any further studies.[7] Because modern practice does not allow for thorough physical examinations of every patient, the practitioner must be adept at picking up subtle findings from observation of the patient. The only laboratory procedures shown to be cost-effective are a hematocrit determination, urinalysis, and a pregnancy test in women of childbearing age.[7]

References

1. Foster E, et al: Risk of noncardiac operation in patients with defined coronary disease: The Coronary Artery Surgery Study (CASS) registry experience. Ann Thorac Surg 41:42, 1986.
2. Goldman L, Caldera D: Risks of general anesthesia and elective operation in the hypertensive patient. Anesthesiology 50:285, 1979.
3. Goldman L, et al: Multifactorial index of risk in noncardiac surgical procedures. N Engl J Med 297:845, 1977.
4. Lind J, Kramhoft M, Bodtker S: The influence of smoking on complications after primary amputations of the lower extremity. Clin Orthop 267:211, 1991.
5. Nolan J, Jenkins R, Kurihara K, Schultz R: The acute effects of cigarette smoke exposure on experimental skin flaps. Plast Reconstr Surg 75:544, 1985.
6. Rees T, Liverett D, Guy C: The effect of cigarette smoking on skin-flap survival in the face lift patient. Plast Reconstr Surg 73:911, 1984.
7. Robbins J, Mushlin A: Preoperative evaluation of the healthy patient. Med Clin North Am 63:1145, 1979.
8. Steen P, Tinker J, Tarhan S: Myocardial reinfarction after anesthesia and surgery. JAMA 239:2566, 1978.

Study Questions

1. Create a medical history form based on the questions you should ask prior to scheduling a patient for implant surgery.

2. What are the systemic effects of diabetes on wound healing and defense of infection?

3. What are the cardiac contraindications to placing implants?

4. How do steroids affect wound healing and what do you do preoperatively for the patient taking steroids?

5. What level of hypertension contraindicates surgery?

6. A patient is taking Coumadin. What do you do to get this patient ready for surgery? Be specific.

CHAPTER 4

Anatomic Considerations

PART 1

Mandible

John Stover
Revised by Michael S. Block

Part I Mandible
  Body Region
  Inferior Alveolar Nerve Location
  Symphysis Region
  References

The mandible, a strong, arched bone fused at the midline mental symphysis, is the only movable bone of the face and performs much of the work of mastication. The dentate mandibular body is basically composed of a thick, rounded lower border and an overlying alveolar process. The loss of teeth is followed by alveolar bone resorption. This dramatically alters mandibular morphology and the relationships between the internal course of the inferior alveolar neurovascular bundle and the external bony contour. The goal of treatment planning for mandibular implant patients is to utilize the existing morphology. To accomplish this, the restorative dentist must have a thorough understanding of the typical anatomic relationships encountered in the mandible and how the loss of teeth affects these relationships.

BODY REGION

Beginning on the inner surface of the mandible in the area adjacent to the roots of the third molar, the often prominent mylohyoid line or ridge (Fig. 4–1H) courses inferiorly and anteriorly. It may continue to the inferior border of the mandible between the genial tubercles (Fig. 4–1F) and digastric fossa (Fig. 4–1G) or may gradually become indistinguishable a variable distance from the inferior border. This ridge,

formed because it is the origin of the mylohyoid muscle, offers important horizontal reinforcement to the mandible. The concavity inferior to the mylohyoid ridge is the submandibular fossa, or fovea (Fig. 4–1D), which is related to the anterior surface of the deep portion of the submandibular gland. The slight depression located superior to the anterior extent of the mylohyoid ridge is the sublingual fossa (Fig. 4–1E), which partially houses the sublingual gland. The mylohyoid ridge of the edentulous posterior mandible is exceptionally variable in shape and strength, largely maintained by the tensions generated by the mylohyoid muscle. Palpation of this region is necessary before implant placement to determine the shape of the ridge and the extent of the underlying submandibular fossa.

Another reason for care while operating in the lingual region of the posterior mandible is the proximity of the lingual nerve. After exiting the pterygomandibular space next to the medial surface of the mandible, the lingual nerve passes superficially under the mucosa and on the periosteum of the lingual alveolar plate.[14] Kiesselbach and Chamberlain[7] reported that in 17.6% of 34 cadaver dissections, the lingual nerve was at the level of the alveolar crest or higher, and in one of these cases the nerve actually passed through the retromolar pad. In 62% of cases the nerve contacted the lingual plate in the horizontal dimension.

INFERIOR ALVEOLAR NERVE LOCATION

The mandibular foramen (Fig. 4–1A), through which the inferior alveolar neurovascular (IAN) bundle enters the mandible, is located on the inner aspect of the ramus at its midpoint in the anteroposterior and the superoinferior dimensions[12, 18, 23] (Figs. 4–2 to 4–5).

Over the past century, many papers have been published describing in great detail the location of the mandibular canal and the many variations in its course and relationships.[1, 17] In 66% of 50

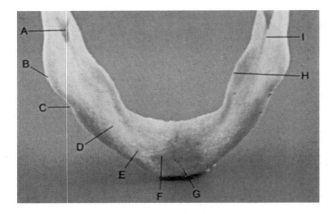

Figure 4–1. Posterior-inferior view of edentulous mandible. *A,* Mandibular foramen. *B,* Mandibular/gonial angle. *C,* Antegonial notch/groove for facial artery. *D,* Submandibular fossa. *E,* Sublingual fossa. *F,* Genial tubercles/mental spines. *G,* Digastric fossa. *H,* Mylohyoid line. *I,* Mylohyoid groove.

adult mandibles, the IAN progressed from the mandibular foramen to the region of the mental foramen, where it bifurcated into distinct mental and incisive branches. In 34% a small plexiform branch given off in the molar region supplied dental structures.[2–5, 15, 16, 19, 21, 24, 28] Carter and Keen[2] confirmed that in up to 60% of specimens, the mandibular canal contains the entire IAN, whereas in 40% the branches may distribute such that a distinct canal is not present. Generally the mandibular canal, between 2.0 and 2.4 mm in diameter,[19] passes from the mandibular foramen inferiorly and anteriorly, then courses horizontally and laterally, usually just below the root

apices of the molar teeth. As the canal approaches the mental foramen, it curves superiorly.[4]

In the vertical dimension, the canal may be in a high, low, or intermediate location within the mandibular body.[16, 17] At the distal aspect of the first molar, the canal is at its lowest point, so this is the safest place in the posterior mandible for implant placement.[13, 19] The mean distance from the inferior border of the mandible to the lowest point along the course of the mandibular canal is 5.9 ± 2.2 mm, with a range of 2 to 11 mm.[20] The canal is rarely greater than 6 mm below the mental foramen.[20]

In the horizontal dimension, the canal begins

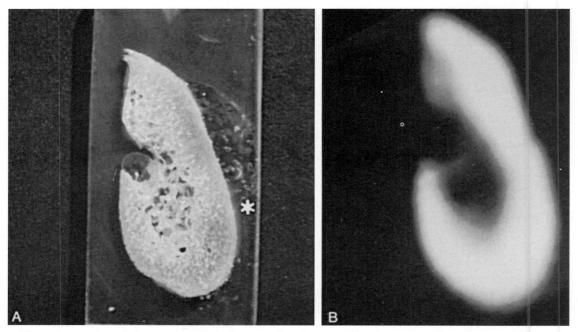

Figure 4–2. *A,* Gross thin cross section from the same edentulous mandible. This section is from the region of the mental foramen. The *asterisk* indicates the lingual cortex, which is generally thicker and stronger than the buccal cortex. *B,* MPR-CT–generated cross section corresponding to the gross specimen seen in *A.*

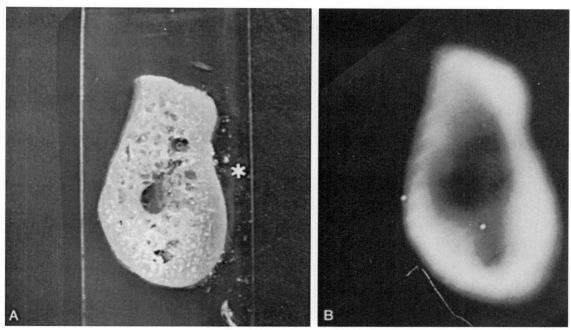

Figure 4–3. *A,* Gross thin cross section from the same edentulous mandible. This section is approximately 6 mm posterior to the mental foramen. Note that the mandibular canal is not uniformly lined with a substantial cortical layer of bone. Note the thick compact layer of lingual cortex *(asterisk). B,* MPR-CT–generated cross section corresponding to the gross specimen seen in *A.*

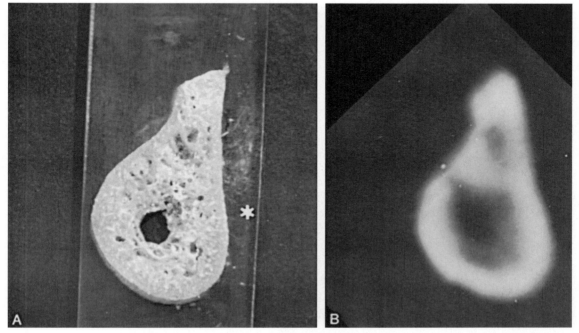

Figure 4–4. *A,* Gross thin cross section from the same edentulous mandible. This section is from approximately 7 mm posterior to the section shown in Figure 4–3. Note the mylohyoid ridge *(asterisk). B,* MPR-CT–generated cross section corresponding to the gross specimen seen in *A.*

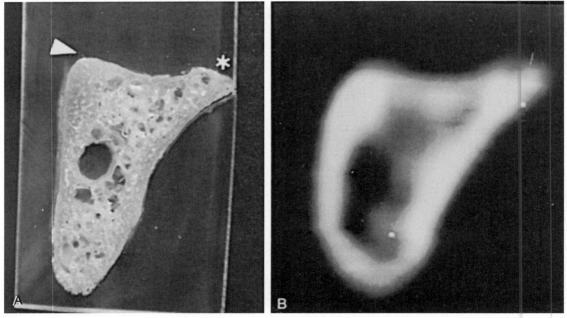

Figure 4–5. *A,* Gross thin cross section from the same edentulous mandible. This section is from the posterior ridge in the retromolar region immediately anterior to the ramus. Note the troughlike ridge formed between the external oblique ridge buccally *(arrowhead)* and the mylohyoid ridge lingually *(asterisk). B,* MPR-CT–generated cross section corresponding to the gross specimen seen in *A.*

posteriorly at the lingual cortical plate and gradually crosses over laterally to the buccal cortex to exit at the mental foramen.[3, 19, 22, 25] It is midway between the two cortical plates in the region of the first molar.[1, 9, 11, 27]

SYMPHYSIS REGION

At the anterior surface of the midline mandibular symphysis, a triangular mental protuberance is prominent (Fig. 4–6). The base of the triangle, continuous with the inferior border of the mandi-

ble, projects laterally on each side as the mental tubercle. Above the mental tubercle and lateral to the mental protuberance lies a small concavity, the mental, which contains several small foramina for the transmission of accessory nerves and blood vessels. Also in this fossa may be seen a small roughened elevation for the attachment of the mentalis muscle. An anterior buccal mandibular depression has also been described extending laterally from either side of the mental protuberance to the area of the mental foramen, inferior to the mental fossa[6] (Fig. 4–7; see also Fig. 4–2).

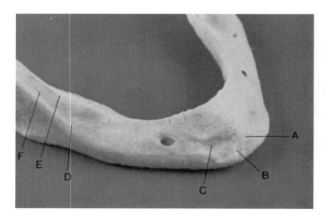

Figure 4–6. Frontal oblique view of edentulous mandible. *A,* Mental protuberance. *B,* Mental tubercle. *C,* Mental fossa. *D,* External oblique ridge blending into the body of the mandible. *E,* Temporal crest. *F,* Retromolar fossa.

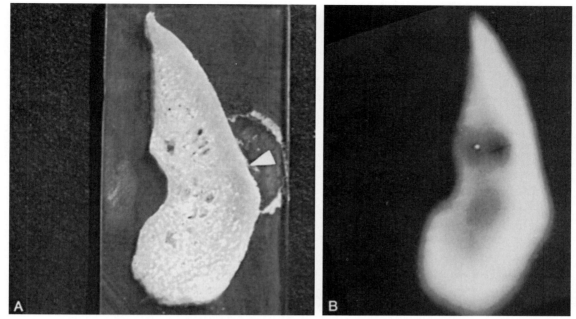

Figure 4–7. *A,* Gross thin cross section of the edentulous mandible shown in Figures 4–1 and 4–6. This section is from the anterior mandibular body between the symphysis region and the mental foramen region. The arrowhead is pointing to the lingual cortex, which is much thicker than the buccal cortical plate. *B,* Multiplanar reformatted computed tomography (MPR-CT)–generated cross section corresponding to the gross cross section shown in *A.* The MPR-CT technique produces images with minimal distortion and magnification that yield valuable information for implant treatment planning. Note the true reproduction of the cortical and cancellous detail.

On the inner surface of the mandibular midline near the inferior border are four distinct or variably fused mental spines, or genial tubercles (see Fig. 4–1F), for the attachment of the right and left genioglossus muscles above and geniohyoid muscles below. In the center of this region, a spinous foramen, or lingual foramen, is often seen for the transmission of communicating accessory nerves and blood vessels. These nerves and vessels apparently supply anterior dental structures.[26] At the inferior mandibular margin, inferolateral to the genial tubercle region bilaterally, is the depression for the origin of the anterior belly of the digastric muscle, the digastric fossa (see Fig. 4–1G). Also on the inner mandibular body in the premolar region, small foramina may be encountered that transmit accessory nerves and vessels.[2]

Extreme caution must be exercised when dissecting on the medial aspect of the mandible and in the floor of the mouth. In this region the sublingual branch of the lingual artery travels medial to the sublingual gland to supply the gland, the mylohyoid muscle, and the soft tissues of the floor of the mouth. It also gives off a medial mandibular branch, which supplies the anterior and lateral surfaces of the lingual cortex.[8] Branches of the sublingual artery can also make important anastomoses with branches of the submental branch of the facial artery through the mylohyoid muscle. Sharp injury to this region can lead to life-threatening hemorrhage, as has been reported after placement of endosteal implants.[10]

References

1. Anderson LC, Kosinski TF, Mentag PJ: A review of the intraosseous course of the nerves of the mandible. J Oral Implantol 17:394, 1991.
2. Carter RB, Keen EN: The intramandibular course of the inferior alveolar nerve. J Anat 108:433, 1971.
3. Cryer MN: Cribriform tube. *In* The Internal Anatomy of the Face. Philadelphia, Lea & Febiger, 1916, p 34.
4. Fawcett E, Edlin MB: The structure of the inferior maxilla with special reference to the position of the inferior dental canal. J Anat 19:355, 1895.
5. Gabriel AC: Some anatomical features of the mandible. J Anat 92:580, 1958.
6. Kaffe I, Littner MM, Arensburg B: The anterior buccal mandibular depression: Physical and radiologic features. Oral Surg Oral Med Oral Pathol 69:647, 1990.
7. Kiesselbach JE, Chamberlain JG: Clinical and anatomic observations on the relationship of the lingual nerve to the mandibular third molar region. J Oral Maxillofac Surg 42:565, 1984.

8. Lasjaunias PL: Craniofacial and Upper Cervical Arteries. Baltimore, Williams & Wilkins, 1983.
9. Littner MM, Kaffe I, Tamse A, et al: Relationship between the apices of the lower molars and mandibular canal—a radiographic study. Oral Surg Oral Med Oral Pathol 62:595, 1986.
10. Mason ME, Triplett RG, Alfonso WF: Life-threatening hemorrhage from placement of a dental implant. J Oral Maxillofac Surg 48:201, 1990.
11. Miller CS, Nummikoski PV, Barnett DA, et al: Cross-sectional tomography. A diagnostic technique for determining the buccolingual relationship of impacted mandibular third molars and the inferior alveolar neurovascular bundle. Oral Surg Oral Med Oral Pathol 70:791, 1990.
12. Miller JA: Studies on the location of the lingula, mandibular foramen and mental foramen. Anat Rec 115:349, 1953.
13. Misch CE, Crawford EA: Predictable mandibular nerve location—a clinical zone of safety. Dent Today 9:32, 1990.
14. Mozsary PG, Middleton RA: Microsurgical reconstruction of the lingual nerve. J Oral Maxillofac Surg 42:415, 1984.
15. Murphy TR, Grundy EM: The inferior alveolar neurovascular bundle at the mandibular foramen. Dent Pract 20:41, 1969.
16. Nortjé CJ, Farman AG, Grotepass FW: Variations in the normal anatomy of the inferior dental (mandibular) canal: A retrospective study of panoramic radiographs from 3612 routine dental patients. Br J Oral Surg 15:55, 1977.
17. Olivier E: The inferior dental canal and its nerve in the adult. Br Dent J 49:356, 1928.
18. Piersol GA: The trigeminal nerve. In Huber G (ed): Human Anatomy. Philadelphia, JB Lippincott, 1903, p 1230.
19. Rajchel J, Ellis E, Fonseca RJ: The anatomical location of the mandibular canal: Its relationship to the sagittal ramus osteotomy. Int J Adult Orthod Orthognath Surg 1:37, 1986.
20. Ritter EF, Moelleken BRW, Mathes SJ, et al: The course of the inferior alveolar neurovascular canal in relation to sliding genioplasty. J Craniofac Surg 3:20, 1992.
21. Rood JP: The organization of the inferior alveolar nerve and its relation to local anesthesia. J Dent 6:305, 1978.
22. Rothman SLG, Chaftez N, Rhodes ML, et al: CT in the preoperative assessment of the mandible and maxilla for endosseous implant surgery. Radiology 168:171, 1988.
23. Shirai M: Contribution to the knowledge of the holes of the lingual surface of the mandible. Yokohama Med Bull 11:541, 1960.
24. Starkie C, Stewart D: The intramandibular course of the inferior dental nerve. J Anat 65:319, 1931.
25. Stella JP, Tharanon W: A precise radiographic method to determine the location of the inferior alveolar canal in the posterior edentulous mandible: Implications for dental implants. Part 1: Technique. Int J Oral Maxillofac Impl 5:15, 1990.
26. Sutton RN: The practical significance of mandibular accessory foramina. Aust Dent J 19:167, 1974.
27. Tammisalo T, Happonen R-P, Tammisalo EH: Stereographic assessment of mandibular canal in relation to the roots of impacted lower third molar using multiprojection narrow beam radiography. Int J Oral Maxillofac Surg 21:85, 1992.
28. Zhang KQ: Anatomical study of the mandibular nerve. Chung Hua Kou Chiang Ko Tsa Chih 20:248, 1985.

Study Questions

1. Describe the course of the inferior alveolar nerve through the mandible. Try to locate the canal in distance measurements in relation to the inferior border of the mandible.

2. What is the significance of the mylohyoid ridge in regard to placing an implant in the second molar location?

3. When placing anterior mandibular implants in the symphysis, do you follow the lingual cortex or the labial cortex? Why?

PART 2

Maxilla

Keith Hoffmann
Revised by Michael S. Block

Part II Maxilla
Osseous Foundation of the Maxilla
Maxillary Alveolar Arch Morphology
Maxillary Sinus
Mucosal Tissues
References

OSSEOUS FOUNDATION OF THE MAXILLA

The osseous foundation of the midface is formed by the paired maxillae and zygomatic bones. These two prominent bones, along with the vomer and palatine bones, contribute structurally to the maxilla, maxillary sinuses, and nasal cavity. The skeletal architecture of the midface reflects the osseous response to the forces of mastication. Three pairs of vertical pillars or buttresses support the maxillary alveolar arch, transferring masticatory forces to the cranial base (Fig. 4–8).

MAXILLARY ALVEOLAR ARCH MORPHOLOGY

The osseous morphology of the dentoalveolar process is influenced by masticatory forces transmitted to the alveolus through the teeth and periodontal ligament. The maxillary posterior teeth are inclined buccally 5 to 10 degrees opposing the mandibular posterior teeth, which are inclined lingually (Fig. 4–9). This transverse curvature of the dental arches, referred to as the curve of Wilson, must be considered when aligning posterior dental implants. As illustrated in Figure 4–9, the discrepancy in arch width progressively worsens with resorption of the alveolus, making it difficult to maintain a normal occlusal relationship. Anteriorly both the maxillary and the mandibular incisors are inclined labially, an orientation that is stable only as long as posterior occlusal stops exist. The inclination of opposing dentition must be considered when planning treatment for implant cases to ensure proper alignment and adequate bone support.

The labial flare of the maxillary anterior teeth and the vector of occlusal force combine to produce a thin labial alveolar plate and a comparatively heavy palatal plate (Fig. 4–10). During mastication the palatal portion of the anterior maxillary alveolus receives osteogenic stimulation through tensional forces transmitted by the periodontal ligament. In contrast, the labial plate receives minimal tensile forces, and in cases lacking posterior occlusal stops, the labial plate is subjected to excessive compressive pressure, leading to resorption. With loss of the maxillary anterior teeth, resorption of the thin labial bony plate progresses disproportionately, accentuating the prominence of the palatal plate (Fig. 4–10E). When palatal migration of the maxillary alveolar crest is combined with the simultaneous resorption of the mandibular alveolus and its associated anterior migration of the alveolar crest, a class III ridge relationship develops, often accompanied by overclosure of the mandible.

In contrast to the mandible, which possesses

Figure 4–8. The osseous buttresses support the maxillary alveolar arch and transfer masticatory forces to the cranial base. The buttresses represent areas of increased bone density and volume, which are useful when placing endosseous implants. The anterior pillar extends superiorly, lateral to the piriform rim. Forces from the first molar region are transferred superiorly through the body of the zygoma. Posterior masticatory forces are transferred from the maxillary tuberosity to the skull base through the pterygoid process of the sphenoid bone and the palatine bone as the posterior or pterygoid pillar.

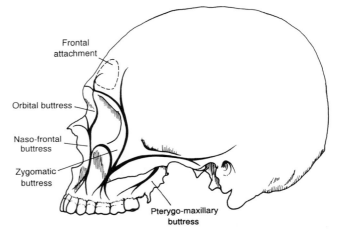

Frontal attachment

Orbital buttress

Naso-frontal buttress

Zygomatic buttress

Pterygo-maxillary buttress

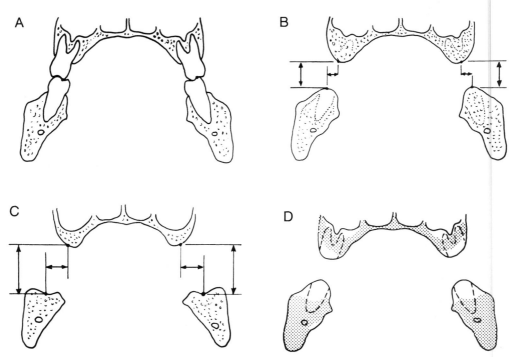

Figure 4–9. *A,* Normal posterior dentition demonstrating buccal inclination of maxillary teeth and lingual inclination of mandibular teeth. *B,* Horizontal and vertical relationships of the alveolar ridges in the early edentulous state. Implants placed perpendicular to the crest would result in posterior crossbite unless hybrid structure or overdenture prosthesis is used. *C, D,* Progressive resorption of the alveolar ridges results in increased interarch space and increasing potential for posterior crossbite. (Adapted from Starshak TJ: Preprosthetic Oral Surgery. St. Louis, CV Mosby, 1971, p 11.)

an alveolar arch of cancellous bone supported by a foundation of dense basal bone, the entire maxillary arch is composed of cancellous or spongy bone extending superiorly to a thin plate of compact bone forming the nasal floor anteriorly and the floor of the maxillary sinus posteriorly. In addition, the maxillary alveolar arch generally exhibits thin buccal/labial and palatal cortical plates (Fig. 4–11).

With progressive bone loss, the functional alveolar ridge may encroach on anatomic structures, complicating implant placement and prosthesis retention. Anteriorly the ridge may resorb to the level of the anterior nasal spine. With palatal migration of the anterior alveolus, the nasopalatine nerve and vessels may eventually emerge from the crest of the alveolus. Laterally the attachment of the buccinator muscle and the

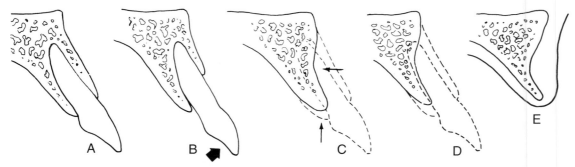

Figure 4–10. *A,* Sagittal view of maxillary incisor tooth and supporting bone in normal healthy state. Note greater bulk of palatal bone compared with the thin labial plate. *B,* With continuous occlusal forces, there is resorption of the thin labial plate. *C, D,* Remodeling and resorption of the alveolar ridges following tooth loss; note the loss of the labial bone. *E,* The natural progression of bone resorption results in a "knife-edge" bony ridge, which can be concealed by the overlying fibrous tissue.

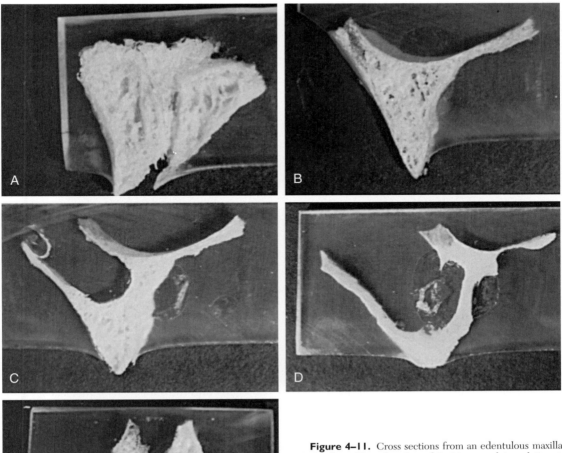

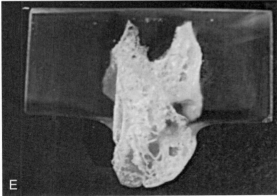

Figure 4–11. Cross sections from an edentulous maxilla. A, Midline. Note location of incisive canal in relation to alveolar crest. B, Canine region. Note presence and concavity of nasal floor and the inclination of the lateral aspect of maxilla to the crest. C, Second premolar region. Note presence of sinus with septal present. The facial resorption places the alveolar crest palatal to the lateral maxillary wall. D, Molar region. Note presence of sinus. The medial wall of the sinus is the lateral wall of the nose. E, The tuberosity region often has sufficient bone for harvesting a graft or placing implants through the tuberosity into the pterygoid plates.

inferior extent of the zygomatic buttress may approximate the crest. Posteriorly the hamular notch may become less distinct following resorption of the tuberosity.

MAXILLARY SINUS

The maxillary sinus is a pneumatic cavity occupying the body of maxilla. In the adult it is the largest of the paired paranasal sinuses with an average capacity of 12 to 15 ml (Fig. 4–12). The average dimensions are 23 mm wide (medial-lateral), 34 mm anterior-posterior, and 33 mm high.[5] The dimensions and capacity vary greatly owing to the variable extent to which the sinus expands into the surrounding bone. Expansion of the maxillary sinus into the alveolus represents a major factor in the amount of vertical bone height available for endosseous implant placement in the posterior maxilla.

The inferior extent of the sinus in the young adult with full dentition is normally in the second

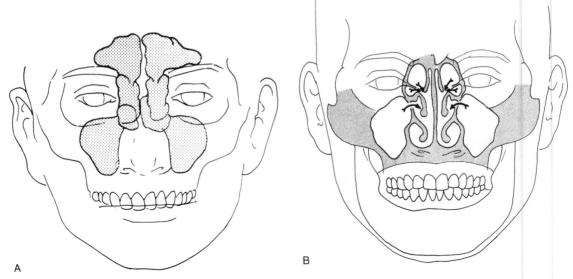

A   B

Figure 4–12. *A, B,* Frontal diagrams illustrating position and relative size of the maxillary sinuses. The actual dimensions are extremely variable depending on the degree of expansion into the surrounding bone. The curved arrows in *B* represent the position of the ostium, which drains the sinus into the nasal cavity located high on the medial sinus wall. Passive drainage through the ostium is nearly impossible because of location.

premolar or first molar region. As teeth are lost, the maxillary sinus may expand into the vacated alveolus. The extent to which the sinus invades the alveolus is impossible to predict, and careful evaluation of radiographs is necessary to avoid violating the sinus membrane during implant placement. The sinus epithelium is thin and tightly bound to the underlying periosteum. Fortunately the periosteum is loosely attached to the bone, and with the exception of antrums with prominent septa, it is readily elevated during sinus grafting procedures. The sinus membrane is composed of pseudostratified ciliated columnar epithelium, with both serous and mucous glands. Studies indicate that the healthy maxillary sinus is sterile.[2, 3] The sinus is maintained free of pathogens by a continuous flow of mucus propelled toward the ostium by the coordinated beating of the cilia. The ostium is positioned high on the medial wall of the sinus, making passive drainage nearly impossible (Fig. 4–12).

An additional hindrance to effective drainage is the configuration of the ostium. The ostium is not a simple orifice through the bony wall into the nasal cavity. This ductlike orifice measures 3.5 to 6.0 mm in length and 3.5 by 6.0 mm in cross section. The ostium emerges into the nasal cavity beneath the middle concha. The dimensions of the opening are frequently reduced during allergic or infectious inflammatory processes, which causes edema of the lining mucosa and constriction or complete obstruction of the ori-

fice. Careful surgical technique must be employed to avoid the introduction of debris and pathogens into the sinus, which may cause acute or chronic sinusitis. Introduction of foreign bodies (dislodged implants) or other surgical debris may lead to chronic suppurative infection with obstruction of the ostium and severe pain requiring surgical debridement and reestablishment of drainage.[6]

MUCOSAL TISSUES

Although implant-retained prostheses are not directly supported by the mucosa, the clinician must be familiar with the characteristics of the different oral tissues to ensure an adequate margin of attached gingiva at the implant site. The mucosal tissues associated with the maxillary alveolus and palate include masticatory and lining mucosa. Keratinized masticatory mucosa covers the alveolar crest and hard palate, whereas nonkeratinized lining mucosa covers the cheeks, vestibule, soft palate, uvula, and basal portion of the alveolar process. Lining mucosa is composed of nonkeratinized stratified squamous epithelium with a distinct submucosal layer of loose connective tissue containing fat, blood vessels, and glandular components. It is the presence and composition of submucosal layer that determines the mobility of the overlying mucosa. In contrast to lining mucosa, masticatory mucosa is generally

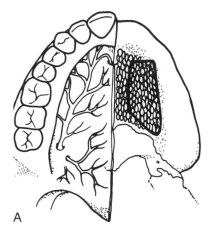
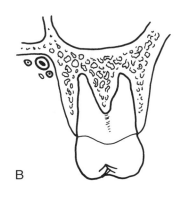

Figure 4–13. *A,* Soft tissue of the palate; the lateral regions exhibit a distinct submucosa containing adipose tissue anteriorly and minor salivary glands posteriorly. This prominent submucosal layer facilitates harvesting of the palatal graft. The lateral regions are separated by the midline palatine raphe, which lacks a defined submucosal layer. Deep to the fatty/glandular layer lie the greater and lesser palatine neurovascular structures. The greater palatine arteries represent potential sites for significant hemorrhage. *B,* The neurovascular structures course deep to the minor salivary glands and adipose tissue within the submucosa of the lateral palate.

immobile, and with the exception of the hard palate, generally lacks a distinct submucosal layer.[1]

The masticatory mucosa covering the alveolar ridge (mucoperiosteum) is firmly bound to the underlying periosteum by heavy collagenous bands extending from the dense lamina propria into the periosteum without an intervening submucosal layer. The transition from attached gingiva to alveolar lining mucosa on the buccal/labial surface of the alveolus is defined by the mucogingival junction. With resorption of the alveolar ridge, the mucogingival junction migrates crestally with a net loss of attached, nonmobile keratinized mucosa. Placement of implants into a severely resorbed ridge may necessitate a palatal or skin graft vestibuloplasty or other graft procedures to regain adequate attached tissue buccally.[6, 7]

The hard palate is lined with keratinized masticatory mucosa and is frequently used as donor site when keratinized tissue is required. The median raphe separates the two lateral regions of the palate extending posteriorly from the incisive papilla to the soft palate. The median raphe represents the site of fusion for the palatine processes, and in contrast to the lateral palatal regions, there is no submucosa. This tightly bound

mucoperiosteum is analogous to the attached mucosa of the alveolar ridge. The lateral regions of the hard palate exhibit a distinct submucosal layer containing a predominance of adipose tissue anteriorly and minor salivary glands posteriorly (Fig. 4–13). This loose submucosal layer provides a cleavage plane that facilitates harvesting palatal mucosal grafts.

References

1. Anderson L, Karring T, Mackenzie I: Oral mucous membrane. *In* Mjor IA, Fejerskov O (eds): Human Oral Embryology and Histology. Copenhagen, Munksgaard, 1986, pp 203–242.
2. Cook HE, Haber J: Bacteriology of the maxillary sinus. J Oral Maxillofac Surg 45:1011, 1978.
3. Evans FO, Sydnor JB, et al: Sinusitis of the maxillary antrum. N Engl J Med 293:735, 1975.
4. Fonseca RJ: Palatal mucosal grafts. *In* Fonseca RJ, Davis WH (eds): Reconstructive Preprosthetic Oral and Maxillofacial Surgery. Philadelphia, WB Saunders, 1986, pp 107–108.
5. Hollinshead WH: Anatomy for Surgeons: The Head and Neck, ed 3. Philadelphia, Harper & Row, 1982, pp 259–262.
6. Quiney RE, Brimble E, Hodge M: Maxillary sinusitis from dental osseointegrated implants. J Laryngol Otol 104:333–334, 1990.
7. Starshak TJ: Preprosthetic Oral Surgery. St Louis, CV Mosby, 1971.

Study Questions

1. Because of resorption patterns, why do patients often need overdentures for the maxilla, instead of a fixed cemented restoration?

2. What are the normal dimensions of the maxillary sinus? Where is the os located in the nose? Based on the above, discuss the ideal location of sinus bone grafts.

3. When bone is harvested from the maxillary tuberosity, what is the location of a blood vessel that the clinician wants to avoid?

CHAPTER 5

Radiologic Planning for Dental Implants

Richard Kraut
Revised by Michael S. Block

Radiologic Methods
  Periapical Radiographs
  Panoramic Radiographs
  Lateral Cephalometric Radiographs

Conventional Tomograms
Computed Tomography
Magnetic Resonance Imaging
References

The first step in formulating a treatment plan for dental rehabilitation using implants must be determination of sufficient bone quantity and quality to support the implants. The choice of radiologic technique appropriate for a given patient depends on a number of factors, including the type of restoration and implants to be used, the position of the remaining dentition, and the extent to which bone quality or quantity is in question. Figures 5–1 and 5–2 demonstrate the decision-making process that the clinician should follow to choose the radiograph necessary for the patient.

RADIOLOGIC METHODS

Periapical Radiographs

Periapical radiographs reveal the location of roots, either from teeth adjacent to the proposed implant site or from teeth that have been lost or extracted without removal of the entire root. They can also reveal the presence of other foreign bodies, such as stainless steel ligatures, bone plates, or screws that might interfere with the placement or osteointegration of an implant. If the maxillary central incisor area is being considered for an implant, periapical radiographs can show the size and location of the incisive canal, which must be avoided because the epithelium within the canal may prevent osteointegration by enveloping the implant. Periapical radiographs are most valuable in monitoring crestal bone maintenance after implants are placed, particu-

larly with superimposed millimeter grid markings.

Advantages of periapical radiographs are: They are available in most dental offices, and all dentists are thoroughly trained to read the resulting radiographs. Disadvantages are: Angulation distortion is present, and determination of actual ridge height is difficult because periapical radiographs do not have one-to-one correspondence with regard to size.[15]

Panoramic Radiographs

The most commonly used radiologic technique for preoperative planning is the panoramic radiograph, because it enables the dentist to visualize the presence or absence of dentition or other implants in both arches. It is also a useful screen for osseous disorders such as residual cysts.

Bone height in the mandible can be accurately assessed using a marker of a known size placed directly on the mucosa when the panoramic radiograph is obtained.[1–3] For example, the markers in Figure 5–3 actually have a diameter of 5 mm; however, on the panoramic film they measure 6 mm—a 20% distortion. Therefore, although the panoramic radiograph in Figure 5–3 shows 22 mm of bone above the inferior alveolar canal in the lower left first molar area, only 18.3 mm is actually available; in the lower right first molar area, 24 mm of bone is measurable above the inferior alveolar canal, but only 20 mm of bone is actually available.

A panoramic radiograph can indicate the anterior-posterior location of the mental foramen

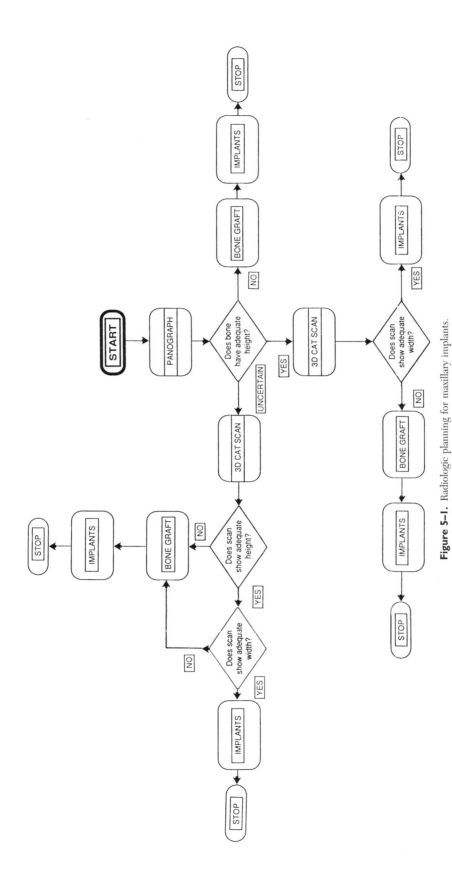

Figure 5–1. Radiologic planning for maxillary implants.

34

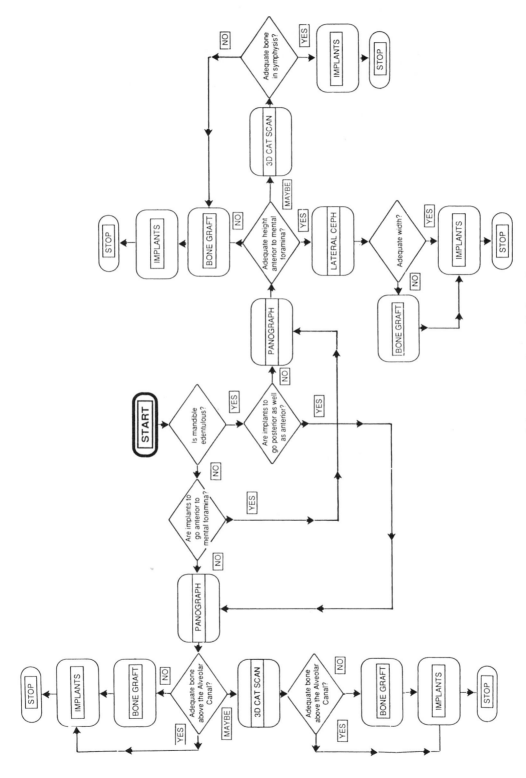

Figure 5–2. Radiologic planning for mandibular implants.

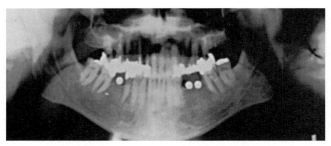

Figure 5–3. Panoramic radiograph with 5-mm markers present at potential implant sites. Owing to distortion, the 5-mm markers measured 6 mm on the radiograph, indicating 20% distortion in the areas being evaluated as implant receptor sites.

relative to the proposed implant site.[15, 16] As long as the proposed implant site is 3 mm or more anterior to the mental foramen, a long endosteal implant that engages the inferior cortical bone of the mandible can be used. If the mental foramina are at the surface of the resorbed mandible, the incision for osseous exposure should be placed toward the lingual aspect of the alveolar process to avoid damaging the mental nerve as the mandibular symphysis is exposed.

Panoramic radiographs provide definitive information regarding the height of the alveolar bone; they do not, however, provide information about the width of bone. Because the maxillary mucosa is of variable thickness, accurate width prediction is problematic. Cross-sectional imaging should be used to confirm anticipated maxillary bone volume before placement of dental implants. When inadequate maxillary bone is available, the patient should be advised of various bone augmentation techniques to restore maxillary bone volume, combined with endosteal implants.

Panoramic radiographs do not provide sufficient diagnostic information about the size and shape of the maxillary sinuses. The concave floor of the sinus results in variable dimensions of the alveolar process anteroposteriorly as well as mediolaterally. Conventional panoramic radiographs show the bone height that is present within the focal trough of the panograph. The paucity of diagnostic information relative to the floor of the maxillary sinus is appreciated when one compares the conventional panograph to the three-dimensional image provided by the special dental processing software that is used to process CT images (Fig. 5–4).

Advantages of panoramic radiographs are that both arches are present on one film, most dental offices are equipped and staffed to obtain panoramic radiographs, and all dentists are thoroughly trained to read the panoramic radiographs. Disadvantages include lack of width determination of the alveolar process and magnification of structures.

Lateral Cephalometric Radiographs

Lateral cephalometric radiographs provide an exact image of the occlusal relationship between the arches and possible skeletal abnormalities. This relationship is important in determining the force that will be applied to any implant-borne restoration. When class I occlusion is not achievable, increased anterior maxillary or mandibular occlusal loading may develop. If the patient's age, general health, or reluctance to undergo orthognathic surgery prevents orthodontic or surgical correction of the skeletal abnormality, the abnormal concentration of forces generated by the alignment of the jaws must be considered when determining the number and size of the implants to support any dental restoration.

For patients who are edentulous in either or both arches, the lateral cephalometric radiograph allows the dentist to evaluate both the soft tissue profile and the relationship between the two arches. After a trial prosthesis is fabricated and coated with radiopaque material, a second cephalometric radiograph can be taken to determine the relationship of the proposed dental restoration to the residual osseous structure (Fig. 5–5) and to demonstrate aesthetics from the facial soft tissue profile generated by the proposed restoration.

The lateral cephalometric radiograph's one-to-one imaging of the buccal and lingual cortical heights of the mandibular symphysis allows the dentist to determine precisely the appropriate length and inclination of implants to be placed.

Advantages of lateral cephalometric radiographs include availability from oral and maxillofacial surgeons and orthodontists, one-to-one im-

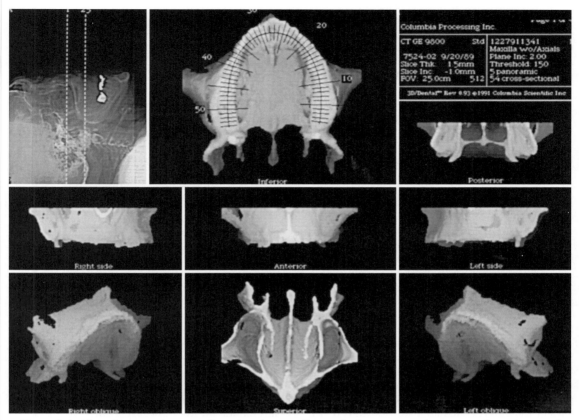

Figure 5–4. Three-dimensional images of an edentulous maxilla provide the surgeon with accurate information regarding the contour of the maxilla.

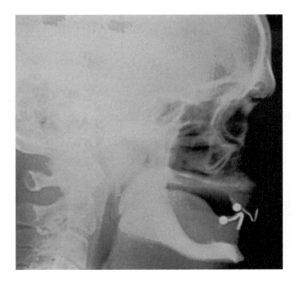

Figure 5–5. Lateral cephalometric radiograph with lead foil placed over the incisal edge of the maxillary and mandibular provisional prosthetic setup. The marking ball is included to verify the one-to-one imaging that is expected on lateral cephalometric radiographs.

ages, and profile prediction. Disadvantages are that the radiographs are not available in general dental offices, and they provide information about the alveolar processes only relative to the midsagittal plane.

Conventional Tomograms

Conventional tomograms provide cross-sectional images that give the dentist precise information about bone volume and the location of vital structures when combined with markers of known size.[8] When tomograms are ordered, communication between the dentist and the radiologist is of utmost importance because the dentist must precisely identify the specific area to be imaged. The dentist must also provide the radiologist with a radiologic marker of known dimension to be placed on the alveolar process in the plane of the tomogram.[9, 13, 14] The advantage of conventional tomograms is reduction of radiation and cost compared with CT.

When radiographs of proposed sites for implant placement reveal inadequate bone volume, the dentist may request images of additional sites. Therefore, although a conventional tomogram results in less radiation exposure for the patient than a CT image, this advantage is diminished when multiple prospective implant sites are to be imaged. Many radiologists no longer maintain conventional tomographic equipment because CT has become the state of the art in tomography.

Computed Tomography

Since 1972, when the first computerized scanner converted x-ray pictures into digital signals, major changes in imaging have occurred. First, CT used computer technology to offer images with dramatically enhanced detail. Conventional diagnostic radiographic techniques provide images with fewer than 30 variations of gray, whereas CT techniques generate images with more than 200 shades of gray. The increased CT gray scale shows subtle variations in tissue density that are not discernible with conventional radiology.[4-7]

Second, special dental processing software programs capable of further enhancing the CT image to show three-dimensional images and one-to-one correspondence were introduced in 1987.[5, 10, 11] These programs provide panoramic and cross-sectional images in addition to three-dimensional images of either the maxilla or the mandible.[2, 6, 10-12] The dentist usually studies the three-dimensional images to gain an overview of the area being considered for implants, especially the contour of the bone being considered for implantation (see Fig. 5-4). Next the dentist studies the panographic views to develop an overall plan for each arch (Fig. 5-6). The panographic image serves as a convenient image for patient counseling. Once the overall plan for each arch has been developed, the dentist uses the cross-sectional images, which include cross references to the panographic images, to determine the width and height of bone at the specific sites selected for individual implants (Fig. 5-7). Knowing the precise height from the alveolar ridge to adjacent vital structures, such as the nasal floor or the inferior alveolar canal, allows the dentist to select the longest implant that will not violate any adjacent vital structure.

Two companies currently market software capable of providing three-dimensional images for dental implant planning. Software from 3D/Dental (Columbia Scientific, Inc, Columbia, MD) provides life-sized (one-to-one) panoramic and cross-sectional images as well as three-dimensional images, and the software from Dent/a/Scan (General Electric Co, Milwaukee, WI) provides a scale that the surgeon can use to convert measurements on the images accurately to actual size.

A CT appliance may be used both to facilitate patient positioning during the scanning process and to simplify correlation of the images at the time of implant placement. The appliance consists of a clear acrylic surgical guide that is modified by placement of a gutta percha line parallel to the proposed occlusal plane and gutta percha lines in the midbuccal facing and central fossa of each tooth that is a proposed implant site. The CT technician uses the occlusal plane marker to ensure that the patient is in the proper position on the scanning gantry before starting the actual scanning process. The surgeon and restorative dentists then modify the appliance after they review the scan so the precise area selected on the scan is the area prepared for implant placement (Fig. 5-8).

SIM/PLANT (Columbia Scientific, Inc, Columbia, MD), an interactive dental implant software package that allows dentists to view and manipulate processed CT images on their office computers, became available in 1993. With SIM/PLANT for Windows (Microsoft Corp, Redmond, WA), dentists can visualize vital structures and judge bone quantity and quality using the life-size panoramic, cross-sectional, and transaxial images produced by CT that are processed on

Text continued on page 43

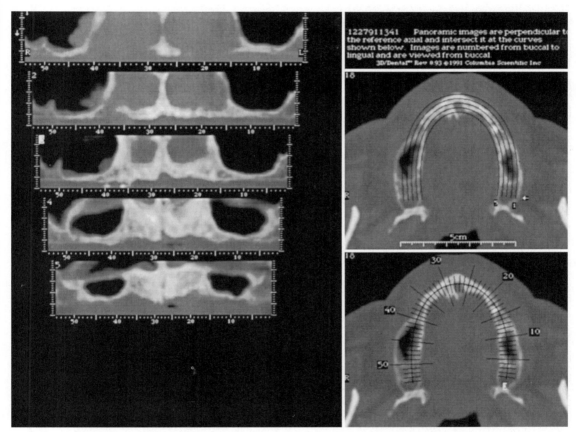

Figure 5–6. Multiple panographic images indicate the presence of adequate bone height in areas 16 through 37.

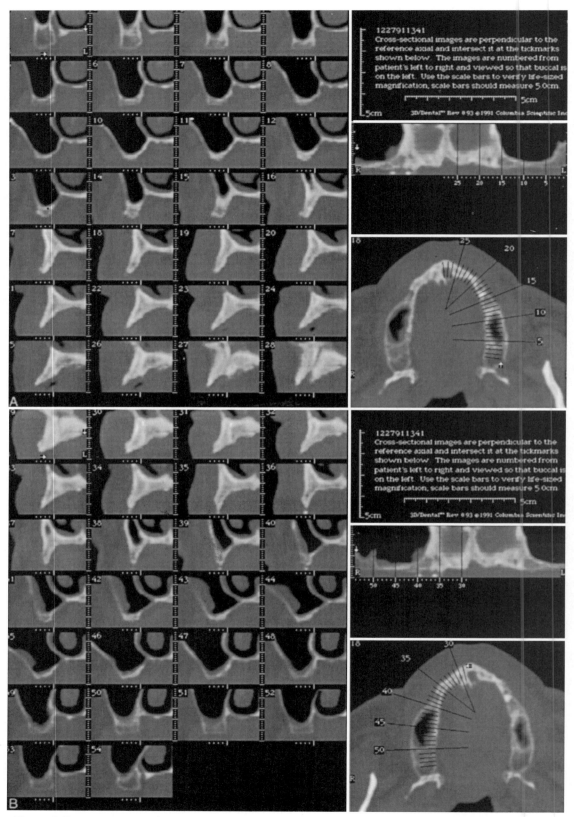

Figure 5–7. *A*, Cross-sectional images of the left side of an edentulous maxilla indicate adequate bone for endosteal implants at areas 20 and 24. *B*, Cross-sectional images of the right side of an edentulous maxilla indicate adequate bone for endosteal implants at areas 31 and 36.

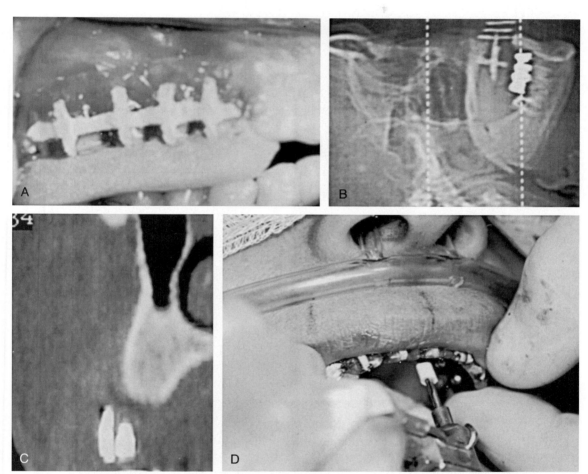

Figure 5–8. *A*, CT appliance for edentulous maxilla, with a horizontal gutta percha line parallel to the proposed occlusal plane and vertical gutta percha lines through the midbuccal facing of each of the teeth that are proposed implant sites. *B*, Scout film in which the technician has positioned the patient so the plane of the scan (indicated by the dotted lines on the film) is parallel to the proposed occlusal plane (indicated by the solid horizontal gutta percha line). *C*, Cross section of the maxilla demonstrating the relationship of the alveolar ridge to the buccal surface of the proposed restoration *(longer radiopaque line)* and the proposed path of insertion of the implant *(shorter radiopaque line)*. *D*, Implant receptor site preparation using the modified CT appliance to position the implant precisely in the area selected. (Courtesy of Dr. Michael Klein.)

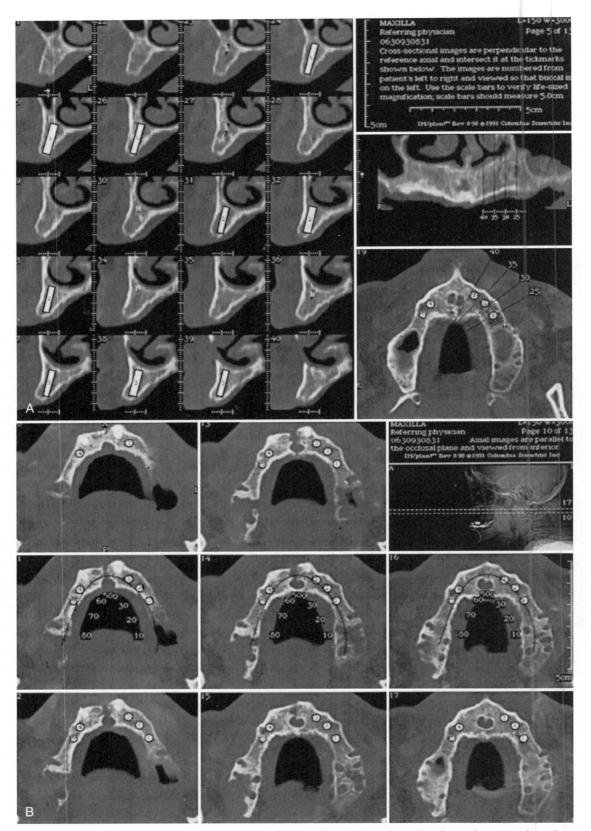

Figure 5–9. *A,* Maxillary CT scan demonstrating the left premaxilla with three planned implants. The proposed angulation of each implant to the alveolar ridge is clearly seen. The panoramic and cross-sectional images at the right facilitate rapid orientation to the location of the cross sections printed on this page. *B,* Axial images of a maxillary CT scan, which provide information relative to the area of the scan referenced in the upper right-hand corner of the page. Images from axial sections 10 through 17 confirm adequate bone in the areas implants are proposed.

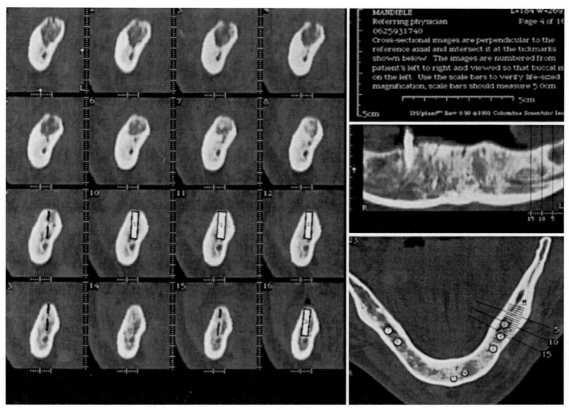

Figure 5–10. Cross-sectional image of the mandible showing the available height and width of bone relative to the planned placement of implants 1 and 2. Implant 1 is placed within the body of the mandible, avoiding perforation into the lingual fossa below the internal oblique ridge. A more cautious approach to proposed implant 2 would be to use a slightly shorter implant and provide a margin of safety relative to the inferior alveolar canal.

Columbia Scientific's Image Master-101 using IM/PLANT software (Figs. 5–9 and 5–10). In addition to using the images to judge bone quality and quantity, dentists can use SIM/PLANT software to superimpose images of actual-size implants on the CT images for treatment planning and presentation purposes.

The advantage of CT is one-to-one imaging with unsurpassed detail relative to all potential implant sites within either the maxilla or the mandible. Disadvantages are that an appointment is necessary at a special facility with the appropriate CT scanner, images are more expensive than routine films, the patient is exposed to more radiation than with other radiologic techniques, and the dentist must be trained to read the resulting images.

Magnetic Resonance Imaging

The physical principle, or effect, that forms the basis of MRI is the interaction of nuclei,

which have a non-zero magnetic moment with a magnetic field. Radiofrequency coils generate a magnetic field that is used to excite the nuclei and detect the signal. Similar to all digital images, magnetic resonance images are displayed via an image processor on a cathode-ray tube.

Tissue with relatively high water content is more precisely imaged with MRI technology than those tissues with relatively low moisture content. At present, bone imaging is not as detailed with MRI as it is with CT.[6] MRI technology is not presently used in assessing the quantity and quality of bone that may be available for placement of dental implants.

References

1. Gallimidi J, Brunel G, Castello J, Ohnona M: A practical method for the determination of the available bone height in oral implantology. Rev Stom Atol Chir Maxillofac 90:357–361, 1989.
2. Jeffcoat M, Jeffcoat RL, Reddy MS, Berland L: Planning

interactive implant treatment with 3-D computed tomography. J Am Dent Assoc 122:40–44, 1991.

3. Jensen O: Site classification for the osseointegrated implant. J Prosthet Dent 61:228–234, 1989.

4. Klinge B, Petersson A, Maly P: Location of the mandibular canal: Comparison of macroscopic findings, conventional radiography, and computer tomography. Int J Oral Maxillofac Impl 4:327–332, 1989.

5. Kraut RA: Selecting the precise implant site. J Am Dent Assoc 122:59–60, 1991.

6. Maher WP: Topographic, microscopic, radiographic and computerized morphometric studies of the human adult edentate mandible for oral implantologists. Clin Anat 4:327–340, 1991.

7. McGivney GP, Haughton V, Strandt JA, Eichholz JE, Lubar DM: A comparison of computer-assisted tomography and data-gathering modalities in prosthodontics. Int J Oral Maxillofac Impl 1:55–68, 1986.

8. Miller CS, Nummikoski PV, Barnett DA, Langlais RP: Cross-sectional tomography. Oral Surg Oral Med Oral Pathol 70:791–797, 1989.

9. Petrikowski CG, Pharoah MJ, Schmitt A: Presurgical radiographic assessment for implants. J Prosthet Dent 61:59–64, 1989.

10. Quirynen M, Lamoral Y, Dekeyser C, Peene P, van Steenberghe D, Bonte J, Baert AL: The CT scan standard reconstruction technique for reliable jaw bone volume determination. Int J Oral Maxillofac Impl 5:384–389, 1990.

11. Shimura M, Babbush CA, Majima H, Yanagisawa S, Sairenji E: Presurgical evaluation for dental implants using a reformatting program of computed tomography: Maxilla/mandible shape pattern analysis (MSPA). Int J Oral Maxillofac Impl 5:175–181, 1990.

12. Smith JP, Borrow JW: Reformatted CT imaging for implant planning. Oral Maxillofac Surg Clin North Am 3:805–825, 1991.

13. Stella JP, Tharanon W: A precise radiographic method to determine the location of the inferior alveolar canal in the posterior edentulous mandible: Implications for dental implants: I. Technique. Int J Oral Maxillofac Impl 5:15–22, 1990.

14. Stella JP, Tharanon W: A precise radiographic method to determine the location of the inferior alveolar canal in the posterior edentulous mandible: Implications for dental implants: II. Clinical application. Int J Oral Maxillofac Impl 5:23–29, 1990.

15. Yosue T, Brooks SL: The appearance of mental foramina on panoramic and periapical radiographs: II. Experimental evaluation. Oral Surg Oral Med Oral Pathol 68:488–492, 1989.

16. Yosue T, Brooks SL: The appearance of mental foramina on panoramic radiographs: I. Evaluation of patients. Oral Surg Oral Med Oral Pathol 68:360–364, 1989.

Study Questions

1. What radiographic methods will provide information on the size and shape of the anterior mandible? Which are available in most oral surgery offices? Which require visits to the radiologist?

2. What radiographs are useful for assessing bone availability for anterior single tooth maxillary implants?

3. What technique is useful to relate available bone to the planned restoration? Describe fabrication of the radiographic stent.

4. If you were concerned with the location of the inferior alveolar nerve, describe two radiographic methods, and their disadvantages and advantages, to determine its specific location.

CHAPTER 6

Healing of Endosseous Implants—The Wound Response

Jozef Zoldos
John N. Kent
Revised by John N. Kent and Michael S. Block

Generalized Surgical Wound Healing
   Bone Healing
   Bone-Implant Interface
   Mucoperiosteal-Implant Interface
   Factors Affecting Healing
Surgical Technique
Premature Loading
Surgical Fit
Bone Quality

Physical Composition of the Patient
   Nutritional Status
   Aging
   Diabetes Mellitus
   Hematologic Derangements
   Corticosteroids
   Radiation
References

During the past two decades, endosseous implants have been used extensively to achieve osseointegration for prosthetic rehabilitation of edentulism. Generally a surgical procedure is performed on a patient to insert a foreign material into bone, and then the body is called on to "heal" the wound. Since the mid-1970s, the general consensus for successful implant healing shifted toward that of a direct bond of the implant to bone with no intervening fibrous tissue, i.e., osseous integration.[1, 2, 4, 5, 11, 14, 43, 49]

There are many requirements for successful osseous integration that must be considered during the placement of endosseous implants. This chapter discusses the general healing of bone and soft tissues around implants, factors influencing healing, biocompatibility of materials, and the healing response of hard and soft tissue with implants.

GENERALIZED SURGICAL WOUND HEALING

The generalized healing of tissues around an implant involves a complex array of events that occur between the initial placement of the implant and the eventual healed result. Wound healing can be broken down into three fundamental phases: inflammation, proliferation, and maturation. There is significant overlap between these three phases, but each one can be noted to be dominant during certain periods of the healing process (Table 6–1).

Replacement of lost or damaged tissues occurs by one of two methods: repair or regeneration.[61] Regeneration results in tissues that are structurally and functionally indistinguishable from their preinjured state. An example of this type of healing is exemplified by normal fracture healing. Not all tissues, however, have the capacity for regenerative healing. Some tissues, for example, skin, heal by the formation of a fibrous connective tissue scar that is structurally and functionally different from the preinjured state, so-called reparative healing. After the surgical placement of implants into their endosteal locations, reparative healing occurs relatively predictably for the mucoperiosteal complex.

Bone Healing

After the surgical placement of implants into endosteal locations, the traumatized bone around

45

Table 6–1. Phases of Generalized Mucoperiosteal Tissue Healing

Phase	Timing	Specific Occurrence
1 Inflammatory phase	Day 1–10	Platelet aggregation and activation
		Clotting cascade activation
		Cytokine release
		Nonspecific cellular inflammatory response
		Macrophage-mediated inflammation
2 Proliferative phase	Day 2–42	Neovascularization
		Differentiation, proliferation, and activation of cells
		Deposition of immature collagen, elastin, and ground substance
3 Maturation phase	After day 21	Connective tissue remodeling

these implants begins the process of wound healing, which can be separated into the inflammatory phase, the proliferative phase, and the maturation phase (Fig. 6–1; Table 6–2).

Bone-Implant Interface

The type of interface that develops between the implant and bone depends on many variables. Ultrastructural investigations between implants and bone in areas of osseous integration reveal a zone of amorphous material between the implant and bone.[6, 17, 34] The exact chemical nature of interface that forms between this amorphous layer and the metallic implant surface is yet to be determined. It has been theorized, however, that weak Van der Waals bonding, direct chemical bonding (i.e., ionic, covalent), or a combination of the two may be present.[36] The implant material in question is the most important factor that determines the chemical nature of this interface. Chemical bonding of the implant material to the surrounding bone is a well-described phenomenon with certain materials, such as calcium phosphate ceramics.[19, 27, 34, 35, 37] Other materials, such as alloys, carbon, aluminum oxide, and most polymers, have a minimal to nonexistent interfacial chemical bond, but they have excellent bone contact.[8, 19, 42] It is controversial, however, whether commercially pure titanium forms a direct chemical bond to bone,

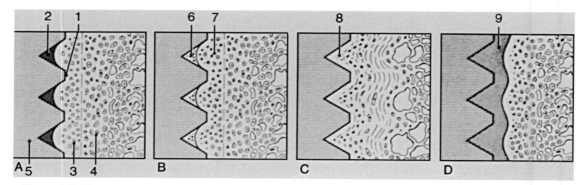

Figure 6–1. Diagrammatic representation of biology of osseointegration. *A,* Threaded bone site cannot be made perfectly congruent to implant. The object of making a threaded socket in bone is to provide immobilization immediately after installation and during the initial healing period. Diagram is based on relative dimensions of fixture and fixture site. 1 = Contact between fixture and bone (immobilization); 2 = hematoma in closed cavity, bordered by fixture and bone; 3 = bone that was damaged by unavoidable thermal and mechanical trauma; 4 = original undamaged bone; and 5 = fixture. *B,* During unloaded healing period, hematoma becomes transformed into new bone through callus formation (6). 7 = Damaged bone, which also heals, undergoes revascularization, demineralization, and remineralization. *C,* After the healing period, vital bone tissue is in close contact with fixture surface, without any other intermediate tissue. Border zone bone (8) remodels in response to masticatory load applied. *D,* In unsuccessful implants, nonmineralized connective tissue (9), constituting a kind of pseudarthrosis, forms in border zone at implant. This development can be initiated by excessive preparation trauma, infection, loading too early in the healing period before adequate mineralization and organization of hard tissue has taken place, or supraliminal loading at any time, even many years after integration has been established. Osseointegration cannot be reconstituted. Connective tissue can become organized to a certain degree, but in our opinion it is not a proper anchoring tissue because of its inadequate mechanical and biologic capacities, which result in creation of locus minoris resistentiae. (From Brånemark P-I: Osseointegration and its experimental background. J Prosthet Dent 50:405, 1983.)

Table 6–2. Phases of Generalized Bone Healing

Phase	Timing	Specific Occurrence
1 Inflammatory phase	Day 1–10	Adsorption of plasma proteins Platelet aggregation and activation Clotting cascade activation Cytokine release Nonspecific cellular inflammatory response Specific cellular inflammatory response Macrophage-mediated inflammation
2 Proliferative phase	Day 3–42	Neovascularization Differentiation, proliferation, and activation of cells Production of immature connective tissue matrix
3 Maturation phase	After day 28	Remodeling of the immature bone matrix with coupled resorption/deposition of bone Bone remodeling in response to implant loading Physiologic bone recession

but it is believed that although a chemical bond may be present, the bond strength is of a lesser magnitude than that experienced with HA.[42] Table 6–3 summarizes some of the commonly used implant materials and their bond type to bone. Table 6–4 describes the degree of compatibility and tissue reaction to specific material.

Mucoperiosteal-Implant Interface

Dental implants have the unique feature of penetrating through lining epithelium.[12, 30, 48] Establishment of an adequate connective tissue seal around an implant provides a barrier to the ingress of oral toxins and bacteria into the internal environment.[48] Some authors[12, 30, 48, 58] believe that maintenance of this seal is essential for preventing the initial peri-implant tissue inflammation that can lead to eventual destruction of implant support. Ten Cate[66] indicates that lack of a biologic seal will not doom implants to failure, but rather the connective tissue response is more likely to be the critical factor involved in implant loss.

Epithelial regeneration around well-integrated implants results in a structure similar to the gingival tissues around natural teeth. The keratin-

Table 6–3. Biomaterial Summary of Surface and Interface Properties

Biomaterial*	Surface	Active (A) or Passive (P)	Bonded (B) or Not (N) to Bone
Metals	Cr_xO_y	P	N
Re-Cr-Ni	TiO_2	A-P	B
Ti and Ti-6Al-4V	Cr_xO_y	P	N
Co alloys			
Ceramics and carbons	Al_2O_3	P	N
Al_2O_3	$Ca_{10}(PO_4)_6(OH)_2$	A	B
HA	$CaPO_4$	A	B
TCP and ALCAP	$CaPO_4$	A	B
Bioglass or Ceravital	C or C-Si	P	N
C and C-Si			
Polymers and composites	Polymer	P	N
PE	Polymer	P	N
Dacron	Polymer	P	N
PTFE	Polymer	P	N
PMMA	Polymer	P	N
Silicone rubber	Polymer	P	N
PS	Polymer	P	N
Composites			

TCP = Tricalcium phosphate; ALCAP = calcium aluminate; PE = polyethylene; PTFE = polytetrafluoroethylene; PMMA = polymethylmethacrylate; PS = polysulfone.

From Lemons JE, Bidez MW: In McKinney RV (ed): Endosteal Implant Biomaterials and Biomechanics. St Louis, Mosby–Year Book, 1991, p 34.

Table 6–4. Grouping of Hard Tissue Replacement Materials According to Their Compatibility to Bony Tissue

Degree of Compatibility	Characteristics of Reactions of Bony Tissue	Materials
Biotolerant	Implants separated from adjacent bone by a soft tissue layer along most of the interface: distance osteogenesis	Stainless steels; PMMA bone cements; CoCrMo and CoCrMoNi alloys
Bioinert	Direct contact to bony tissue: contact osteogenesis	Alumina ceramics, zirconia ceramics, titanium, tantalum, niobium, carbon
Bioactive	Bonding to bony tissue: bonding osteogenesis	Calcium phosphate–containing glasses, glass-ceramics, ceramics, titanium (?)

From Heimke G: The aspects and modes of fixation of bone replacements. *In* Heimke G (ed): Osseo-Integrated Implants. Vol I. Basics, Materials, and Joint Replacements. Boca Raton, FL, CRC Press, 1990, p 4. Copyright CRC Press, Boca Raton, Florida.

ized oral epithelium is continuous with nonkeratinized sulcular epithelium adjacent to the implant in the peri-implant sulcus. This sulcus is analogous to the periodontal sulcus around natural teeth and is approximately 3 to 4 mm deep in healthy sites.[7] Junctional epithelium is located in the apical portion of the sulcus, and this portion of the epithelium is adherent to the implant surface.[9, 45] Ultrastructural investigations of this attachment reveal that the junctional epithelial cells attach to the implant surface with a basal lamina and hemidesmosomes in the same way that they would attach to teeth (Fig. 6–2).[30, 44, 48, 59, 64] The basal lamina–hemidesmosomal complex is thought to be chemically bonded to the implant surface by a 10- to 20-nm amorphous glycoprotein layer similar to that found at the bone-implant interface.[1, 5, 69] These hemidesmosomes become evident 2 to 3 days after implant insertion.[69]

Factors Affecting Healing

There are many factors that can affect the healing process. Some of these factors deal with surgical technique and treatment protocol, whereas others deal with patient selection, hygiene, loading pattern, and site selection.

SURGICAL TECHNIQUE

All surgical procedures are considered to be traumatic to the host tissues, but the level of trauma induced is one of the critical factors that determines whether healing will progress toward fibrous or osseous integration. Studies by Albrektsson[2] reveal that all surgical preparations on hard tissue cause a necrotic zone of bone at the implant bone interface owing to cutting of blood vessels, frictional heat generated during instrumentation, and vibrational trauma. Excessive trauma, however, invariably leads to fibrous encapsulation of the implant.[10] Surgical trauma must be minimized during all aspects of implant surgery to optimize success rates.

Surgical instrumentation of bone produces heat that can elevate the local temperature of bone. Rotary instruments used during preparation of an implant site can cause bone necrosis that can impair local bone viability and eventually lead to fibrous encapsulation of the implant.[2, 22, 24, 25, 31, 41, 71] In vivo studies have shown that traumatic surgical manipulation of bone causes poor vascularization of the implant border zone with delay or absence of ossification.[2] The effect of elevated temperature on bone tissue has been postulated to cause denaturation of alkaline phosphatase, which occurs at 56°C.[23] The crucial threshold temperature for impaired bone regeneration, however, has been shown to be as low as 44°C to 47°C when applied to the bone for periods of 1 minute.[18] Possible explanations for this lower critical temperature threshold could possibly be interference with local circulation, capillary leakage, and dehydration and osmotic changes that occur with traumatic manipulation of bone.[23, 40, 41, 46, 55] These effects could cause enough of a change in bone physiology to result in altered differentiation of local progenitor cells, leading to fibrous encapsulation.[33]

Bone temperatures of 60°C can be found during bone surgery using conventional instrumentation even with copious external irrigation.[25, 40, 67] It has been shown, however, that gentle surgical technique using a graduated series of sharp drills run intermittently at low speeds with copious amounts of internal and external irrigation can help to maintain the local bone temperature below the crucial threshold.[2, 22, 31, 40, 41] This allows for the escape of debris from the bur flutes

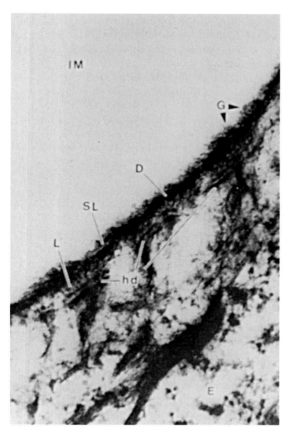

Figure 6–2. Electron micrograph of implant-junctional epithelium interface. A cryofracture electron micrograph specimen revealing the plasma membrane edge of the gingival epithelial cell (E) with hemidesmosomes (hd) and the lamina lucida (L), lamina densa (D), and sublamina lucida (SL) layers of the basal lamina. The outer layer, which interfaced the implant (IM), reveals some remnants of the glycocalyx (G). (Original magnification × 108,200.) (From McKinney RV, et al: The biological tissue response to dental implants. *In* McKinney RV [ed]: Endosteal Dental Implants. St. Louis, Mosby–Year Book, 1991, p 42.)

during preparation, which minimizes frictional heat and enables the irrigant to control local temperatures effectively.[40] It is probably most critical that ultraslow rotary instrumentation (15 to 30 rpm) be used for the final phase of implant site preparation (tapping).[2] Other mechanisms for minimizing operative trauma summarized by Lindström et al[44] include the use of drills with suitable instrument topography, constant profuse irrigation during drilling, adequate drill speed, and careful tapping techniques.

Delicate manipulation of soft tissue around the implant site must also be observed during implant placement. Maintenance of periosteal integrity allows for preservation of local osteoblastic function[50] and maximization of local bone

vascularity, which is essential for implant healing to occur.[3]

PREMATURE LOADING

As mentioned previously, surgical preparation of bone for the placement of implants inevitably causes a zone of necrotic bone around the implant as a result of the surgical procedure. This zone of dead bone must be resorbed and replaced by new vascularized bone for osseous integration to occur. Significant movement of implants during this healing phase has been shown to result in fibrous encapsulation by inhibiting new bone formation and by inhibiting revascularization of necrotic bone.[15, 57] Implant motion has been shown to activate local macrophages, causing them to release cytokines, eicosanoids, and metalloproteinases. It can also create conditions that promote wear and corrosion of the implant material, yielding particulate debris and metal ions.[63] This can further activate inflammatory cells to elaborate other cytokines and enzymes, with the net effect being altered differentiation of local mesenchymal cells, leading to bone resorption and fibrous encapsulation.[70]

In an investigation comparing titanium blade-type implants that were either unloaded or loaded during the third implantation day, Brunski et al[13] demonstrated significantly different interface morphology between these two groups. The loaded implants seemed to demonstrate a fibrous type of encapsulation, whereas the unloaded implants attained direct bone contact. In a series of animal experiments, Pilliar et al[53] have shown that micromovement in the magnitude of 28 μm can allow for bone ingrowth into porous-surfaced implants, whereas excess movement (150 μm or more) results in attachment by mature connective tissue ingrowth. This bone remodeling that occurs during the healing phase occurs at different rates, depending on the amount of local bone necrosis, local bone physiology, and generalized physical composition of the patient. For this reason, it is recommended that these implants remain in an unloaded state for a period of 2 to 8 months, depending on the clinical situation, implant material used, location of implantation, and whether the implant is placed into bone grafts.[38]

SURGICAL FIT

Technical difficulties and inconsistencies between an implant and instrument diameter make it virtually impossible to obtain perfect microscopic contact between bone and implants. Even in the best situation, bone contacts only portions of the implant.[62, 70] When implants are placed into fresh extraction sockets, inconsistencies between the implant diameter and the tooth root diameter at the crest of the alveolar ridge create the potential for a significant space between the residual bone and the implant surface. Successful integration of the implant requires that bone be deposited in these areas for implant support.

With the lack of significant initial bone contact comes the potential for micromotion between the implant and bone. As discussed earlier, it can be seen how this situation might prevent osseous integration of the implant. Cameron et al[15] have demonstrated that with implant stabilization, bone generation can occur around porous-surfaced chromium-cobalt alloy implants in situations with an interfacial gap of 1.5 mm, but it appears that smaller gaps were filled by bone earlier. This has significant implications with respect to timing of implant loading in situations with imprecise implant fit. Carlsson et al[16] studied bone regeneration around titanium implants with interfacial gaps of 0, 0.35, and 0.85 mm. They demonstrated that even after 6 weeks the only implants to achieve significant osseous integration were the ones without interfacial gaps. In an animal investigation examining the healing of a 1-mm interfacial gap with HA-coated implants and titanium implants, Søballe et al[62] demonstrated that there was significantly more bone contact with HA-coated implants than with titanium implants at a 4-week interval. These results would seem to indicate that longer healing periods may be required before loading implants when surgical fit is less than optimal and that earlier loading may be possible when using HA-coated implants.

BONE QUALITY

Bone quality and quantity are factors that can affect implant integration. There are significant differences between bone of the mandible and that of the maxilla. Within each of these bones, different bone quality is seen in different locations. The mandible generally has a denser cortex and coarser, thicker cancelli than does the maxilla. Bone in more posterior locations of both jaws tends to have a thinner, more porous cortex and finer cancelli.[1, 31, 38] If implants are placed in bone with a dense cortex and a thick cancellous component, initial stabilization is more likely to be obtained when compared with implants placed in areas of thinner cortex with fine cancelli. As already seen, stable implants are more likely to heal with osseous integration than implants that are mobile. In addition, regeneration of a cortical rim of bone around the implant from the surrounding cancellous bone is more likely to progress at a faster rate if the surrounding bone is more dense.[31] Thus, before functional loading, it is recommended that the implant healing period be anywhere from 2 to 8 months, depending on the quality of bone at the surgical site, implant material used, and whether the implant is placed into bone grafts.[38] Differences in bone architecture are one of the reasons for the differences in success rates experienced between mandibular and maxillary implants.

PHYSICAL COMPOSITION OF THE PATIENT

The healing of implants involves a dynamic process in which the physical composition of a patient may alter the course of events. There are certain local and systemic conditions that have been implicated in causing impaired implant healing.

Nutritional Status. A patient's nutritional status could be of paramount importance in determining whether implants will heal. Certain vitamins, trace elements, and amino acids are critical for healing to occur. Amino acids are the building blocks for protein and enzyme synthesis, and it would thus stand to reason that a deficiency in these building blocks would prevent appropriate wound healing.[52, 54, 56] Vitamin C is required for the hydroxylation of proline and lysine during collagen synthesis.[20, 56, 60] Collagen is produced by the osteoblasts and fibroblasts during the healing of implants, and a deficiency in vitamin C, called scurvy, is associated with inefficient collagen synthesis with resultant poor wound healing.[39, 51, 56] Vitamin D, together with parathyroid hormone, calcitonin, glucocorticoids, thyroid hormone, estrogen, and possibly other peptides and hormones, is critical for calcium and phosphorus homeostasis.[32, 39] Altered calcium and phosphorus homeostasis can lead to impaired mineralization of the deposited osteoid with resultant implant failure.

Aging. Edentulism commonly occurs in the aging patient. Along with increasing age, changes occur in mineral composition, matrix, and cellular constituents of the skeletal system.[21, 68] Osteoporosis is also a condition of the elderly that results in decreased mineral composition of bones.[26] The rate of calcium exchange between bone and serum in nontraumatized bones is significantly decreased with increasing age.[29] Fracture healing has also been demonstrated to be delayed with increasing age,[21, 68] and aged bones do not appear to be able to form an external callus as readily as do younger bones.[68] In addition, the ability of bone matrix to induce heterotopic bone formation also diminishes with advancing age.[65] Although endosseous implants are not contraindicated in the elderly, one must realize that success rates may be less than optimal with advancing age because of the changes discussed above. Special consideration should thus be placed on timing of initial loading when determining implantation protocol because of the potential for delayed healing in aged bone.

Diabetes Mellitus. Diabetes mellitus is a systemic disease that may alter the healing capacity of the host. Diminished neutrophil chemotaxis and decreased phagocytic activity are responsible for the increased susceptibility to infection in diabetic patients.[56] Microvascular and macrovascular abnormalities may alter local circulation and lead to impaired healing. Diabetes is not a specific contraindication to implant therapy, but it must be considered in therapeutic planning.

Hematologic Derangements. Wounds in patients with acquired or hereditary coagulopathies can be complicated with excessive extravasation of blood into the surgical site. This blood, being an excellent bacterial culture medium, would also increase the susceptibility to wound infections. Aside from the delayed healing associated with wound infections, implant success is severely compromised.

Corticosteroids. Long-term therapy with high doses of steroids has been shown to inhibit formation of granulation tissue (i.e., inhibit capillary proliferation and fibroplasia); retard mesenchymal cell differentiation; inhibit epithelial regeneration; inhibit collagen and ground substance production; inhibit macrophage migration and fibroblast proliferation; and inhibit leukocyte chemotaxis, phagocytosis, and intracellular killing.[51, 52] Many of these effects are likely related to the impaired inflammatory cell function, particularly the macrophage, with resultant decrease in the release of cytokines and growth factors.[52] Single-dose steroid therapy probably has no effect on wound healing.[51]

Radiation. Implants are often used for the reconstruction of maxillofacial defects resulting from surgical ablation of malignant tumors. Radiation to the head and neck region can produce both early and late changes in tissues. Early clinical changes usually involve the intrinsic soft tissues in the field of radiation and include mucositis, dermatitis, and xerostomia. The delayed effects of radiation are demineralization of bone, fibrosis, increased susceptibility to infection, delayed wound healing, and avascular necrosis.[28] The end results of radiotherapy are hypocellular, hypovascular, and hypoxic tissues.[47] Delayed bone healing is thought to result from damage to osteoprogenitor cells or reduced neovascularization.[28]

Preliminary results indicate that significant improvement in integration can be obtained when patients are pretreated with hyperbaric oxygen (HBO).[28] It is thus recommended that implant insertion be delayed for a period after radiation therapy and that patients be pretreated with an HBO regimen before the procedure.

The value of using relatively atraumatic surgical technique cannot be overstated when dealing with irradiated tissues. These tissues do not have the capacity to respond to significant surgical manipulation, and implant failure would be inevitable. Traumatizing irradiated bone can also lead to osteoradionecrosis.

References

1. Adell R, et al: A 15-year study of osseointegrated implants in the treatment of the edentulous jaw. Int J Oral Surg 10:387–416, 1981.
2. Albrektsson T: Direct bone anchorage of dental implants. J Prosthet Dent 50:255–261, 1983.
3. Albrektsson T: Bone tissue response. *In* Brånemark P-I, Zarb GA, Albrektsson T (eds): Tissue Integrated Prostheses—Osseointegration in Clinical Dentistry. Chicago, Quintessence Publishing Co, Inc, 1985, pp 129–144.
4. Albrektsson T, Sennerby L: Direct bone anchorage of oral implants: Clinical and experimental considerations of the concept of osseointegration. Int J Prosthet 3:30–41, 1990.
5. Albrektsson T, et al: Osseointegrated titanium implants. Requirements for ensuring a long-lasting direct bone-to-implant anchorage in man. Acta Orthop Scand 52:155–170, 1981.
6. Albrektsson T, et al: Osseointegration dental implants. Dent Clin North Am 30:151–174, 1986.
7. Apse P, et al: Microbiota and crevicular fluid collagenase activity in the osseointegrated dental implant sulcus: A comparison of sites in edentulous and partially edentulous patients. J Periodont Res 24:96–105, 1989.
8. Beirne OR: Osseointegrated implant systems. *In* Peterson LJ, Indresano AT, Marciani RD, Roser SM (eds): Principles of Oral and Maxillofacial Surgery. Philadelphia, JB Lippincott, 1992, pp 1133–1154.
9. Berglundh T, et al: The soft tissue barrier at implants and teeth. Clin Oral Impl Res 2:81–90, 1991.
10. Brånemark P-I, et al: Intra-osseous anchorage of dental prostheses. Scand J Plast Reconstr Surg 3:81–100, 1969.
11. Brånemark P-I, et al: Osseointegrated implants in the treatment of the edentulous jaw. Experience from a 10-year period. Scand J Plast Reconstr Surg 11(suppl 16):1–132, 1977.

12. Brånemark P-I, et al: Osseointegrated titanium fixtures in the treatment of edentulousness. Biomaterials 4:25–28, 1983.

13. Brunski JB, et al: The influence of functional use of endosseous dental implants on the tissue-implant interface: I. Histological aspects. J Dent Res 58:1953–1969, 1979.

14. Brunski JB, et al: The influence of functional use of endosseous dental implants on the tissue-implant interface: II. Clinical aspects. J Dent Res 58:1970–1980, 1979.

15. Cameron HU, et al: The rate of bone ingrowth into porous metal. J Biomed Mater Res 10:295–302, 1976.

16. Carlsson L, et al: Implant fixation improved by close fit. Acta Orthop Scand 59:272–275, 1988.

17. Clark AE, et al: The influence of surface chemistry on implant interface histology: A theoretical basis for implant materials selection. J Biomed Mater Res 10:161–174, 1976.

18. Clarke EGC, Hickman J: An investigation into the correlation between the electric potential of metals and their behavior in biological fluids. J Bone Joint Surg 35B:467, 1953.

19. Cook SD, Kay JF, Thomas KA, Jarcho M: Interface mechanics and histology of titanium and hydroxylapatite-coated titanium for dental implant applications. Int J Oral Maxillofac Impl 2:16, 1987.

20. Deporter DA: Collagen and mineralization. In Ten Cate AD, Stites DP, Stobo JD, Fundenberg HH, Wells JV (eds): Oral Histology. St. Louis, CV Mosby, 1980, pp 94–109.

21. Ekeland A, et al: Influence of age on mechanical properties of healing fractures and intact bones in rats. Acta Orthop Scand 53:527–534, 1982.

22. Eriksson RA, Adell R: Temperatures during drilling for the placement of implants using the osseointegration technique. J Oral Maxillofac Surg 44:4–7, 1986.

23. Eriksson RA, Albrektsson T: Temperature threshold levels for heat-induced bone tissue injury: A vital-microscopic study in the rabbit. J Prosthet Dent 50:101–107, 1983.

24. Eriksson RA, et al: The effect of heat on bone regeneration. An experimental study in the rabbit using the bone growth chamber. J Oral Maxillofac Surg 42:705–711, 1984.

25. Eriksson RA, et al: Heat caused by drilling cortical bone. Acta Orthop Scand 55:629–631, 1984.

26. Fox SI: Endocrine control of metabolism. In Jaffe ET (ed): Human Physiology. Dubuque, Iowa, William C. Brown Publishers, 1984, pp 596–625.

27. Friedenstein AJ, et al: Osteogenesis in transplants of bone marrow cells. J Embryol Exp Morphol 16:381–390, 1966.

28. Granstrom G, et al: Titanium implants in irradiated tissue: Benefits from hyperbaric oxygen. Int J Oral Maxillofac Impl 7:15–25, 1992.

29. Hansard SL, et al: Effects of aging upon the physiological behaviors of calcium in cattle. Am J Physiol 177:383–389, 1954.

30. Hansson H-A, et al: Structural aspects of the interface between tissue and titanium implants. J Prosthet Dent 50:108–113, 1983.

31. Hobos S, Ichida E, Garcia LT: Osseointegration and Occlusal Rehabilitation. London, Quintessence Publishing Co, Inc, 1989, pp 33–54.

32. Holick MF, et al: Calcium, Phosphorous, and bone metabolism: Calcium regulating hormones. In Braunwald E, et al (eds): Harrison's Principles of Internal Medicine, ed 11. New York, McGraw-Hill, 1987, pp 1857–1870.

33. Hulth A: Fracture healing. Acta Orthop Scand 51:5–8, 1980.

34. Jarcho M: Biomaterial aspects of calcium phosphates—properties and applications. Dent Clin North Am 30:25–47, 1986.

35. Jarcho M: Retrospective analysis of hydroxyapatite development for oral implant applications. Dent Clin North Am 36:19–26, 1992.

36. Kasemo B: Biocompatibility of titanium implants: Surface science aspects. J Prosthet Dent 49:832–837, 1983.

37. Kay JF: Calcium phosphate coatings for dental implants. Current status and future potential. Dent Clin North Am 36:1–18, 1992.

38. Krauser JT: Hydroxylapatite-coated dental implants. Biologic rationale and surgical technique. Dent Clin North Am 33:879–903, 1989.

39. Lake FT: Basic bone biology in implants. In McKinney RV (ed): Endosteal Dental Implants. St. Louis, Mosby–Year Book, 1991, pp 52–62.

40. Lavelle C, et al: Effect of internal irrigation on frictional heat generated from bone drilling. J Oral Surg 38:499–503, 1980.

41. Lavelle CLB, et al: Some advances in endosseous implants. J Oral Rehabil 8:319–331, 1981.

42. Lemons JE, Bidez MW: Endosteal implant biomaterials and biomechanics. In McKinney RV (ed): Endosteal Implants, Biomaterials, and Biomechanics. St. Louis, Mosby–Year Book, 1991, pp 28–36.

43. Linder L, Lundskog J: Incorporation of stainless steel, titanium and vitallium in bone. Injury 6:277–285, 1975.

44. Lindström J, et al: Mandibular reconstruction using the preformed autologous bone graft. Scand J Plast Reconstr Surg 15:29–38, 1981.

45. Listgarten MA, et al: Periodontal tissues and their counterparts around endosseous implants. Clin Oral Impl Res 2:1–19, 1991.

46. Lundskog J: Heat and bone tissue. An experimental investigation of the thermal properties of bone tissue and threshold levels or thermal injury. Scand J Plast Reconstr Surg (Suppl) 9:1–132, 1972.

47. Marshall TS, et al: Matrix vesicle enzyme activity in endosteal bone following implantation of bonding and non-bonding implant materials. Clin Oral Impl Res 2:112–120, 1991.

48. McKinney RV, et al: The biological tissue response to dental implants. In McKinney RV (ed): Endosteal Dental Implants. St. Louis, Mosby–Year Book, 1991.

49. Meffert RM, et al: What is osseointegration? Int J Periodont Restor Dent 4:9–21, 1987.

50. Melcher AH, Accursi GE: Osteogenic capacity of periosteal and osteoperiosteal flaps elevated from the parietal bone of the rat. Arch Oral Biol 6:573–580, 1971.

51. Peacock EE: Collagenolysis and the biochemistry of wound healing. In Wound Repair, ed 3. Philadelphia, WB Saunders, 1984, pp 56–101.

52. Peacock JL, Lawrence WT, Peacock EE Jr: Wound healing. In O'Leary JP (ed): The Physiologic Basis of Surgery. Baltimore, Williams & Wilkins, 1993, pp 112–136.

53. Pilliar RM, et al: Observations on the effect of movement on bone ingrowth into porous-surfaced implants. Clin Orthop Rel Res 208:108–113, 1986.

54. Rae T: A study on the effects of particulate metals of orthopaedic interest on murine macrophages in vitro. J Bone Joint Surg 57:444, 1975.

55. Rhinelander FW: The normal circulation of bone and its response to surgical intervention. J Biomed Mater Res 8:87–90, 1974.

56. Robbins SL, et al: Inflammation and repair. In Robbins SL (ed): Robbins Pathological Basis of Disease, ed 4, Philadelphia, WB Saunders, 1989, pp 39–86.

57. Schatzker J, et al: The effect of movement on the holding

power of screws in bone. Clin Orthop Rel Res 111:257–262, 1975.

58. Schroeder A: Preconditions for long-term implantological success. *In* Schroeder A, Sutter F, Krekeler G (eds): Oral Implantology: Basics—ITI Hollow Cylinder System. New York, Thieme Medical Publishers, 1991, pp 2–10.

59. Schroeder A: Tissue reactions. *In* Schroeder A, Sutter F, Krekeler G (eds): Oral Implantology: Basics—ITI Hollow Cylinder System. New York, Thieme Medical Publishers, 1991, pp 91–117.

60. Schwesinger WH, Moyer PM: Cell biology. *In* O'Leary JP (ed): The Physiologic Basis of Surgery. Baltimore, Williams & Wilkins, 1993, pp 1–45.

61. Shetty V, Bertolami CN: The physiology of wound healing. *In* Peterson LJ, Indresano AT, Marciani RD, Roser SM (eds): Principles of Oral and Maxillofacial Surgery. Philadelphia, JB Lippincott, 1992, pp 3–18.

62. Søballe K, et al: Hydoxyapatite coating enhances fixation of porous coated implants. Acta Orthop Scand 61:299–306, 1990.

63. Spector M, et al: Advances in our understanding of the implant-bone interface: Factors affecting formation and degeneration. *In* Tullos HS (ed): Instructional Course Lectures. American Academy of Orthopedic Surgeons, Vol 40, 1991.

64. Steflik DE, et al: Ultrastructural investigations of the bone and fibrous connective tissue interface with endosteal dental implants. Scanning Microsc 4:1039–1048, 1990.

65. Syftestad GT, Urist MR: Bone aging. Clin Orthop Rel Res 162:288–297, 1982.

66. Ten Cate AR: The gingival junction. *In* Bränemark P-I, Zarb GA, Albrektsson T (eds): Tissue Integrated Prostheses—Osseointegration in Clinical Dentistry. London, Quintessence Publishing Co, Inc, 1985, pp 145–153.

67. Tetsch P: Development of raised temperature after osteotomies. J Maxillofac Surg 2:141–145, 1974.

68. Tonna EA, Cronkite EP: Histochemical and autoradiographic studies of the effects of aging on the mucopolysaccharides of the periosteum. J Biophys Biochem Cytol 6:171–183, 1959.

69. Toth RW, et al: Soft tissue response to endosseous titanium oral implants. J Prosthet Dent 54:564–567, 1985.

70. Uhthoff HK, Hans K: Mechanical factors influencing the holding power of screws in compact bone. J Bone Joint Surg 55B:633–639, 1973.

71. Weiss CM: Tissue integration of dental endosseous implants: Description and comparative analysis of the fibro-osseous integration and osseous integration systems. J Oral Implantol 12:169–214, 1986.

Study Questions

1. What are the steps of wound healing after drilling of the hole and placing an endosseous implant?

2. What are the most important factors related to proper healing of implants and achieving osseointegration?

3. How do different materials affect healing of implants?

4. How long does the maturation phase last? What are the results—bone and soft tissue—of the maturation phase?

5. Taking into consideration the wound healing response, discuss your postoperative instructions to the patient.

CHAPTER 7

Biocompatibility, Biofunctionality, and Biomechanics of Dental Implants

PART 1

Tissue Response to Implanted Materials

Stephen D. Cook
Jeanette E. Dalton
Revised by Luis R. Guerra

Tissue Response to Implant Materials
    Titanium and Titanium-Based Alloys
    Surface-Active Ceramics
Implant Design and Biomechanical
    Properties
    Direct Bone Apposition
    Porous Ingrowth Attachment
    Calcium Phosphate Ceramic Coatings
Optimizing Biologic Attachment Methods
    Motion at Bone-Implant Interface
    Surgical Fit
References

The body is a harsh chemical environment for foreign materials. An implanted material can have its properties altered by body fluids. Degradation mechanisms, such as corrosion or leaching, can be accelerated by ion concentrations and pH changes in body fluids. The body's response to an implant can range from benign to a chronic inflammatory reaction, with the degree of biologic response largely dependent on the implanted material. For optimal performance, implanted materials should have suitable mechanical strength, biocompatibility, and structural biostability in physiologic environments.[17] The development of biomaterials science has resulted in classification schemes for implantable materials according to chemical composition and biologic response.

Biologic classification is based on tissue response and systemic toxicity effects of the implant and is divided into three classes of biomaterials: biotolerant, bioinert, and bioactive. In terms of the long-term effects at the bone-implant interface, biotolerant materials, such as polymethylmethacrylate (PMMA), are usually characterized by a thin fibrous tissue interface. The fibrous tissue layer develops as a result of the chemical products from leaching processes, leading to irritation of the surrounding tissues. Bioinert materials, such as titanium and aluminum oxide, are characterized by direct bone contact, or osseointegration, at the interface under favorable mechanical conditions. Osseointegration is achieved because the material surface is chemically nonreactive to the surrounding tissues and body fluids. Finally, bioactive materials, such as glass and calcium phosphate ceramics, have a bone-implant interface characterized by direct chemical bonding of the implant with surrounding bone. This chemical bond is believed to be caused by the presence of free calcium and phosphate compounds at the implant surface.

Minimizing the local and systemic response to an implanted material through improved biocompatibility is only one engineering concern for reconstructive implant surgery. A prosthetic implant must be capable of tolerating adequate stress transfer at the bone-implant surface to ensure long-term implant stability. Nonphysiologic stress transfer may cause pressure necrosis or resorption at the bone-implant interface. Necrotic and resorbed bone may lead to implant loosening and migration, thus compromising implant longevity. Finally, material properties capable of sustaining the cyclic body forces to which the implant will be subjected are essential. For example, if the material properties are not adequate for load-sharing, the implant may fail owing to fracture. If the material properties are such that stress shielding of the bone occurs, however, bone resorption and implant loosening are sure to occur.

TISSUE RESPONSE TO IMPLANT MATERIALS

The most commonly used biomaterials for dental implants are metals and their alloys. Commercially pure (CP) titanium and titanium-aluminum-vanadium (Ti-6Al-4V) alloy are most often used for endosseous implants, whereas cobalt-chromium-molybdenum (Co-Cr-Mo) alloy is most often used for subperiosteal implants. Calcium phosphate ceramics, particularly hydroxyapatite (HA), have been used in monolithic form as augmentation material for alveolar ridges and as coating on metal devices for endosseous implantation.

Titanium and Titanium-Based Alloys

CP titanium and titanium-based alloys are low-density metals that have chemical properties suitable for implant applications. Titanium has a high corrosion resistance attributed to an oxide surface layer, which also creates a chemically nonreactive surface to the surrounding tissues. The modulus of elasticity is half the value for cobalt-based alloys but still at least five times greater than bone. The higher the impurity content of the metal, the higher the strength and brittleness. Owing to the low density, titanium and titanium-based alloys have superior specific strength (strength per density) over all other metals. Titanium has poor shear strength and wear resistance, however, making it unsuitable for articulating surface or bone screw applications.

Surface-Active Ceramics

Glass ceramics, such as Bioglass and Cervital, are polycrystalline ceramics produced by the controlled crystallization of glasses. Table 7–1 shows the chemical composition of glass ceramic materials. Glass ceramics have poor mechanical

Table 7–1. Chemical Composition of Glass Ceramic Materials

	Amount		
	Mole%		Weight
Compound	Bioglass 42S5.6	Bioglass 45S5	Cervital Bioactive
SiO_2	42.1	46.1	40.0–50.0
CaO	29.0	26.9	30.0–35.0
NaO_2	26.3	24.4	5.0–10.0
P_2O_5	2.6	2.6	10.0–15.0
MgO	–	–	2.5–5.0
K_2O	–	–	0.5–3.0

properties for load-carrying applications because they are extremely brittle. Controlling grain size, however, increases both tensile strength by a factor of two (from 100 to 200 MPa) and abrasion resistance. The implant surface responds to local pH changes by releasing sodium ions in exchange for phosphorus or hydrogen ions. A calcium phosphate layer forms on the surface. Osteoblasts proliferate at the surface, and collagen fibrils become incorporated into the calcium phosphate–rich layer.

Calcium phosphate ceramics, classified as polycrystalline ceramics, have a material structure derived from individual crystals that have become fused at the grain boundaries during high-temperature sintering processes.[22] Hydroxylapatite (HA), $[Ca_{10}(PO_4)_6(OH)_2]$, commonly called tribasic calcium phosphate, is a geologic mineral that closely resembles the natural mineral in vertebrate bone tissue. Tribasic calcium phosphate should not be confused with other calcium phosphate ceramics, especially tricalcium phosphate (TCP), $[Ca_3(PO_4)_2]$, which is chemically similar to HA but is not a natural bone mineral.

The biocompatibility of the calcium phosphate ceramics is well documented. The body's typical response to these implanted ceramics is:

1. No local or systemic toxicity.
2. No inflammatory or foreign body reaction.
3. Functional integration with bone.
4. No alteration to natural mineralization processes.
5. Chemical bonding to bone via natural bone cementing mechanisms.[23]

The biocompatibility and close chemical composition to natural bone mineral are factors that make the calcium phosphate ceramics desirable bioactive materials. HA implant surfaces have been characterized as being capable of forming direct, intimate bonds with the surrounding bone (Fig. 7–1). The bonding area (approximately 500 to 2000 Å) contains biologic apatite crystals that are highly oriented at the interface with a 100 Å periodicity similar to that of calcified tissue, as determined by electron diffraction studies.[24] The bone apatite crystals are arranged against the implant surface in a palisade fashion, resembling the natural bonding between two bone fragments.[17] The bonding area contains a ground substance that is heavily mineralized, although devoid of collagen fibrils,[23] and has been likened to the natural bone-cementing substance. The natural bone-cementing substance is amorphous in structure, heavily mineralized, and rich in mucopolysaccharides.[22] Because the bond area contains a substance biologically similar to the natural bone cement substance, it is reasonable that the bond between bone and the calcium phosphate ceramic is strong.

IMPLANT DESIGN AND BIOMECHANICAL PROPERTIES

A common method of implant fixation is impaction into the alveolar ridge. The implants are held in place by compressive stress interaction, and the devices are designed to remain in compression relative to the surrounding tissue. Static and dynamic masticatory forces are then transmitted from the implant to the surrounding tissues. The precision required to obtain uniform contact between the device and surrounding

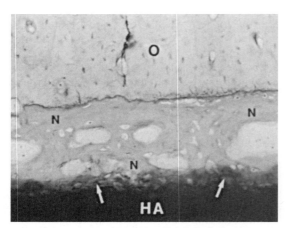

Figure 7–1. Photomicroradiograph from a histologic section of an HA-coated implant demonstrating the osteoconductive nature of HA coatings. O = Old bone; N = new bone; H = HA coating.

bone is limited by the skills of the surgeon and design of the instrumentation with which the site is prepared. The surface area of actual contact is probably small relative to the implant surface area. These contact points tend to induce areas of stress concentrations rather than an even distribution of stresses. Bone maintains its structural integrity by responding to stress; high areas of stress concentration are often associated with bone resorption. Additionally, fibrous encapsulations of varying thicknesses are common occurrences that further alter the ability of the implant to distribute stress uniformly. This situation often manifests itself in eventual implant loosening and migration, leading to patient discomfort and the need for eventual removal.

Several types of implant fixation methods and surface texture designs have been investigated to obtain better surgical fit and stress distribution at the implant-bone interface. These methods include direct bone apposition to the implant surface, bone growth into porous-surfaced implants, and chemical bonding between bone and surface-active chemical implant coatings.

Direct Bone Apposition

Optimal osseointegration at the bone-implant interface is affected by the material properties and design of the implant. Implant design encompasses both the surface texture and geometry of the implant. The mechanical properties of the implant-bone interface have been investigated with various surface preparations: smooth finish, roughened or grit-blasted finishes, and grooved surfaces (Fig. 7–2). Histologically, implants with smooth finishes have interfaces characterized by fibrous encapsulation, whereas implants with grit-blasted finishes have interfaces characterized by areas of direct bone apposition. Several studies[33] determined that surface texture is a significant factor in obtaining adequate implant fixation with direct bone apposition methods.

The effects of implant diameter and length on direct bone apposition have been studied using a dental implant model.[1]

Mechanical results indicate a statistical correlation with implant length and no correlation with implant diameter. Implications of factors involving cortical and cancellous bone structural differences are attributed to some of the mechanical differences between implant lengths.

Porous Ingrowth Attachment

It is generally accepted that an implant can achieve stabilization by tissue growth into the

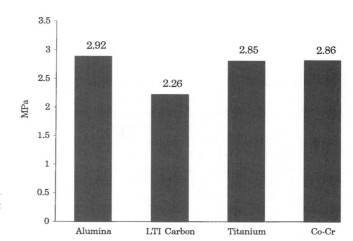

Figure 7–2. Histogram plot of the mean interface attachment strength for grit-blasted implant materials after 32 weeks in situ.

surface porous structure if the material is bioinert, if there is direct apposition of the bone at the implant interface, if there is minimal or no movement at the implant site, and if the porous structure has appropriate pore size and morphology. The effectiveness of porous coatings as a means of biologic fixation becomes apparent when considering interfacial mechanical properties. The interface attachment strength of porous implants relying on bone ingrowth for fixation are at least an order of magnitude higher than that of nonporous implants relying on direct bone apposition for fixation.[33] Several different porous structures have been evaluated: irregular, fiber mesh, and bead; however, bead porous coatings have been studied in more detail than the other types. An example of bone growth into beaded and irregular porous structures is illustrated in Figure 7–3.

To maintain optimal bone growth into a porous

structure, the pores must be large enough to accommodate bone tissue development. Several investigators have studied the degree and rate of bone ingrowth for several different pore size ranges.[3, 21] They concluded that a pore size range of 50 to 400 μm obtained the maximum attachment strength in the shortest time. Histologically, however, it was observed that osteon formation was not observed and did not appear to be a prerequisite to attain maximum attachment strength.

Besides a minimal pore size, an effective porous coating must also have appropriate pore morphology. The available porous layer for bone growth must be large enough to accommodate enough bone for adequate fixation without compromising the mechanical properties necessary for a load-bearing prosthesis. A volume fraction porosity of 35% to 40% is accepted as optimum for effective biologic fixation for a strongly

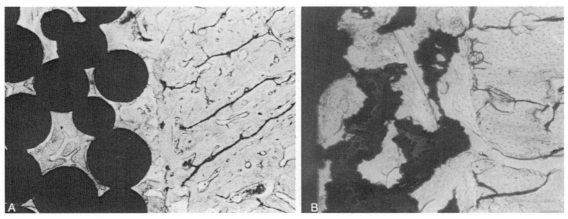

Figure 7–3. Photomicroradiographs from histologic sections demonstrating bone growth in beaded *(A)* and irregular *(B)* porous surfaced implants after 12 weeks in situ.

bonded porous layer.[15] The volume fraction porosity is related to the interconnection pore size, particle interconnectivity, and particle size of the porous coating. Particle interconnectivity is important for ensuring adequate strength within the coating and between the coating and substrate. Too much particle interconnectivity, however, can decrease the interconnection pore size and restrict the amount and type of ingrown tissue.[9] It is accepted that a two-layer porous surface creates an interconnected and open porosity that is effective in creating a three-dimensional mechanical interlock of the ingrown bone.[3]

Calcium Phosphate Ceramic Coatings

Studies with plasma-sprayed HA coatings onto metal implants have been conducted using a variety of implant models in dogs.[2, 6–12, 14, 16, 18, 29, 34] For femoral transcortical models, mechanical strengths for the HA-coated implant were significantly higher than the uncoated strengths for nonporous implants and were greater, but not significantly, for porous-coated implants. The attachment strengths for HA-coated implants varied greatly among the studies (Table 7–2).

HA-coated and uncoated macrotextured titanium implants were evaluated from 3 to 32 weeks by Thomas et al.[34] Histologically the HA-coated implants demonstrated direct bone mineralization on the coating surface, whereas the uncoated implants often demonstrated areas of fibrous tissue at the interface (Fig. 7–4).

HA-coated and uncoated dental implants have been evaluated in dog models to compare both mechanical and histologic response.[2, 6, 7] The grit-blasted implants demonstrated osseointegration after 4 months' implantation. Even at 10 months, however, the bone was not continuous at the implant interface. The HA-coated implants exhibited direct bonding of bone to the HA surface at 1 month. By 4 months, lamellar bone was observed at the HA-bone interface.

HA-coated and grit-blasted titanium dental implants were evaluated 6 weeks after implantation into healed extraction sites.[6] Implants were mechanically tested to determine interface torsional strength. Mechanical results demonstrated an interface torsional strength of 3.98 ± 0.93 MPa for HA-coated implants and 2.25 ± 0.65 MPa for grit-blasted implants. The difference in torsional strength was statistically significant. Histologically, HA-coated implants exhibited direct bone apposition with no intervening fibrous tissue at

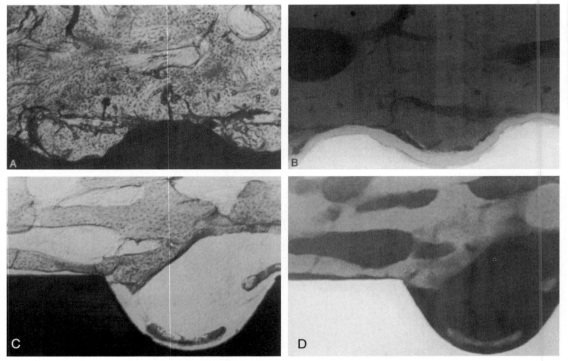

Figure 7–4. Photomicroradiographs from histologic and corresponding microradiographic sections of mechanically tested HA-coated (A and B) and uncoated (C and D) macrotextured femoral transcortical implants.

Table 7–2. Summary of Mechanical Testing Results for Hydroxylapatite-Coated Implants

Interface Attachment Strength (MPa)

Times (weeks)	Cook et al°		Thomas et al†		Cook et al‡		Dalton§	
	HA-Coated	Uncoated	HA-Coated	Uncoated	HA-Coated	Uncoated	HA-Coated	Uncoated
2					5.04 ± 1.79 (9)	3.11 ± 1.60 (9)		
3	3.99 ± 2.06 (21)	1.44 ± 1.00 (9)	6.05 ± 1.94 (8)	4.43 ± 1.32 (9)				
4					9.17 ± 4.20 (9)	6.95 ± 2.17 (9)	1.88 ± 0.68 (4)	1.12 ± 0.38 (4)
5	6.96 ± 3.22 (40)	0.93 ± 0.57 (19)	9.56 ± 3.55 (18)	4.88 ± 1.01 (9)				
6	7.00 ± 2.31 (22)	1.54 ± 1.18 (7)			12.80 ± 2.30 (9)	10.50 ± 2.68 (9)		
8					12.60 ± 2.72 (9)	10.52 ± 2.26 (9)	5.83 ± 1.61 (8)	2.61 ± 1.10 (8)
10	7.27 ± 2.08 (44)	0.98 ± 0.73 (21)	14.17 ± 4.87 (16)	10.53 ± 3.29 (12)				
12					15.73 ± 2.36 (9)	11.10 ± 1.46 (9)	4.91 ± 4.56 (4)	3.01 ± 1.21 (4)
18					23.15 ± 3.64 (9)	17.58 ± 3.10 (9)		
24							8.08 ± 3.54 (11)	3.87 ± 2.15 (11)
26					27.06 ± 2.36 (8)	22.08 ± 3.88 (8)		
32	6.07 ± 1.29 (31)	1.21 ± 0.77 (11)	12.12 ± 2.43 (12)	—				
52					21.21 ± 3.80 (9)	18.71 ± 3.74 (9)	11.44 ± 5.82 (12)	5.88 ± 3.13 (12)
Implant details	HA-coated titanium alloy; bead-blasted CP titanium		Surface macrotextured HA-coated titanium alloy and CP titanium		Porous cobalt-chromium alloy; half HA-coated		Titanium alloy HA-coated and uncoated implants; 0-mm initial gap	

°Cook SD, et al: Interface mechanics and histology of titanium and hydroxylapatite-coated titanium for dental implants. J Oral Maxillofac Impl 2:15, 1987.
Cook SD, et al: Hydroxylapatite-coated porous titanium for use as an orthopedic biologic attachments system. Clin Orthop Rel Res 230:303, 1988.
†Thomas KA, et al: The effect of surface macrotexture and hydroxylapatite coating in the mechanical strengths and histologic profiles of titanium implant materials. J Biomed Mater Res 21:1395, 1987.
‡Cook SD, et al: Enhanced bone ingrowth and fixation strength with hydroxylapatite-coated porous implants. Semin Arthroplasty 2:268, 1991.
Cook SD, et al: Hydroxylapatite coating of porous implants improves bone ingrowth and interface attachment strength. J Biomed Mater Res 26:989, 1992.
§Dalton JE: The effects of surgical fit and hydroxylapatite coating on the mechanical and biological response to porous implants. Master's Thesis, Tulane University, New Orleans, 1991.

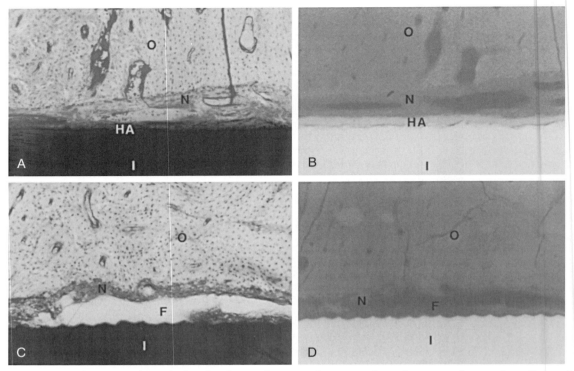

Figure 7–5. Photomicroradiographs from histologic and corresponding microradiographic sections from mechanically tested HA-coated *(A and B)* and grit-blasted *(C and D)* dental implants after 6 weeks in situ. O = Old bone; N = new bone; F = fibrous tissue; HA = HA coating; and I = implant.

the implant interface. Although the grit-blasted implants also exhibited regions of direct bone apposition, these regions were limited to a small percentage of the implant surface (Figs. 7–5 and 7–6).

OPTIMIZING BIOLOGIC ATTACHMENT METHODS

Optimal attachment at the bone-implant interface is affected by the material properties and

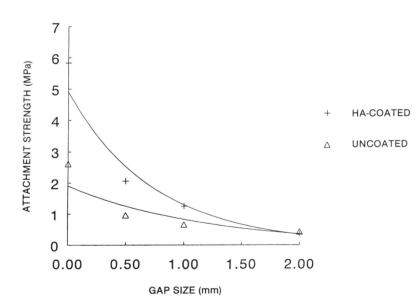

Figure 7–6. Plot of attachment strength versus implant-bone interface gap size for HA-coated and uncoated porous femoral intramedullary implants after 8 weeks in situ.

design of the implant. Other conditions that affect osseointegration are instrumentation design, surgical technique, initial implant stability, and direct contact with the surrounding bone.

Motion at Bone-Implant Interface

Initial implant stability and apposition with bone are not always achievable, but are vital for implant longevity. Persistent micromotion at the bone-implant interface has been an established cause of bone resorption and necrosis. Necrosis and destructive bone remodeling often result in fibrous tissue infiltration at the interface and may cause implant loosening.[14] Also, any initial gap between the implant and surrounding bone may adversely alter the amount and rate at which osseointegration occurs. Initial implant stability is essential for early tissue infiltrate within the porous structure to differentiate into bone by either direct bone formation or appositional bone growth.[28] When excessive early movement occurs at the bone-implant interface, bone formation within the pores is inhibited.[28] The majority of research concerning motion at the interface has involved porous implants; however, the findings are applicable for press-fit implant systems.

It is generally accepted that micromotion of 150 μm is the upper limit of acceptable motion. In a carefully controlled study, Bragdon et al[4] determined that 150 μm of implant motion did not allow bone ingrowth.

Surgical Fit

The technical difficulties in cutting bone precisely to provide an exact fit around the implant often result in a poor surgical fit. Difficulties in achieving initial implant-bone interface apposition are due to implant and instrumentation design and surgical technique. Numerous researchers have investigated the effect of interface gap spaces on the histologic response to implants.[5, 13, 20, 25, 30–32] These studies demonstrate that the closer the fit between the bone and the implant (< 0.5 mm) the earlier osseointegration is achieved, and the quality of bone is superior.

Surgical fit is also a concern for HA-coated prostheses because HA coatings do not make up for improper surgical placement of the implant. The concentrations of the physiologic components necessary for bone formation are decreased across large interfacial gaps as compared with concentrations for press-fit situations. Therefore the rate of gap filling, and subsequent ingrowth, is delayed. Large gaps may reduce the quality of bone at the interface as compared with that of press-fit interfaces.

In summary, the mechanical and chemical properties of metals, such as titanium and titanium-based alloys and cobalt-based alloys, and ceramics, such as glass and calcium phosphate, make them suitable for implant applications. Several factors, however, affect the biologic response to these implanted materials. The predominant tissue found at the implant interface is affected by implant stability, material biocompatibility, and implant design and placement into the surgical site. Improvements in implant design and surface preparation may increase implant longevity and fixation for all implant materials.

References

1. Block MS, Delgado A, Fontenot MG: The effect of diameter and length of hydroxyapatite-coated dental implants on ultimate pullout force in dog alveolar bone. J Oral Maxillofac Surg 48:174, 1990.
2. Block MS, Kent JN, Kay JF: Evaluation of hydroxyapatite-coated titanium dental implants in dogs. J Oral Maxillofac Surg 45:601, 1987.
3. Bobyn JD, Pilliar RM, Cameron HU, Weatherly GC: The optimum pore size for the fixation of porous-surfaced metal implants by the ingrowth of bone. Clin Orthop Rel Res 150:263, 1980.
4. Bragdon CR, Burke D, O'Connor DO, Jasty M, Haire T, Harris WH: Dynamic measurement of interface mechanics and the effect of micromotion on bone ingrowth into a porous surface device under controlled loads in vivo. Transactions of the 17th Annual Meeting of the Society for Biomaterials 17:100, 1991.
5. Cameron HU, Pilliar RM, Macnab I: The rate of bone ingrowth into porous metal. J Biomed Mater Res 10:295, 1976.
6. Cook SD, Baffes GC, Burgess A: In vivo study of the torsional strength of HA-coated and grit-blasted implants. J Oral Implantol 18:354, 1992.
7. Cook SD, Baffes GC, Thomas KA: Comparison of models for evaluating interface characteristics of HA-coated implants. J Dent Res 70:530, 1991.
8. Cook SD, Thomas KA, Dalton JE, Kay JF: Enhanced bone ingrowth and fixation strength with hydroxyapatite-coated porous implants. Semin Arthroplasty 2:268, 1991.
9. Cook SD, Thomas KA, Dalton JE, Volkman TK, Whitecloud TS: Hydroxyapatite coating of porous implants improves bone ingrowth and interface attachment strength. J Biomed Mater Res 26:989, 1992.
10. Cook SD, Kay JF, Thomas KA, Jarcho M: Interface mechanics and histology of titanium and hydroxyapatite-coated titanium for dental implant applications. Int J Oral Maxillofac Impl 2:15, 1987.
11. Cook SD, Thomas KA, Kay JF, Jarcho M: Hydroxyapatite-coated porous titanium for use as an orthopedic bio-

logic attachments system. Clin Orthop Rel Res 230:303, 1988.

12. Cook SD, Thomas KA, Kay JF, Jarcho M: Hydroxyapatite-coated titanium for orthopedic implant applications. Clin Orthop Rel Res 232:225, 1988.

13. Dalton JE: The Effects of Surgical Fit and Hydroxyapatite Coating on the Mechanical and Biological Response to Porous Implants. Master's Thesis, Tulane University, New Orleans, 1991.

14. deGroot K, Geesink R, Klein CP, Serekian P: Plasma sprayed coatings of hydroxyapatite. J Biomed Mater Res 24:1375, 1987.

15. Engh CA, Bobyn JD: Biologic Fixation in Total Hip Arthroplasty. Thorofare, NJ, Slack Inc, 1985.

16. Galante JO, Rivero DP: The biologic basis for bone ingrowth in titanium fiber composites. *In* Harris WH (ed): Advanced Concepts in Total Hip Replacement. Thorofare, NJ, Slack Inc, 1985.

17. Geesink RG: Hydroxy-Apatite Coated Hip Implants. Doctoral Thesis, University of Limburg, Maastricht, Netherlands, 1988.

18. Geesink RG, deGroot K, Klein CP: Bonding of bone to apatite-coated implants. J Bone Joint Surg 70B:17, 1988.

19. Haddad RJ, Cook SD, Thomas KA: Biological fixation of porous-coated implants. J Bone Joint Surg 69A:1459, 1987.

20. Harris WH, Jasty M: Bone ingrowth into porous coated canine acetabular replacements: The effect of pore size, apposition, and dislocation. *In* The Hip: Proceedings of the Thirteenth Open Scientific Meeting of the Hip Society, St. Louis, CV Mosby, 1985.

21. Hulbert SF, Cooke FW, Klawitter JJ, Leonard RB, Sauer BW, Moyle DD, Skinner HB: Attachment of prostheses to the musculoskeletal system by tissue ingrowth and mechanical interlocking. J Biomed Mater Res Symp 4:1, 1973.

22. Jarcho M: Calcium phosphate ceramics as hard tissue prosthetics. Clin Orthop Rel Res 157:259, 1981.

23. Jarcho M: Biomaterial aspects of calcium phosphates:

Properties and applications. Dent Clin North Am 30:25, 1986.

24. Jarcho M, Kay JF, Gumaer KI, Doremus RH, Drobeck HP: Tissue, cellular and subcellular events at a bone-ceramic hydroxyapatite interface. J Bioeng 1:79, 1976.

25. Jones LC, Opishinski DF, Kay JF, Hungerford DS: Enhancement of osteogenesis across an interface gap by hydroxyapatite. Transactions of the 17th Annual Meeting of the Society for Biomaterials 17:88, 1991.

26. Ogino M, Ohuchi F, Hench LL: Compositional dependence of the formation of calcium phosphate film on Bioglass. J Biomed Mater Res 14:55, 1980.

27. Park JB: Biomaterials Science and Engineering. New York, Plenum Press, 1984.

28. Pilliar RM, Lee JM, Maniatopoulas C: Observations on the effect of movement on bone ingrowth into porous-surfaced implants. Clin Orthop Rel Res 208:108, 1986.

29. Rivero DP, Skipor AK, Urban RM, Galante JO: Calcium phosphate-coated porous titanium implants for enhanced skeletal fixation. J Biomed Mater Res 22:191, 1988.

30. Sandborn PM, Cook SD, Spires WP, Kester MA: Tissue response to porous-coated implants lacking initial bone apposition. J Arthroplasty 3:337, 1989.

31. Søballe K, Hansen ES, Brockstedt-Rasmussen H, Pedersen CM, Bünger C: Hydroxyapatite coating enhances fixation of porous coated implants: A comparison in dogs between press fit and noninterference fit. Acta Orthop Scand 61:299, 1990.

32. Stephenson PK, Freeman MAR, Revell PA, Germain J, Tuke M, Pirie CT: The effect of hydroxylapatite coating on ingrowth of bone into cavities in an implant. J Arthroplasty 6:51, 1991.

33. Thomas KA, Cook SD: An evaluation of variables influencing implant fixation by direct bone apposition. J Biomed Mater Res 19:875, 1985.

34. Thomas KA, Kay JF, Cook SD, Jarcho M: The effect of surface macrotexture and hydroxylapatite coating in the mechanical strengths and histologic profiles of titanium implant materials. J Biomed Mater Res 21:1395, 1987.

Study Questions

1. Be able to discuss the classic bone-implant interface of titanium and hydroxylapatite.

2. What are the effects of surface roughness on mechanical strength of the bone-implant interface?

3. What do you think is the ideal implant design, based on the mechanical testing results discussed in this chapter? Be able to defend your ideas.

4. How does surgical fit affect osseointegration?

PART 2

Biomechanics of Dental Implants

John Brunski
Revised by Michael S. Block
and Luis R. Guerra

Biomechanics of Dental Implants
  Biting Forces
  Forces on Implants Supporting Bridgework
  Edentulous Mandible
  Partial Edentulousness
  Effects of Implant Angulation
  Definition of Stiffness
  Tooth Connected to an Implant
  Mechanics of Implant System
  References

An implant is subjected to mechanical forces because of the loading placed on the prosthesis. There is a corresponding biologic response to this loading and the implant itself by the hard and soft tissues involved.[2] The following are topics that will define the biomechanics of dental implants: (1) biologic responses and systemic toxicity effects of implants; (2) the number and placement of implants in a patient's mouth; (3) the significance of implant angulation with respect to the occlusal plane; (4) the fracture of prosthetic parts, such as gold screws, abutment screws, or metal frameworks; (5) the propriety of connecting natural teeth to implants; (6) the pros and cons of screw-shaped versus cylindrical-shaped implants; (7) the clinical significance of misfit of metal frameworks; and (8) the role of mechanical loading on the status of bone around an implant.

Dental implants can experience *tensile* as well as *compressive* forces. Under certain conditions, the forces can exceed the value of the biting force on the restoration by factors of $2\times$ or $3\times$, owing to leverage effects. Moreover, implants are ordinarily exposed to lateral as well as axial force components. Finally, there can be moments on implants.

Biting Forces. Under normal circumstances, a single freestanding tooth or implant is commonly exposed to chewing forces that are usually, but certainly not exclusively, compressive. This becomes evident by considering how the jaw works, mechanically, and how a biting force is exerted on the inclined surfaces of the crown of a natural tooth or implant restoration.

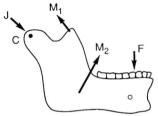

Figure 7–7. Simplified model of the jaw as a class 3 lever. The fulcrum is at the condyle (C), whereas the two major muscle forces (M_1 and M_2) act nearer to the fulcrum than the biting force (F). (J is the joint reaction force.) (From Brunski JB, Skalak R: Biomechanics of osseointegration and dental prostheses. *In* Naert I, et al [eds]: Osseointegration in Oral Rehabilitation. London, Quintessence, 1993, pp 133–156.)

To begin with, the simplest mechanical model of the jaw is to idealize it as a so-called class 3 lever (Fig. 7–7). The forces from the muscles of mastication (M_1, M_2) contract during mastication and cause the mandible to close, producing a biting force F on a bolus of food at a certain location in the arch and a reaction force J at the temporomandibular joint. F acts on the food particle and in turn on the occlusal surface of the restoration connected to a tooth or implant. To a first approximation, the direction of F is perpendicular to the plane of occlusion, but in reality this is an oversimplification. Owing to the inclined occlusal surfaces of the crown, a food particle typically does not make contact with the crown in such a way that the contact force acts perfectly parallel to the long axis of the tooth or implant. This can be appreciated by a more detailed look at what is happening in Figure 7–8. Here a freestanding implant is shown being

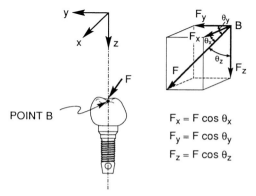

$$F_x = F \cos \theta_x$$
$$F_y = F \cos \theta_y$$
$$F_z = F \cos \theta_z$$

Figure 7–8. A force F acting on the pontic at point B may be resolved into components directed along the x-, y-, and z-axes. (From Brunski JB, Skalak R: Biomechanics of osseointegration and dental prostheses. *In* Naert I, et al [eds]: Osseointegration in Oral Rehabilitation. London, Quintessence, 1993, pp 133–156.)

acted on by F, which is slightly angled with respect to the long axis of an implant. The axial component of the force (F_z) tends to compress, or "push," the implant into the bone. At the same time, however, lateral force components (F_x and F_y) also exist, tending to push the tooth sideways and tip it about a point.

In most instances, the axial component of biting force on a single tooth or implant is the largest. Data from bite force experiments with human patients show that axial forces during biting can range from low values such as 77 N to much higher values such as 2440 N.° The lateral force components are much less, e.g., less than 100 N.

Many factors influence biting forces in the human mouth. These factors include the location where food is masticated in the mouth and prosthetic conditions. Completely edentulous patients with soft tissue–supported dentures in both arches tend to bite with less axial force than patients with natural teeth or with a denture opposing natural teeth. For edentulous patients with full-arch prostheses supported by Brånemark implants, the axial forces of biting were approximately equal to the forces in the normal dentate patient. Generally speaking, it is difficult to arrive at a single, average bite force value that would represent the forces in various patients' mouths under all conditions. Consequently, one might select an intermediate value such as about 250 N (56.2 lb) as a typical value for the axial component, but with the understanding that any given patient might exert significantly more or less force.

Another important issue with freestanding teeth or implants is that teeth and implants often have to support moments as well as forces. A moment (also called a torque) tends to produce rotation of a rigid body.

The case of an implant experiencing a moment is shown in Figure 7–9. The freestanding implant is being loaded by a purely vertical F, but F acts eccentrically, i.e., it acts at point C, which is not along the centerline of the implant. The effect is to produce a tendency for the implant to tip, or rotate, in a counterclockwise sense. Two clinically significant points about this are: (1) The bone-implant interface has to supply the counterbalancing moment to keep the implant in static equilibrium, and (2) the implant hardware, such

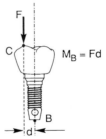

Figure 7–9. A moment being produced on a fixture owing to so-called eccentric loading: The point at which the force is applied (C) is at a distance (d) from the centerline of the fixture. (From Brunski JB, Skalak R: Biomechanics of osseointegration and dental prostheses. *In* Naert I, et al [eds]: Osseointegration in Oral Rehabilitation. London, Quintessence, 1993, pp 133–156.)

as the screw joint, must be able to withstand the moment without failing. Obviously the interface and the implant hardware both have their limits.

Forces on Implants Supporting Bridgework. So far we have discussed loading of freestanding teeth and implants. Let us now consider the simple case of just two implants supporting a bridge with a cantilever section (Fig. 7–10). Assume a downward force P acts at the end of the bridge with a cantilever section of length a. The distance between the line of action of P and the nearest implant (#2 in Fig. 7–10) is a. The bridge is assumed to be a rigid beam, i.e., it does not deform. The beam is supported by two implants, #1 and #2, spaced apart by distance b. The problem is to predict the forces on implants #1 and #2.

The beam is isolated (separated from the implants), and all forces acting on the beam are shown in the free body diagram; these forces are P and the implant forces (the beam is assumed to have a negligible weight). The forces F_1 and F_2 are the forces that the implants exert on the beam. The actual directions of these two forces—whether they act in the positive or negative y-direction—do not have to be known at this stage of the problem. The correct directions emerge from the solution. Force P is the biting force on the bridge.

The second step in the analysis is to recognize that the beam is in static equilibrium, which means, according to Newton's laws, that the sum of all forces acting on the beam as well as the sum of all moments equals 0. This allows us to solve for the two unknown forces F_1 and F_2. The result is that:

$$F_2 = (1 + a/b)P$$
$$F_1 = (a/b)P$$

°A Newton (N) is the unit of force in the metric, or SI, system. There are 4.448 N per pound. Therefore, the quoted range of axial bite forces corresponds to about 27 to 550 lb in the English system of units. An easy way to appreciate the size of 1 N is to realize that 1 N is about the weight of one apple (such as the proverbial apple that fell from the tree and hit Sir Isaac Newton). There are about four apples—about 1 N each—per pound.

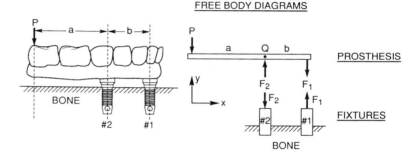

Figure 7–10. A method for predicting the forces on two fixtures supporting a cantilever portion of a prosthesis. See text for explanation. (From Brunski JB, Skalak R: Biomechanics of osseointegration and dental prostheses. *In* Naert I, et al [eds]: Osseointegration in Oral Rehabilitation. London, Quintessence, 1993, pp 133–156.)

These two equations show that although the biting force on the bridge is P, the forces on implants #1 and #2 exceed P, depending on the ratio a/b. For instance, suppose the ratio a/b is 2, e.g., the cantilever length is 20 mm and the interimplant spacing is 10 mm. (This is not an unusual clinical situation.) Then in this case, the forces on the implants would be 3P and 2P. Where P = 250 N, the forces would be 750 N and 500 N on implants #2 and #1, respectively. Note that the 750 N force on implant #2 is compressive, tending to push it into the bone, and the 500 N force on implant #1 is tensile, tending to pull it out of the bone. The force *on the bridge from each implant* is equal and opposite from the force *on the implant from the bridge.* The implants are in static equilibrium because the interfacial bone supplies the balancing forces.

An important message from this analysis is that the forces on the implants increase rapidly as the interimplant spacing, b, decreases and the cantilever length, a, increases. For instance, if a = 25 mm and b = 5 mm, the forces become 1500 N and 1250 N. These forces are large relative to danger levels for implant hardware and the interfacial bone, as discussed later.

To utilize this analysis when there are more than two implants, one must make the questionable assumption that is okay to ignore the remaining implants in the distribution. In effect, one assumes that the two implants nearest the loading point "do all the work" (Fig. 7–11).

Edentulous Mandible. Consider the edentulous mandible. Suppose a patient has an edentulous jaw having enough space to allow four or six implants in the anterior (Figs. 7–12 to 7–14). Consider the case of four versus six implants symmetrically distributed about the midline of a mandible over the same arc of 112.5 degrees. The radius of the mandible is taken to be 22.5 mm. The arc of 112.5 degrees represents a distance roughly equal to that between the mental foramina in the human mandible. Does it make any difference if we use four or six implants?

To compare a six-implant case with a four-implant case, first let us consider the case of four implants *distributed over the same arc as six implants* (112.5 degrees). The results show that the magnitudes of the forces on the most distal implants are similar in the four-implant and the six-implant cases. This means that there is only a slight difference between using four implants instead of six to support a prosthesis, *as long as the four implants are spaced out over the same arc as the six implants.*

If the two most distal implants are removed from the six-implant case, *keeping the interimplant spacing the same,* the four implants are not spread over the same arc length as the six implants. Now the forces on the four remaining implants become much larger than in the original six-implant case. Here one could argue that this is worse than the six-implant case because the forces per implant are larger. Although not analyzed here, an even worse situation would be to place the four implants in a straight line rather than an arc across the anterior of the mandible.

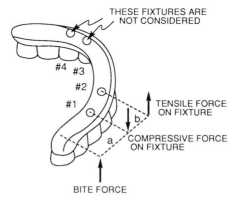

Figure 7–11. A maxillary prosthesis loaded by a biting force. Forces at implant locations #1 and #2 can be predicted approximately by the method used in Figure 7–5, provided that implants at locations #3 and #4 are neglected. (From Brunski JB, Skalak R: Biomechanics of osseointegration and dental prostheses. *In* Naert I, et al [eds]: Osseointegration in Oral Rehabilitation. London, Quintessence, 1993, pp 133–156.)

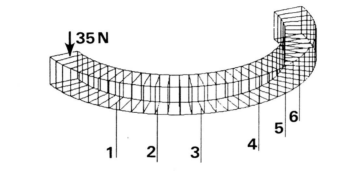

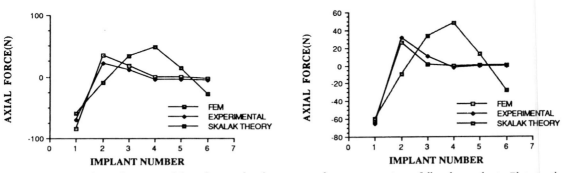

Figure 7–12. A finite element model used to predict forces on six fixtures supporting a full-arch prosthesis. Plots on the left and right show axial forces on the implants when the prosthesis is metal versus acrylic. (From Brunski JB, Skalak R: Biomechanics of osseointegration and dental prostheses. *In* Naert I, et al [eds]: Osseointegration in Oral Rehabilitation. London, Quintessence, 1993, pp 133–156.)

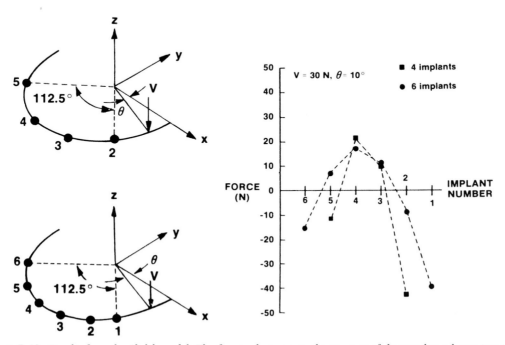

Figure 7–13. Results from the Skalak model. The four-implant case in the top part of diagram has a larger interimplant spacing than the six-implant case. The plots on the graph show that the magnitude of the forces on the implants is about equal in the six-implant and four-implant cases. (From Brunski JB, Skalak R: Biomechanics of osseointegration and dental prostheses. *In* Naert I, et al [eds]: Osseointegration in Oral Rehabilitation. London, Quintessence, 1993, pp 133–156.)

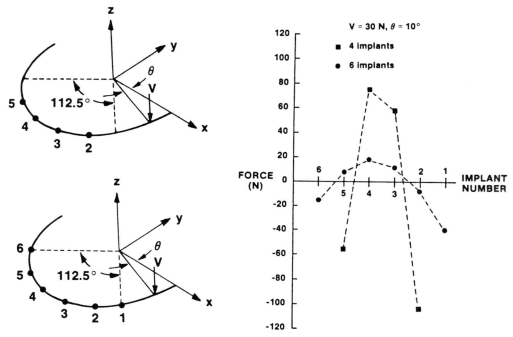

Figure 7–14. Results from the Skalak model. Implants #1 and #6 have been removed from the six-implant arrangement, yielding a four-implant arrangement with the same interimplant spacing as the original six-implant case. The plots on the graph show that the forces are higher in the four-implant case. (From Brunski JB, Skalak R: Biomechanics of osseointegration and dental prostheses. *In* Naert I, et al [eds]: Osseointegration in Oral Rehabilitation. London, Quintessence, 1993, pp 133–156.)

A fundamental problem in making firm conclusions based on these types of comparisons is incomplete information on loading limits for implant hardware and interfacial bone. Obviously if one knew the loading capabilities for the many different implant systems as well as the loading capabilities of the interfacial bone, one could develop guidelines for how best to use implants. But to date, data of this type are sparse. We do know that the Brånemark system's screw joint is held together with a preload of about 300 N. That is, when the gold screw is torqued to the nominal value of 10 N·cm, the gold cylinder and abutment are compressed together by about 300 N. It follows that one should avoid conditions that produce more than 300 N tension on the screw joint. The reason is that at a tensile force of about 300 N on a Brånemark fixture, the screw joint could begin to open, in turn increasing the tensile force on the abutment screw. On the biologic side, animal experiments suggest that bone around fixtures may be damaged to the point of requiring repair when exposed to controlled loading, consisting of 500 cycles per day for 5 days of 300 N tensile force.[5] Overall, until we know exactly what the danger limits are for various implant systems, it will remain difficult to make firm rules about the allowable loading per implant.

Partial Edentulousness. Consider now partially edentulous cases. From experience in replacing natural teeth with implants, many clinicians have come to adopt the following rule of thumb: It is better to use one implant per 1 to 1½ teeth to be restored. In other words, it seems presumptuous to expect more from an implant than the natural tooth it is replacing. Following this line of thinking, more implants may well be better in the case of partial edentulousness.

Effects of Implant Angulation. The previously mentioned models for predicting forces on implants did not specifically take into account the effects of implant angulation. For example, in the simple, two-dimensional problem of a bridge supported by two implants, the analysis assumed that both implants were perpendicular to the bridge and the occlusal plane (see Fig. 7–10). Now we can ask: What happens if one of the implants is inclined to the plane of the prosthesis (Fig. 7–15); does this make any difference in the forces on each implant?

The answer is no, at least as far as the force calculations are concerned. The analysis works out the same as before; the bridge has to be supported by the same distribution of vertical forces F_1 and F_2, regardless of how the implants happen to be oriented with respect to the bridge. When implant #1 is inclined to the plane of the

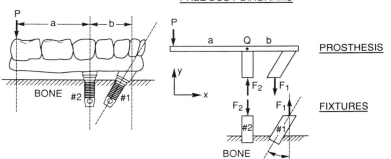

FREE BODY DIAGRAMS

Figure 7–15. Same diagram as Figure 7–10 except that one of the implants here has a 30-degree inclination. There are significant lateral components on the implant. (From Brunski JB, Skalak R: Biomechanics of osseointegration and dental prostheses. *In* Naert I, et al [eds]: Osseointegration in Oral Rehabilitation. London, Quintessence, 1993, pp 133–156.)

bridge, however, the force F_1 now acts at an angle to the long axis of the implant. By resolving the force F_1 into components, it can be shown that the component of F_1 acting parallel to the axis of the implant is $F_1 \cos (30°) = 0.866 F_1$, whereas the component of F_1 acting perpendicular to the long axis of the implant is $F_1 \sin (30°) = 0.5 F_1$. In such cases, the effect of the perpendicular component ($0.5 F_1$) is to produce bending stresses in the implant as well as high stresses at some locations in crestal bone around the implant.

Note that the notion of *stress* comes into play. For the purposes of our discussion, stress can be defined as force per unit area. For example, a force of 10 lb acting vertically on a screw-type implant produces different stresses in the bone than a 10-lb force applied perpendicular to the long axis of the implant; the area for support differs in the two cases. The story is actually more complicated in that there are different types of stress: tensile, compressive, and shear stresses. Moreover, the stresses typically vary from place to place in bone around a loaded implant, i.e., the stress distribution is generally nonuniform. For the same downward force on the implant, however, the stresses in bone are different around a straight versus an inclined implant. A major unsolved problem in implant biomechanics is to unravel the biologic significance of this fact and to determine exactly when the stresses in bone around an implant exceed danger limits. Similar analyses could be made to account for implant angulation when it comes to results from calculations for multiple, angulated implants supporting a bridge.

Definition of Stiffness. The stiffness of a tooth or implant is related to the clinical term *mobility*. Mobility means relatively small (e.g., tenths to thousandths of a millimeter), reversible (approximately elastic) displacements of teeth or implants that are proportional to the applied forces.

When testing tooth mobility, a dentist typically applies a lateral force to a tooth with a dental instrument (e.g., a mirror handle) and then estimates the movement of the tooth by eye. Movement greater than 1 mm is easily detected and would suggest an advanced degree of breakdown in the periodontal support system of the tooth.

A short review of literature on tooth and implant mobility leads to a definition of stiffness. First, teeth and implants can move (or displace) in different directions: intrusively, extrusively, laterally, mesiodistally, or combinations thereof. Sometimes there can be tooth displacements in more than one direction even when the applied force acts only in one direction, but this can be ignored as a secondary effect. Second, when a constant force is applied to a tooth or implant, the displacement of a tooth or implant may increase slowly with time; this phenomenon is called *creep*. Third, intrusive tooth displacement is not linear with intrusive force. Data for maxillary incisors show that there is an approximately bilinear relationship between intrusive displacement and intrusive force.

In arriving at a definition of stiffness, it is necessary to define *displacement*. In mechanics, displacement is a vector quantity, having both magnitude and direction. For example, if one pushes laterally with a 1 N force on the tip of a tooth, the tip of the tooth might move (displace) 0.2 mm in a direction parallel to the applied force. Alternatively, one might apply the 1 N force in a different direction—parallel to the tooth's long axis, i.e., an intrusive force—causing an intrusive displacement measuring 0.1 mm. In either case, a coordinate system is needed to describe both the force and the displacement. Typically, one picks an x-y-z coordinate system that is *fixed* with respect to some reference point, such as nearby bone of the jaw. In defining stiffness, we refer to the relationship between the force and related displacement parallel to the line of action of the force.

Values of about 3 to 5 N/μm have been determined for the net spring stiffness of an IMZ system, including an intramobile element. Most implants in bone produce a net stiffness greater than that for natural teeth; the largest value (10 N/μm) is for an alumina (Al_2O_3) implant in bone. If there is a soft tissue interface around an implant, however, as around the blade-vent implants tested by Brunski and Schock,[1] or as found around the cylindrical implants tested by Weinstein et al,[9] the stiffness values are less than for natural teeth or for implants with an osseointegrated interface.

Tooth Connected to an Implant. Based on the stiffness concept just discussed, analyses can be done for (1) a prosthesis supported by a natural tooth and one implant with or without an *intramobile element* (IME) and (2) a prosthesis supported by two implants and one natural tooth.

Based on a finite element model[4] and studies by Rangert et al,[6] there does not appear to be strong evidence that a major biomechanical problem exists in connecting an implant with a natural tooth, at least for the prosthetic situations described. The need for an IME inside an implant in this case is questionable from a biomechanical view.

Prosthesis Supported by Several Abutments Having Different Stiffnesses. When several abutments support a prosthesis, and the abutments do not have equal stiffnesses, the force distribution among the abutments can still be predicted theoretically. It is necessary, however, to use a modified version of the original Skalak model discussed earlier in this chapter (Figs. 7–12 to 7–14). The original Skalak model assumes all of the implants have the same stiffness, whereas the modified version of the model allows for unequal stiffnesses of the abutments.[8]

This modified theory demonstrates an important result—that the force distribution among the abutments depends strongly on the relative values of the abutment stiffnesses.

It would be desirable to have a way of knowing the stiffnesses of the implants in a given distribution before making final decisions about how to design the prosthesis. The stiffness data could be employed as input to the modified Skalak model, allowing more accurate prediction of the expected forces on each implant in various loading conditions.

Mechanics of Implant System. It is necessary to start with the specific mechanics of each implant system. To use the familiar example of the Brånemark system, a fundamental concept is the operation of a *screw joint*. This joint involves the abutment, abutment screw, gold cylinder, and gold screw. The system is designed to work as follows: As the gold screw is torqued into the abutment screw to a torque of T, a compressive clamping force of F is generated in the titanium abutment and gold cylinder. In turn, an equal but opposite tensile force is generated in the gold screw and abutment screw. This force F is sometimes referred to as the joint preload, or simply the preload. This situation can be described by an equation from machine theory:[7]

$$T = \kappa\,DF$$

where D is the screw diameter, F is the joint preload, T is the torque, and κ is a constant whose value depends on factors such as the smoothness, accuracy, and degree of lubrication at mating surfaces in the joint. The last is an important point, as explained next.

Under ideal conditions of the screw joint in the Brånemark system, e.g., with perfectly machined components that mate well with one another, measurements with strain-gauged abutments and abutment screws show that a 300 N preload is generated when the gold screw is torqued to the prescribed 10 N·cm value.[3, 6]

A little thought, however, shows that there are ways in which nonideal conditions can arise clinically. Two problems are described:

The first problem stems from variations in the value of the constant κ owing to prosthetic/casting techniques and the subsequent effects on the joint preload F. For instance, imperfections at the mating surfaces between the head of the gold screw and the inside of the gold cylinder (e.g., casting debris or metallic burs) increase the value of κ and thereby decrease F according to the equation:

$$F = T/\kappa D$$

In fact, direct measurements using strain-gauged abutments and abutment screws have demonstrated that joint preloads can be lower than the ideal 300 N value owing to various types of imperfection in the joint surfaces between the gold screw (tapered versus flat-headed) and gold cylinder (Fig. 7–16).[3]

The clinical significance of lower preload values is that the screw joint tends to open at lower applied forces during function. Tensile forces can arise on some of the abutments supporting a loaded prosthesis. If the tensile force on an abutment exceeds the joint preload—nominally 300 N, but possibly less, as just explained—the joint tends to open, i.e., contact is lost between the gold cylinder and abutment. This means that the

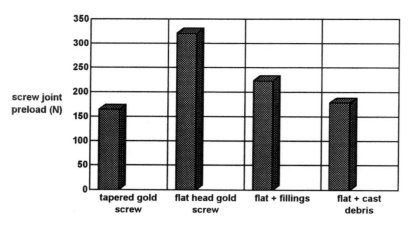

Figure 7–16. Mean values of screw-joint preloads in the Bråne-mark system under different conditions. Tapered gold screw refers to the older, first-generation gold screw that was used with the Bråne-mark system. Flat head gold screw refers to the newer Brånemark gold screw design. Flat and fillings refers to an experiment in which metal fillings were introduced into the joint. Flat and casting debris refers to casting defects (e.g., metal spill-age) on the inner surfaces of the gold cylinder.

abutment screw and gold screw then must take all of the imposed tensile load, which *adds to the already-present tensile preload.* In turn, the gold screw and abutment screws become more liable to fail by yielding or fatigue. For example, it is estimated that the stresses in the abutment screw exceed the ultimate tensile stress of titanium when the tensile force in the screw exceeds about 600 N.[6] This suggests that tensile forces on any abutment owing to biting activities should be kept below 300 N. This might be difficult. Higher than expected tensile forces on abutment screws may help explain the cause of reported screw failures.

The second problem is physical misfit of a prosthesis and one (or more) of its abutments. Consider a schematic diagram of five abutments supporting a prosthesis (Fig. 7–17). Suppose four of the five abutments mate perfectly with the gold cylinders in the framework. When each of the gold screws is torqued down onto these four well-fitting abutments, the ideal joint preload of 300 N should be achieved at each location. Sup-pose one of the five abutments, however, does not fit well; suppose there is a gap between the top of the middle abutment and the bottom of the middle gold cylinder (exaggerated in Fig. 7–17A). If this joint's gold screw is then torqued down to the target value of 10 N·cm, the tension that develops in the gold screw and abutment screw still tends to be 300 N and tends to draw together the gold cylinder and the abutment un-til the 10 N°cm torque value is reached. If the original gap between the gold cylinder and abut-ment is small, it might be possible to close the joint completely, with a negligible effect on the other four abutments. If the gap is large, how-ever, it might not be possible to close the joint via the 300 N preload that develops when the 10 N·cm torque is applied. For this "worst-case scenario," a free-body diagram of the situation

(see Fig. 7–17C) indicates that a force of about 300 N would develop on the prosthesis and the abutment (plus the implant) at the location of the misfit. In turn, this 300 N force would have to be balanced by an appropriate distribution of forces among the other four abutments. In principle, the distribution of forces should be predictable via the Skalak model. This means that the middle abutment as well as the other four abutments would be loaded by virtue of misfit at the middle abutment. Assuming that this degree of misfit was not sensed by the patient or

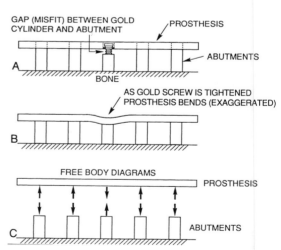

Figure 7–17. How a misfitting framework can cause loads on fixtures even before any biting force is applied to the prosthesis. *A,* Four well-fitting joints and one (middle) joint with a gap between the gold cylinder and abutment. *B,* Exaggerated view of bending of the prosthesis when the gold screw is tightened and the joint closes. *C,* Free body diagrams of the prosthesis and abutments corresponding to the situa-tion in *B.* Forces develop on all abutments as a result of misfit at only one. (From Brunski JB, Skalak R: Biomechanics of osseointegration and dental prostheses. *In* Naert I, et al [eds]: Osseointegration in Oral Rehabilitation. London, Quintessence, 1993, pp 133–156.)

the dentist installing the prosthesis, each abutment would be loaded by constant forces before any biting forces occurred. Subsequent biting forces on the prosthesis would produce forces on each abutment that would be superimposed on the forces, owing to the misfit. Such a situation could cause problems with the hardware or bone around the implants or with both.

In conclusion, in the same way that medical sciences, including basic physiology and anatomy, provide a foundation for dentistry, basic principles of biomechanics must be respected when doing oral implants, or else the case may fail. Although the design of implants and prostheses is not yet an exact science, many biomechanical aspects can be explained quantitatively. Although a reasonable amount is known about the biomechanical aspects relating to abutments and bridgework "above the bone," perhaps the biggest remaining challenge is to understand fully the loading limits of bone as they exist at the bone-implant interface.

References

1. Brunski JB, Schock RB: Mechanical behavior of a fibrous tissue interface of an endosseous dental implant. Transactions of the 5th Annual Meeting of the Society for Biomaterials, 41, 1990.
2. Brunski JB, Skalak R: Biomechanics of osseointegration and dental prostheses. *In* Naert I, van Steenberghe D, Worthington P (eds): Osseointegration in Oral Rehabilitation. London, Quintessence, Inc, 1993, pp 133–156.
3. Carr AB, Brunski JB, Labishak J, Bagley B: Preload comparison between as-received and cast-to-implant cylinders. J Dent Res 73:190, 1993.
4. El Wakad M: Measurement and Prediction of Loading on Dental Implants: Transducer Design and Finite Element Modeling. Dissertation, Department of Biomedical Engineering, Rensselaer Polytechnic Institute, Troy, NY, 1988.
5. Hoshaw SJ, Brunski JB, Cochran GVB: Mechanical loading of Brånemark fixtures affects interfacial bone modeling and remodeling. Int J Oral Maxillofac Implants 9:345–360, 1994.
6. Rangert B, Gunne J, Sullivan DY: Mechanical aspects of a Brånemark implant connected to a natural tooth: An in vitro study. Int J Oral Maxillofac Implants 6:177–186, 1991.
7. Shigley JE, Mischke CR: Mechanical Engineering Design, ed 5. New York, McGraw-Hill, 1989, pp 325–382.
8. Skalak R, Brunski JB, Mendelson M: A method for calculating the distribution of vertical forces among variable-stiffness abutments supporting a dental prosthesis. *In* Langrana NA, Friedman MH, Grood ES (eds): Am Soc Mechan Engin (BED) 24:347–350, 1993.
9. Weinstein AM, Klawitter JJ, Cook SD: Implant-bone characteristics of bioglass dental implants. J Biomed Mater Res 14:23–29, 1980.

Study Questions

1. Be able to explain how the mandible acts as a class III lever.

2. Describe the forces placed on a freestanding mandibular premolar tooth or implant restoration.

3. If you plan on restoring the posterior two premolars and two molars with a four-unit, splinted-implant–supported prosthesis, describe how many implants would be placed from a mechanical point of view.

4. Given the situation as described in question 3, why not place two implants in the molar locations and cantilever the two premolar pontics?

5. Describe the mechanical difference in placing four implants versus five or six implants in the anterior mandible for a full arch hybrid prosthesis.

6. Be able to discuss the effects of debris in the screw-abutment interface.

SECTION 2

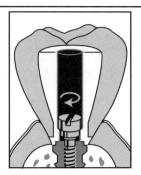

Restorative
Considerations

CHAPTER 8

Principles of Implant Prosthodontics

Luis R. Guerra
Israel M. Finger
Revised by Luis R. Guerra

Team Approach
Clinical Evaluation
    Chief Complaint
    General Physical Evaluation
    Psychological Evaluation
    Dental Evaluation
    Bone
    Soft Tissue
    Ridge Relationships
    Radiographic Evaluation
    Prosthodontic Options
    Prosthesis Required
    Number of Implants Required
    Aesthetics
    Phonetics
    Occlusal Surface Materials

Occlusion
Diagnostic Casts
    Width of the Arch
    Width of the Ridge
    Length of the Arch
    Interarch Space
    Maxillomandibular Relationships
Diagnostic Wax-up
Surgical Stent
References

Implants have added options to successful prosthodontic rehabilitation formerly unavailable.[2–4, 7, 9, 13] A global statement can be made in relation to implants: *Any edentulous space is a potential implant site.* This is obviously a broad statement that must be modified. However, if the full potential of implant therapy is to be reflected in improved prosthodontic restorations, the consideration of implants must be incorporated into every treatment plan. There are many patients for whom both conventional removable and fixed prosthodontic procedures are compromised owing to a lack of adequate support, retention, and stability of the resultant prosthesis. Implants offer the restorative dentist additional options to obtain these necessary requirements for a successful restoration.[35] Conventional prosthodontic procedures have been successfully employed to meet functional and aesthetic requirements. These unfortunately have often required the alteration of intact tooth structure to achieve their ends. Implants can be used to prevent or minimize this unnecessary loss of tooth or supporting structures. There must be a clear understanding of the rationale for this point of view. It must be conceded that fixed restorations are more desirable than removable restorations. Removable partial dentures that are supported by implants are superior to those supported by the residual alveolar ridges and the remaining dentition alone. Complete dentures that are more retentive and stable and relieve the load on the residual alveolar ridge by means of implants are superior to those that rely on the residual alveolar ridge alone for support, stability, and retention.

The main focus then must be on establishing the need, desire, and feasibility of the use for implants in the restorative effort.[14, 18, 29–31] The clinical examination must elicit information regarding various aspects of the ultimate proposed treatment plan. There are certain principles and philosophies that must be clearly understood before initiation of any dental examination when dental implants are considered.

TEAM APPROACH

Some authors believe that the same person should place and restore the implants.[23] The rationale is that it is more efficient from a patient's point of view. It also allows the practitioner more latitude in changing the predetermined position of the implants at the time of surgery. Because the same individual is responsible for the prosthetic treatment, these changes can be incorporated into the treatment plan more readily.

Others believe that a team approach is the more appropriate method to follow.[26] A surgeon should place the implants, and a restorative dentist should complete the restoration. Because it allows for the utilization of the expertise of the two individuals, there is a built-in second opinion in this approach. Additionally, there is shared responsibility and shared liability. Regardless of the philosophy followed, it is well to delineate the responsibilities at each stage of implant therapy.

The restorative dentist should:

1. Perform the initial clinical evaluation.
2. Perform the initial radiographic evaluation.[1, 39, 42]
3. Obtain the diagnostic casts.
4. Obtain the diagnostic wax-up.
5. Determine the location and number of implants and fabricate a surgical template.[48]
6. Select the proper abutments following implant exposure.
7. Design and fabricate prosthesis.[22, 46-48]
8. Provide oral hygiene care and instructions.[28]
9. Ensure recall of the patient to evaluate maintenance and provide care as required.

The surgeon's responsibilities include:

1. Confirmation of the radiographic evaluation.
2. Confirmation of the physical evaluation.
3. Determination of the location and number of implants within limits set by the restorative dentist.
4. Placement of the implants.
5. Uncovering of the implants.
6. Confirmation of integration of the implants.

CLINICAL EVALUATION

Chief Complaint

The reason the patient is seeking treatment must be carefully determined. Often patients are not forthcoming with the true motive in seeking dental care. The areas of function and aesthetics can often become blurred in the mind of the patient. The practitioner must determine which is most important for the patient. It requires careful listening and acute questioning on the part of the practitioner to make this determination. Generally, both areas play a role in the seeking of dental care. The patient's emphasis on one area or the other, however, has a significant bearing on the final treatment plan proposed. It must be recognized that determining the chief complaint is the crucial point of interaction between the patient and the practitioner. Sufficient time must be allowed to get the required information. Although this may not appear any different than for those patients requiring extensive conventional prosthodontic restorations, the use of implants introduces an entire new dimension to the overall care of the patient. Not only is there additional expense, but it involves more complicated treatment that requires that implants be placed in an accurate, restorable position. Once placed, the implants represent an irreversible aspect of the restorative process. The challenge is to elicit carefully from the patient the information that can be used to formulate the best treatment plan, taking into consideration patient needs and desires.

General Physical Evaluation

The medical history normally taken in a modern dental office often suffices for the implant patient. It must be kept in mind that there are few contraindications to the use of dental implants. This topic is addressed in Chapter 3 as well as reviewed by Misch.[36]

The restorative dentist must be familiar with the surgical procedures involved in placement of implants. In this manner, a proper evaluation can be made whether the patient can tolerate the planned procedures.[16] Consultation with the surgeon at this point may be necessary to arrive at a proper evaluation in patients with a complicated medical history.

From a prosthodontic point of view, the patient's physical ability to maintain the restoration and the implants is a most significant consideration.[21] The physical ability or limitations of the patient also play a part in the design of the prosthesis, the selection of the type of retentive devices used, and the materials used in the fabrication of the prosthesis.

Psychological Evaluation

Although the medical history and physical evaluation must be thoroughly performed, they do rely in large measure on recordable signs and symptoms. This is not the case in assessing the patient's desires and expectations. One must realize that, for many patients, the perception of what constitutes implant therapy has been formed from information provided by friends, lay publications, and other mass media. This is not necessarily all negative, because it results in the patient seeking implant therapy. Many times, however, the information cannot be properly evaluated by the patient, and limitations of therapy are not clearly understood. Therefore, it is necessary to educate the patient concerning the necessity of specific procedures for his or her particular case.

Probably the most frequent misconceptions expressed by patients concerning the use of implants are the time involved to complete the treatment, the techniques used to achieve integration of the implants to bone, the effects of resorption of the residual alveolar ridge on the final restoration, the requirement for maintenance of the restoration, and the cost involved.

These are all issues that must be resolved before the initiation of treatment to ensure long-term success in the area of patient relations. Patients must realign their expectations to the reality of the conditions present. This often leads to confusion on the part of patients because in their minds the placement of implants is often synonymous with fixed restorations. The education of the patient should begin at the first appointment and continue throughout the treatment. Visual aids can be of tremendous help in assisting the patient to understand the treatment plan proposed based on the clinical findings.

Dental Evaluation

In addition to the usual comprehensive dental evaluation, the practitioner must incorporate into this evaluation the effects of the conditions present in the oral cavity on implants placed in this environment. There are many questions that must be addressed at this initial evaluation. The condition of the remaining dentition in regard to the implants must be evaluated. Will the implants be used to support the remaining dentition? The periodontal condition of the remaining dentition and the effect on the peri-implant health must be determined. Although it has been stated that there are in fact few contraindications to the use of implants, some factors must be addressed. Lack of maintenance and overloading have been cited as the most frequent reasons for implant loss.[41] Therefore, a history of bruxism, malaligned dentition, and extruded teeth, which preclude the development of a harmonious occlusion and a hygienic restoration, should alert the practitioner to problems in this area. The patient's commitment to a long-term maintenance program must also be evaluated. The patient with a less than desirable level of oral hygiene should not be automatically excluded from receiving implant prostheses. Many of these patients have never been informed about the effects of poor oral hygiene, nor have they been shown effective methods of maintaining their dentition. These patients often respond to the educational effort of the dental team and become ideal candidates for implant therapy.

The most important aspect of this initial dental evaluation is that a decision about the appropriateness of the use of implants cannot be made based on this initial evaluation alone. It requires further evaluation of radiographs, mounted diagnostic casts, and the diagnostic wax-up.

Implants represent only a part of the overall treatment of a patient. The entire dentition must be considered in the treatment plan. Restoration of carious lesions, elimination of spaces by conventional fixed restorations, elimination of periodontal disease, and restoration of a harmonious occlusion in the partially edentulous patient are all requisites for successful implant therapy.[31] It is recognized that active periodontal disease has the potential to spread to the peri-implant tissues causing peri-implantitis.[5, 25, 27, 32, 33]

Bone

The age of the patient[38] and the amount and type[6] of bone available to support the implants must be determined.[37] The usual method of accomplishing this is by means of radiographs. The types of radiographs used depend on the number of implants to be placed, their location in the jaws, and the availability of equipment with which to take the radiographs, as is discussed in Chapter 5.

Another method often overlooked in determining the amount of bone available is palpation. This method is particularly useful in the mandible. It is often possible to encircle the mandible completely with forefinger and thumb and obtain an indication of the size and shape of the arch at a particular point. This method is much less useful in the maxilla. Dense fibrous tissue over the ridges prevents palpation of the maxillary bone itself, and a misdiagnosis is often made from relying on palpation in the maxilla.

Soft Tissue

The soft tissue through which the implant-abutment head–complex exits into the oral cavity is a critical area in terms of long-term success.[45] This is the area that the patient must maintain to ensure gingival health and therefore must be capable of withstanding the hygiene regimen performed. Fixed keratinized tissue is the preferred tissue in this area. This is the only type of tissue that has the ability to form a tight collar of tissue around the implant necks. It can also withstand the trauma of brushing and flossing or whatever hygiene regimen is used. Every effort should therefore be made to obtain fixed keratinized tissue around the implants.

If soft tissue grafting procedures are anticipated, these are probably best done before implant placement, because it is difficult to graft soft tissue around exposed implants. Israelson and Plemons[20] have described techniques that can be used to improve the quality and aesthetics of the soft tissues at the peri-implant site.

Ridge Relationships

The relationship of the maxilla to the mandible plays an important role in determining the type of prosthesis that can be fabricated and is a deciding factor in the type of occlusion that can be achieved. Occlusion plays a pivotal role in the manner in which the forces are directed to the implants at the bone-implant interface. Although ridge relationships can often be determined by visual examination, the best observation of this relationship is accomplished from mounted diagnostic casts.

RADIOGRAPHIC EVALUATION

A variety of dental radiographs can be used to determine the quality and quantity of bone available and to determine the location of anatomic structures at the implant site. Panoramic, lateral cephalometric and periapical radiographs have specific uses in the pretreatment evaluation. Additionally, tomography, computerized tomography (CT), and magnetic resonance imaging offer additional information.

The length of the implants to be used can also be determined by radiograph. Although the option of using the longest implant by placing it where the bone exists is tempting, it is more advantageous to place the implant perpendicular to the plane of occlusion. This may result in the use of a shorter implant, but this disadvantage is offset by having the forces exerted on the implant along its long axis (Fig. 8–1).

PROSTHODONTIC OPTIONS

Prosthesis Required

The type of prosthesis required depends on a large measure on the patient's desires and chief complaint. Every effort must made to meet the patient's needs. When these desires are unwarranted owing to the conditions present, the patient must be educated as to other treatment options available to provide a stable, retentive, supported, and aesthetic restoration. This requires an empathetic and knowledgeable practitioner. Visual aids that illustrate similar cases

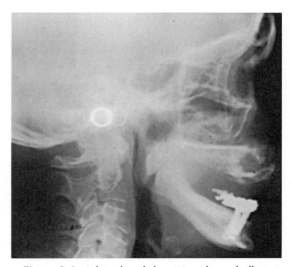

Figure 8–1. A lateral cephalometric radiograph illustrating the correct placement of implants to support a hybrid prosthesis. The implants are vertical to the occlusal plane. Owing to the normal maxillomandibular relationship, placement of the anterior maxillary teeth is not compromised.

from previous patients can be of great help in assisting the patient to understand the situation.

It should be apparent that the decision of which type of restoration is best suited for the individual patient cannot be made after a perfunctory examination. It requires a complete diagnostic workup. This is the only manner in which a proper diagnosis can be made and greatly enhances the patient's ability to understand why a particular treatment plan is being proposed.

Implants can also be used to improve conventional prostheses. This is particularly evident when removable partial dentures are planned. Not infrequently there is only the remaining anterior natural dentition in the mandible. These patients are generally edentulous in the maxillary arch; the occlusal forces from the anterior mandibular teeth overstress the opposing edentulous residual ridge resulting in its extreme resorption. This condition could be alleviated if the occlusal loading could occur more posteriorly on the ridges. Implants can be placed distal to the remaining mandibular cuspids to allow for a design that incorporates posterior stops on the implants and relieves some of the load on the anterior maxillary ridge. The number of implants can vary from one to several, but it becomes obvious that if a removable partial denture is the final prosthesis of choice in a situation in which only anterior teeth are present in an arch, it can be better designed with the use of implants (Figs. 8–2 and 8–3).

Implants placed in strategic positions in the partially edentulous residual ridge can also be used to support removable partial dentures. In situations in which there is insufficient bone for placement of the required number of implants

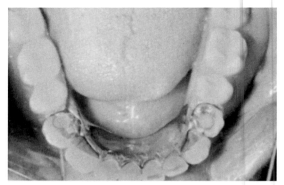

Figure 8–3. Removable partial denture in place. The use of attachments (ASC-52) on the implant crowns eliminates the use of rests, clasps, and reciprocal arms.

to support a fixed prosthesis, it is often possible to place fewer implants to help support a removable partial denture. The implants can be used individually with a variety of abutment heads with attachments incorporated into the design of the abutments or can be splinted with superstructures to provide the required retention, stability, and support (Figs. 8–4 and 8–5).

Number of Implants Required

The number of implants required depends on the type of prosthesis to be placed. This can vary from two implants for an overdenture to a greater number for a fixed type of restoration. The key factors in determination of the number of implants that can be placed are the quality and quantity of bone available.

The following are general observations about the number of implants required for various types of prostheses:

Two to four implants in the anterior mandible

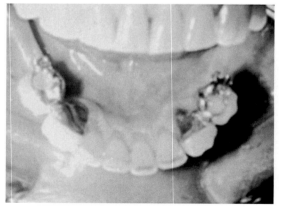

Figure 8–2. Bilateral placement of implant crowns distal to the cuspids. The crowns are joined to the crowns on the cuspids by means of attachments.

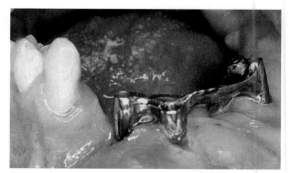

Figure 8–4. Implant-supported bar assembly placed to support a removable partial denture and eliminate torquing forces on the remaining dentition.

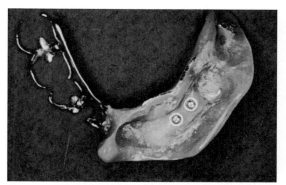

Figure 8–5. Tissue side of removable partial denture used in Figure 8–4. The Ceka attachments, which provide the retention to the prosthesis over the bar assembly, are visible.

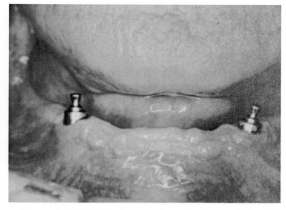

Figure 8–7. Two implants in the anterior mandible with O-ring abutments. The implants are not splinted together.

can be used for tissue-supported overdentures. This allows for the use of bar and clip or other vertical stress-breaking types of attachments (Fig. 8–6). If the bone is of good quality and implants of sufficient length, attachments can be placed over the individual implants without the use of a splinting bar (Fig. 8–7).

A minimum of four implants in the anterior mandible can be used for an implant-supported, implant-retained prosthesis (hybrid). In an attempt to gain added support for this type of prosthesis, it is preferred that five or six implants be utilized. Obviously, this has a great deal to do with the opposing occlusion and the anticipated forces to be placed on the implants.

In a totally implant-supported overdenture, the number of implants required is the same as in a hybrid denture. The forces exerted on the implants are essentially the same except that in the case of the overdenture, the prosthesis is patient removable and the

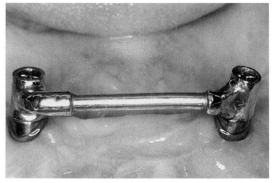

Figure 8–6. Two implants in the anterior mandible used to retain a coping bar assembly.

hybrid denture is removable only by the dentist or other trained staff.

In patients with an edentulous space distal to the natural dentition in whom a single implant is to be placed, it is recommended that the restoration be attached to the distal remaining tooth by means of a mortise-type attachment if a retrievable prosthesis is desired. If the prosthesis is cemented to place, it should be splinted to the distal natural tooth. This aids the implant in resisting the torquing forces, which may ensue as the result of occlusal loading. The use of a system providing nonrotational capability for the prosthesis placed over it is highly recommended in these cases.

Two implants can support a freestanding bridge replacing three teeth in a quadrant. As long as 3 to 4 mm of space is available between implant bodies, one implant per tooth replacement is preferred.

In situations in which there are teeth remaining on the mesial and distal sides of the space, single implants can be used to replace a single tooth. The use of a nonrotational implant system is essential to prevent rotation of the single crown placed over the implant and to provide orientation for the single tooth restoration.

In the maxilla, it is best to maximize the number of implants. The nature of the bone in the maxilla generally requires that the per unit area of the implants be increased to support the occlusal loading.[37]

Aesthetics

Aesthetics is an area in which the practitioner can encounter a great deal of problems. The prosthetic options to ensure an aesthetic result depend on implant placement. It is obvious that the restorative dentist has limited options when trying to restore a malpositioned implant. Four solutions to the problem of malpositioned implants are:

> 1. Proper treatment planning
> 2. Communication with the surgeon
> 3. Use of surgical stents to ensure proper placement of the implants
> 4. Communication with the patient about potential problems and anticipated results along with alternative treatment plans

Aesthetics has become an important issue in implant dentistry.[43] As a result of increased emphasis on aesthetics, the various implant companies have responded with a variety of components to ensure more aesthetic restorations. It is important that the practitioner stay abreast of these new components to provide state-of-the-art care to the patient. The role of the laboratory cannot be overemphasized. The laboratory technician must also be current with present-day technology. To achieve the maximal aesthetic result, there must be close communication between the restorative dentist and the laboratory technician.[11]

Phonetics

Phonetics is an area of dentistry that is often neglected. This becomes an important consideration in implant dentistry.[24] This is more frequently a problem in the maxilla than in the mandible owing to the articulatory importance of the maxilla.[34]

It is most often the patient with a severely resorbed maxilla who is likely to complain of phonetic difficulties. This is due to the encroachment that occurs to the tongue. As the maxilla resorbs, the anterior portion moves posteriorly and superiorly. This means that implants placed in the anterior resorbed maxilla are more palatal than were the natural teeth. When the thickness of the prosthesis is added to cover the implants and any superstructures used, the problem of encroachment on tongue space becomes critical. A solution to this problem is to use a diagnostic wax-up that includes the anticipated thickness of the prosthesis. This discloses potential problems and leads to alternate solutions. When fixed restorations are considered for the severely re-

sorbed maxilla, the aesthetic placement of the teeth results in the creation of a space between the prosthesis and the crest of the residual alveolar ridge. This may result in problems with plosive sounds and with proper soft tissue support. The use of a diagnostic wax-up reveals this inordinate space between the teeth and the crest of the ridge and provides the patient with evidence of the problem. In most of these cases the treatment plan can be altered from a fixed prosthesis to an overdenture. This provides the correct lip support and eliminates the space between the crest of the ridge and the prosthesis.

Severe resorption of the residual ridge can often be corrected by grafting with bone or allogeneic materials to rebuild the residual ridge to a more favorable contour. This requires proper soft tissue management to ensure coverage of the graft and acceptable soft tissue contours around the restorations and adjacent teeth.

Occlusal Surface Materials

There are essentially three materials used on the occlusal surfaces of prostheses: (1) porcelain, (2) metal, and (3) acrylic resin. All three are used on prostheses placed over implants.[12]

Some authors[17] have stated that porcelain is the hardest of the materials and thus leads to an abrupt, sharp stressing of the implants at the bone-implant interface. Some other objections to porcelain are that it is extremely difficult to achieve a finely refined occlusion owing to the nature of its processing and the loss of the glaze when adjusted in the mouth.

Metal has been a standby in fixed restorations for decades. It can be cast and adjusted quite easily and thus can be used to achieve a finely refined occlusion by most practitioners. It is also somewhat less hard than porcelain and thus may moderate the loading at the implant-bone interface. The most severe drawback to the use of metal is its appearance, and with today's demands by the public for cosmetic results, it is often rejected by patients.

Acrylic resin is the least hard of the materials. The hardness can vary, depending on the type of resin used and how it is processed. It has been stated that resin acts as a buffer to absorb some of the shock of occlusal loading at the implant-bone interface. The disadvantages for the use of resins, despite dramatic improvements in their manufacture, is that resins still exhibit a greater degree of wear and are more susceptible to staining than either porcelain or metal.

Long-term beneficial results of one material

over the other have not been evident.[19] Until further evidence becomes available, the use of any of these materials cannot be condemned. Progressive loading of the implants may improve long-term survival of the implants.[37] This does involve the use of a longer period of temporization using acrylic resin as the material of choice on the occlusal surface. This material readily allows for the modification of the occlusal surface to increase the loading of the implants gradually. After a time, the final restoration using porcelain or metal as the occlusal surface can be completed. Depending on the opposing occlusion, the prolonged use of acrylic resin may be contraindicated because if rapid wear occurs, this may result in increased loading, particularly lateral stresses, on the implants.

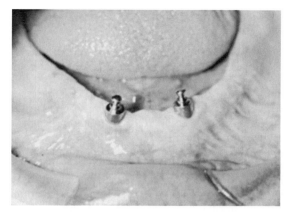

Figure 8–8. A V-shaped arch demonstrating the implants placed close together as a result of the anatomy of this type of jaw.

OCCLUSION

Occlusion is a complex subject and is covered in detail in Chapter 13 and in chapters dealing with specific types of restorations. Some general occlusal requirements, however, must be entertained at the time of treatment planning. Occlusion is an individual requirement. That is, each patient brings with him or her unique occlusal determinants that guide in developing a unique harmonious occlusion for that particular patient. We should not attempt to bring all patients into a particular philosophy of occlusion.

The manner in which the occlusion is developed determines how occlusal forces are directed to the implant and how these are distributed at the implant-bone interface. In general, lateral forces must be avoided, and all efforts must be made to direct the forces along the long axis of the implant. The loading on the implants must be minimized to the greatest extent possible. This requires evaluation of the following.

DIAGNOSTIC CASTS

The value of obtaining diagnostic casts has been emphasized in the restorative literature.[8, 10, 15, 40] The mounted casts enable the practitioner to plan the restorative procedure carefully. This is particularly important when the diagnostic casts play such an important role in not only the restorative phase of treatment, but also in the surgical placement of the implants. There is a pivotal relationship between the placement of the implants and the design and fabrication of the final prosthesis.

Width of the Arch

The width of the arch relates to the horizontal distance between the quadrants in the same jaw. This plays a role in determining the position of the implants and the distance between the implants. This distance must be considered in designing the prosthesis and is linked closely to the shape of the arch. Implants placed in the anterior of a V-shaped arch may result in a short distance between the implants limiting the type of support or retention that can be used (Fig. 8–8). Implants placed in a square-shaped arch are more easily placed an ideal distance apart, resulting in optimal support or retention (Fig. 8–9). The shape of the arch can be viewed clinically, but diagnostic casts allow for a more accurate assessment of the shape of the arch.

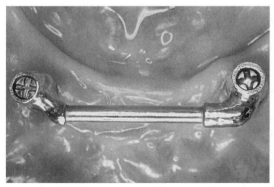

Figure 8–9. A U-shaped arch requiring the placement of the bar anterior to the implants to avoid intrusion into the tongue space.

Width of the Ridge

The width of the ridge is a limiting factor in the diameter or width of an implant that can be placed. Palpation is an excellent method of determining the width of the mandibular ridge. It is difficult, however, to determine ridge width in the maxilla. CT and routine tomography, corrected for magnification, although adding expense to the treatment plan, are excellent methods of determining the width of the available ridge. Mounted diagnostic casts provide visualization of the width of the arch and its relation to the opposing arch and the remaining dentition in the same arch. These relationships play a role in determining the position of the implant in a horizontal plane.

Length of the Arch

The length of the arch is a measurement of the arch from a coronal or occlusal view. This measurement includes all the areas into which an implant can be placed. This usually includes the distance from the first molar on one side to the position of the first molar on the opposite side. The length of the arch determines the number of implants that can be placed. Sufficient bone (4 mm) must remain between the implants to allow for the normal reaction of the bone to stress. This physiologic response must not be compromised by crowding of the implants, or loss of bone around the implants results.

It is useful to view each arch as having three lengths. The area in the anterior between the mental foramina is often used to support hybrid dentures and overdentures. The other two lengths involve the areas between mental foramen and the first molars bilaterally. The length of the edentulous space to be employed as the site of implant placement is used to determine the number of implants to be placed in the posterior mandible. This is particularly meaningful when restoring relatively small spaces, such as are encountered in designing a prosthesis for single missing posterior teeth. The space may not be of sufficient length to place the proper number of implants to distribute the load adequately. In these cases, it is often necessary to incorporate adjacent natural teeth into the design of the prosthesis. Mounted diagnostic casts can be utilized to plan the case correctly and avoid costly mistakes of choosing the incorrect number of implants.

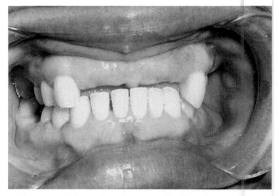

Figure 8–10. Reduced interarch distance resulting in minimal space for the placement of an abutment head and a fixed prosthesis over the implants.

Interarch Space

Interarch space can be a limiting factor in the design of a prosthesis. The interarch space is the space that exists at the site of implant placement between the mandibular and maxillary arch. Often extrusion of teeth occurs from one arch into an edentulous space of the opposing arch (Fig. 8–10). This must be correctly evaluated not only to ensure sufficient space to place the restoration with its attendant components, but also to evaluate the effect of this space limitation on the occlusion that must be developed.

Maxillomandibular Relationships

Discrepancies in the horizontal relationship of the maxillary arch and mandibular arch can lead to difficulty in attempting to develop a harmonious occlusion to avoid overloading the implants. This horizontal relationship must be viewed in both the sagittal (anteroposterior) and the frontal planes. Miscalculations in the anterior relationship may result in serious mistakes, which may preclude a satisfactory aesthetic result. Errors in the frontal plane can lead to occlusal discrepancies, which can lead to implant failure. Mounted diagnostic casts are an essential aid in determining the correct maxillomandibular relationships.

DIAGNOSTIC WAX-UP

The diagnostic wax-up is an essential portion of the evaluation of the patient.[10, 44] The diagnostic wax-up accomplishes the following:

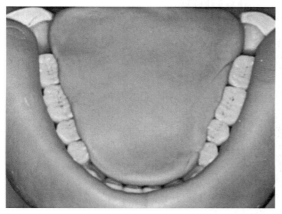

Figure 8–11. A mandibular cast with a polyvinylsiloxane index molded over the diagnostic wax-up.

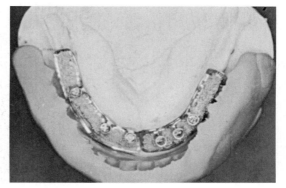

Figure 8–13. The mandibular cast with the completed framework in place.

1. Accurately reflects the final prosthesis
   A. Tooth position
   B. Denture base
2. Aids in determining the position of the implants
   A. Cingulum
   B. Central fossa
3. Aids in determining the length of the abutment heads
   A. Interarch distance
   B. Opposing occlusion
4. Can be used to optimize aesthetic results
   A. Tooth position
   B. Soft tissue support
5. Used in fabrication of indices
   A. Buccal-labial
   B. Lingual
6. Used in the fabrication of radiographic stent
   A. Measure horizontal dimensions
   B. Measure vertical dimensions
7. Used in the fabrication of the surgical stent
   A. Partially edentulous patients
   B. Edentulous patients

It is imperative that both the dentist and the patient have a visualization of the expected final prosthesis. By providing the diagnostic wax-up, the final tooth position and the required soft tissue support can be anticipated. It can also lead to modifications of the treatment plan. An overdenture may be required to provide the proper soft tissue support versus a fixed restoration. The length of the abutment heads can be predetermined from the diagnostic wax-up on the diagnostic casts. The space between the residual ridge and the opposing ridge or dentition can be accurately measured and accounted for in the selection of the abutment heads. To facilitate the final aesthetic result, it has been observed that implants that exit the jaws in the cingulum area of anterior teeth and the central fossa of posterior teeth offer the best opportunity for achieving this goal.

The fabrication of an index deserves special attention. An index can be fabricated around the

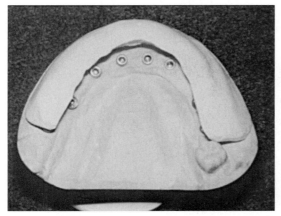

Figure 8–12. The mandibular cast and index with the wax-up removed. Note the space available for the waxing of the framework.

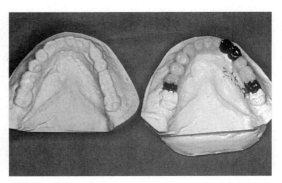

Figure 8–14. The diagnostic wax-up on the right and the duplicated wax-up on the left.

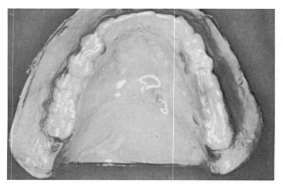

Figure 8–15. A clear resin "temporary" stent adapted to the cast shown in Figure 8–14.

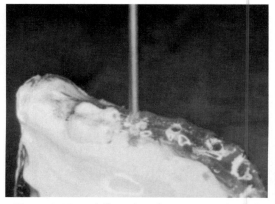

Figure 8–17. A drill in place demonstrating the drilling of holes through the central fossa of the occlusal surfaces of the teeth duplicated in the "temporary" stent. The holes are drilled into the stone of the cast so they are clearly visible.

diagnostic wax-up made of a pliable material. This is accomplished after the border area of the casts has been scored to allow repositioning of the index. The index is used to ensure that the superstructures that are fabricated are restricted to the volume of the fabricated prosthesis (Fig. 8–11).

After the index is fabricated, the diagnostic wax-up is removed and the indices replaced on the diagnostic casts (Fig. 8–12). This allows visualization of the space available for the superstructures without exceeding the volume of the anticipated prosthesis (Fig. 8–13).

SURGICAL STENT

Once the position of the implants is determined by palpation and clinical, radiographic, and diagnostic cast examinations, the surgical stent is then fabricated. An impression is made of the diagnostic wax-up on the master cast (Fig. 8–14). On the resultant cast, a "temporary" stent is fabricated using a heat-vacuum–forming machine (OmniVac) (Fig. 8–15). Care is taken to ensure that the occlusal surfaces are impressed on the temporary stent. In edentulous patients, this step is omitted, and an acrylic resin surgical stent resembling a base plate is fabricated on the master cast without the wax-up.

The temporary stent is then placed on the master cast with the wax-up removed (Fig. 8–16). The temporary stent should seat on the occlusal surfaces of the remaining dentition, and the ridge should be clearly visible through the occlusal surfaces where the wax-up has been removed. Holes are then drilled through the temporary stent on the cingulum of anterior teeth and the central fossa of posterior teeth (Fig. 8–17). This is done ensuring that the drill used is held vertical to the crest of the ridge and parallel from one hole to the other.

The surgical stent can be fabricated using a clear heat-cured or autopolymerized acrylic resin

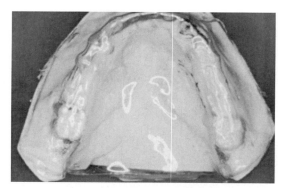

Figure 8–16. The "temporary" stent placed over the master cast with the wax-up removed. The temporary is keyed to the remaining teeth.

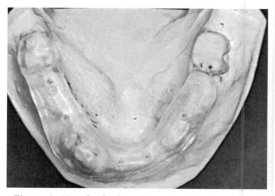

Figure 8–18. The final acrylic resin stent placed over the master cast with the wax-up removed. The holes drilled into the cast should be visible.

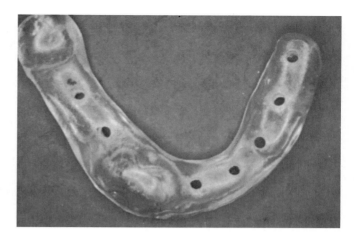

Figure 8–19. The completed resin stent with the holes drilled in to ensure the proper placement of the implants.

(Fig. 8–18). The stent should be approximately 4 mm in thickness. A stent that is too thick prevents the various drills that are used at the time of placement of the implants from seating all the way down, resulting in holes that are of insufficient depth. When the surgical stent has cured, the holes scored on the cast should be clearly visible. A pilot or intermediate-size drill, depending on the surgeon's choice, is then used to drill through the surgical stent directly over the holes previously scored on the cast. The drill should be vertical to the residual ridge, and the preparations should be parallel to each other (Fig. 8–19).

In the edentulous patient the cast is scored over the areas where the implants are to be placed. In cases in which two implants are to be used for an implant-retained, tissue-supported overdenture, these are usually placed at the cuspid area 20 mm apart. Where several implants are to be placed to support a hybrid denture, the holes are drilled over the central fossa of posterior teeth and the cingulum or lingual to the anterior teeth. These positions are determined from the diagnostic wax-up.

References

1. Abrahams JJ: The role of diagnostic imaging in dental implantology. Radiol Clin North Am 31:163–180, 1993.
2. Adell R, Eriksson B, Lekholm U, et al: A long-term follow-up study of osseointegrated implants in the treatment of totally edentulous jaws. Int J Oral Maxillofac Impl 5:347–359, 1990.
3. Adell R, Lekholm U, Rockler B, et al: A 15-year study of osseointegrated implants in the treatment of the edentulous jaw. Int J Oral Surg 10:387–416, 1981.
4. Albrektsson T, Dahl E, Enhom L, et al: Osseointegrated oral implants. A Swedish multicenter study of 8,139 consecutive inserted Nobelpharma implants. J Periodont 59:287–296, 1988.
5. Apse R, et al: Microbiota and crevicular fluid collagenase activity in the osseointegrated dental implant sulcus: A comparison of sites in edentulous and partially edentulous patients. J Periodont Res 24:96–105, 1989.
6. Baxter JC, Fattore LD: Osteoporosis and osseointegration of implants. J Prosthodont 2:120–125, 1993.
7. Block MS: Cylindrical HA coated implants—8 year observation. Comp Contin Educ 15:526–532, 1993.
8. Boersma H: Placement of teeth on a model as an aid in prediction of therapy results. Quintessence Int 1:45–48, 1970.
9. Brånemark P-I, Hansson BO, Adell R, et al: Osseointegrated implants in the treatment of the edentulous jaw. Experience from a 10-year period. Scand J Plast Reconstr Surg Suppl (16):1–132, 1977.
10. Carlyle LW, Richardson JT: The diagnostic wax-up: An aid in treatment planning. Texas Dent J 102:10–12, 1985.
11. Chiche GJ, Pinault A: Considerations for fabrication of implant-supported posterior restorations. Int J Prosthodont 4:37–44, 1991.
12. Cibirka RM, Razzoog ME, Lang BR, Stohler CS: Determining the force absorption quotient for restorative materials used in implant occlusal surfaces. J Prosthet Dent 67:361–364, 1992.
13. Cranin AN, Rabkin MF, Garfinkle L: A statistical evaluation of 952 endosteal implants. J Am Dent Assoc 94:315–320, 1977.
14. Eckert SE, Laney WR. Patient evaluation and prosthodontic treatment planning for osseointegrated implants. Dent Clin North Am 33:599–618, 1989.
15. Ferraro EF: Study models in general practice. J Conn Dent Assoc 43:126–129, 1969.
16. Gilbert GH, Minaker KL: Principles of surgical risk assessment of the elderly patient. J Oral Maxillofac Surg 48:972–979, 1990.
17. Gracis SE, Nicholls JI, Chalupnik JD, Youdelis RA: Shock-absorbing behavior of five restorative materials used on implants. Int J Prosthodont 4:282–291, 1991.
18. Henry PJ: Treatment planning for tissue integrated prosthesis. Int Dent J 39:171–182, 1989.
19. Hobkirk JA, Psarros KJ: The influence of occlusal surface material on peak masticatory forces using osseointegrated implant-supported prostheses. Int J Oral Maxillofac Impl 7:345–352, 1992.
20. Israelson H, Plemons JM: Dental implants, regenerative techniques, and periodontal plastic surgery to restore maxillary anterior esthetics. Int J Oral Maxillofac Impl 8:555–561, 1993.

21. Jemt T: Implant treatment in elderly patients. Int J Prosthodont 6:456–461, 1993.
22. Jemt T, Carlsson GE: Aspects of mastication with bridges on osseointegrated implants. Scand J Dent Res 94:66–71, 1986.
23. JOMI Current Issues Forum: Should there be a specialty of oral implantology? Int J Oral Maxillofac Impl 7:268–273, 1992.
24. Karlsson S, Carlsson GE: Oral motor function and phonetics in patients with implant-supported prostheses. *In* Naert I, van Steenberghe D, Worthington P (eds): Osseointegration in Oral Rehabilitation: An Introductory Textbook. London, Quintessence Publishing, 1993, p 123.
25. Klinge B: Implants in relation to natural teeth. J Clin Periodontol 18:482–487, 1991.
26. Kohner JS: Implant team: Problems and solutions with osseointegrated implants. Pract Peridont Aesthet Dent 4:27–32, 1992.
27. Koka S, Razzoog ME, Bloem TJ, Syed S: Microbial colonization of dental implants in partially edentulous subject. J Prosthet Dent 70:141–144, 1993.
28. Koumjian JH, Kerner J, Smith RA: Hygiene maintenance of dental implants. J Calif Dent Assoc 18:29–33, 1990.
29. Langer E, Sullivan DY: Osseointegration: Its impact on the interrelationship of periodontics and restorative dentistry: I. Int J Periodont Restor Dent 9:85–105, 1989.
30. Langer E, Sullivan DY: Osseointegration: Its impact on the interrelationship of periodontics and restorative dentistry: II. Int J Periodont Restor Dent 9:165–183, 1989.
31. Langer E, Sullivan DY: Osseointegration: Its impact on the interrelationship of periodontics and restorative dentistry: III. Int J Periodont Restor Dent 9:241–261, 1989.
32. Langer IS: Dental implants used for periodontal patients. J Am Dent Assoc 121:505–508, 1990.
33. Lundgren D: Prosthetic reconstruction of dentitions seriously compromised by periodontal disease. J Clin Periodontol 18:390–395, 1991.
34. Lundqvist S, Haraldson T, Lindblad P: Speech in connection with maxillary fixed prostheses on osseointegrated implants: A three-year follow-up study. Clin Oral Impl Res 3:176–180, 1992.
35. Meffert RM, Langer B, Fritz ME: Dental implants: A review. J Periodont 63:859–870, 1992.
36. Misch CE: Medical evolution of the implant candidate. J Oral Implantol 9:556–570, 1981.
37. Misch CE: Density of bone: Effect on treatment plans, surgical approach, healing and progressive bone loading. Int J Oral Implantol 6:456–461, 1993.
38. Oesterle IJ, Cronin RJ, Ranly DM: Maxillary implants and the growing patient. Int J Oral Maxillofac Impl 8:377–387, 1993.
39. Petersson A, Lindh C, Carlsson LE: Estimation of the possibility to treat the edentulous maxilla with osseointegrated implants. Swed Dent J 16:1–6, 1992.
40. Rudd KD: Making diagnostic casts is not a waste of time. J Prosthet Dent 20:98–100, 1968.
41. Saadoun AP, LeGall M, Kricheck M: Microbial infectious and occlusal overload: Causes of failure in osseointegrated implants. Pract Periodontics Aesthet Dent 5:11–20, 1993.
42. Steele J, Khan Z, Steiner N, Farman AG: Stent-aided imaging for osseointegrated implants. Oral Surg Oral Med Oral Pathol 70:243, 1990.
43. Sullivan DY, Sherwood RL: Considerations for successful single tooth implant restorations. J Esthetic Dent 5:118–124, 1993.
44. Tarantola GJ, Becker IM: Definitive diagnostic waxing with light-cured composite resin. J Prosthet Dent 70:315–319, 1993.
45. van Steenberghe D: Periodontal aspects of osseointegrated oral implants modum Brånemark. Dent Clin North Am 32:355–370, 1988.
46. Watson RM, Davis DM, Forman GH, Coward T: Considerations in design and fabrication of maxillary implant supported prostheses. Int J Prosthodont 4:232–239, 1991.
47. White SN, Lewis SG: Framework design for bone-anchored fixed prostheses. J Prosthet Dent 67:264–268, 1992.
48. White GE: Osseointegrated Dental Technology. London, Quintessence Books, 1993.

Study Questions

1. Which factors must be considered for the use of implants in dentate and edentulous patients?

2. In the clinical evaluation of a patient for whom implant prosthetic rehabilitation is contemplated, which factors must be considered?

3. What is the minimum number of implants required for the following cases:
   a. Tissue-supported implant overdentures.
   b. Implant-supported, implant-retained overdentures.
   c. Mandibular hybrid prosthesis.
   d. Edentulous spaces distal to the remaining dentition.
   e. Replacement of three teeth in a quadrant.

4. Which elements must be evaluated prior to determining the occlusal scheme for a particular patient?

5. What does a diagnostic wax-up accomplish?

CHAPTER 9

Implant Screw Mechanics

Edwin A. McGlumphy
Aydogan Huseyin
Revised by Luis R. Guerra

Screw Mechanics
Application to Dental Implants
Minimize Clinical Joint-separating Forces
Maximize Clinical Resistance to Joint
    Separation
References

Retrievability is the major advantage of screw-retained implant restorations. However, implant screw-loosening continues to be a frequently cited disadvantage of this technique in both the segmented and the nonsegmented implant restorations (Fig. 9–1).

Loosening of implant prosthetic components has been cited by multiple authors.[3, 7, 9, 12] The advantages of prosthesis retrievability afforded by screw retention, however, are multiple. Retrievability facilitates individual implant evaluation, soft tissue inspection, calculus debridement, and any necessary prosthesis modifications. Additionally, future treatment considerations can be made more easily and less expensively. Porcelain repair, changing the shade of a restoration, and creating additional access for oral hygiene become minor issues if the prosthesis can be easily unscrewed. Screw connections, however, need to remain tight during function to realize these advantages and to avoid the clinical problems.

Potential advantages of screw retention are lost when abutments are cemented into the implant. The disadvantages of cemented abutments are several. Improperly cemented components may not be safely retrieved without damage to the implant (Fig. 9–2). In the event of component fracture, a cemented abutment is likely to render the implant unusable. Also, removable abutments may be necessary for subgingival calculus removal and implant revision surgery.

Once the abutment is screwed into the implant, some clinicians prefer to cement the prosthesis in place. This may provide an optimal aesthetic result because screw access holes can be avoided. With this practice, abutment screws must stay tight because a loose screw cannot be easily accessed. A cemented prosthesis may require sectioning to tighten a loose abutment. Provisional cement could make retrieval possible without damage to the unit, but this is not always predictable.

Screw loosening seems to occur most often with single-tooth implant restorations[3] but has also been reported to occur in multiple-unit situations.[7, 12] Joining individual implants to natural

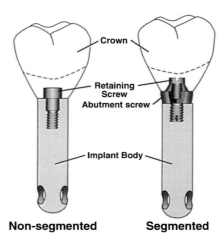

Figure 9–1. Types of implant restorations and component definitions as used in this chapter.

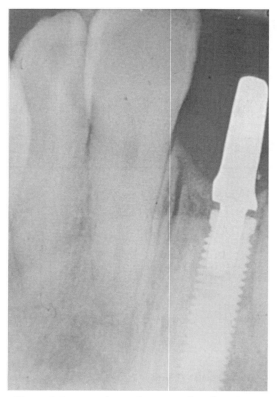

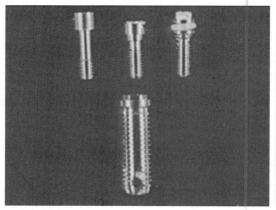

Figure 9–4. The gold single tooth *(left)*, titanium UCLA abutment screw *(center)*, and the standard abutment screw *(right)*, which are all designed to fit in the Brånemark implant system. Changing the shape of the screw head or the screw metal can have an effect on the antirotational properties.

changes (Fig. 9–4), and torque-controlling mechanisms (Fig. 9–5). All of these approaches have helped minimize the screw-loosening problem in some instances. None, however, has eliminated the problem completely. For example, in one single-tooth implant study, 65% of the screws loosened over a 3-year period, even though the crowns directly engaged the external implant hexagon.[3]

Figure 9–2. An inadequately cemented implant abutment that resulted in implant removal.

teeth or extending long cantilevers from the implant prosthesis may exacerbate any screw-loosening problem. Many products, components, and techniques have been suggested for maintaining a tight screw connection. These suggestions include antivibrational thread compounds, direct mechanical interlocks (Fig. 9–3), screw design

SCREW MECHANICS

When two parts are tightened together by a screw, this unit is called a *screw joint*. The screw loosens only if outside forces trying to separate the parts are greater than the force keeping them together (Fig. 9–6). Forces attempting to disengage the parts are called *joint separating forces*. The force keeping the parts together can be called the *clamping force*.

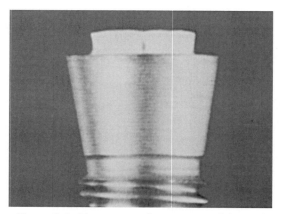

Figure 9–3. The most popular antirotational feature has been an external hex. Internal hexes have also been used effectively in this regard. Most implant systems on the market use a version of these methods.

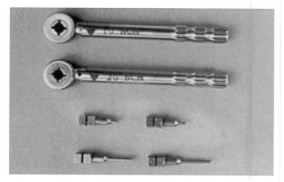

Figure 9–5. Mechanical torque wrenches, which can increase the amount of torque applied to an implant screw but also limit the maximum amount applied. (Courtesy of Implant Technologies Limited.)

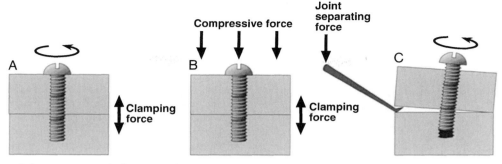

Figure 9–6. *A,* Torque applied to screw develops clamp load. *B,* Vertical forces maintain component connection. *C,* If a force separates the joint, the screw will loosen.

Joint-separating forces do not have to be eliminated to prevent screw loosening. The separating forces must only remain below the threshold of the established clamping force. If the joint does not open when a force is applied, the screw does not loosen (Fig. 9–7). Therefore there are two primary factors involved in keeping implant screws tight: (1) maximize clamping force, and (2) minimize joint-separating forces.

To achieve secure assemblies, screws should be tensioned to produce a clamping force greater than the external force tending to separate the joint. In the design of a rigid screw joint, the most important consideration from a functional standpoint is the initial clamping force developed by tightening the screw. Joint strength is affected more by clamp force than by tensile strength of the screws. Clamp load is usually proportional to tightening torque.

Torque is a convenient, measurable means of developing desired tension. Too small a torque may allow separation of the joint and result in screw fatigue failure or loosening. Too large a torque may cause failure of the screw or stripping of the screw threads. Applied torque develops a force within the screw called *preload.* Preload is the initial load in tension on the screw.[2] This tensile force on the screw develops a compressive clamping force between the parts. Therefore the preload of the screw is equal in magnitude to the clamping force. Preload is determined by the following factors:

1. Applied torque
2. Screw alloy
3. Screw head design
4. Abutment alloy
5. Abutment surface
6. Lubricant

In general, the more torque applied, the more preload generated. Two factors limit the amount of torque that may be applied. The mechanical limit is the strength of the screw. The amount of torque is also limited by how it is applied. Screwdrivers with larger handles can generally apply more torque than those with small handles. A wrench can be used if larger torques are needed (Fig. 9–8).

In theory, the maximum preload is developed just before torsional fracture of the screw occurs. Therefore, to increase preload and minimize the risk of screw fracture during use, a safety margin is established. Simplistically, optimum tightening torques can be calculated using 75% of the ulti-

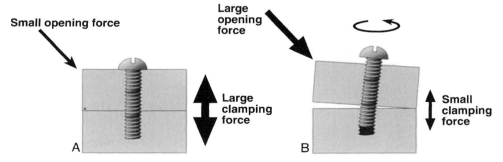

Figure 9–7. *A,* Separating force < clamping force = stable connection. *B,* Separating force > clamping force = loose screw.

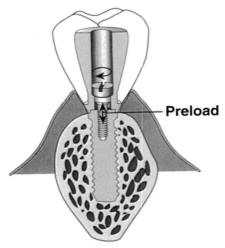

Figure 9–8. Torque applied to the implant screw develops the preload.

mate torque to failure values.[11] In other words, the optimal torque value can be calculated by tightening a screw until it fails; 75% of this value is the optimum torque to place on the screw. In this manner, a significant clamping force can be developed with minimum risk of screw fracture.

In industry, bigger screws are made to allow more torque to be applied. In this way, clamping force can be developed to resist nearly any joint-separating force. It is not that easy in the mouth. The size of the screws is limited by tooth size. The strength of the bone implant interface is the biologic limit of applied torque. If these engineering principles are applied to dental implants within the limitations of the oral cavity, clinical decision making and problem solving should be improved.

APPLICATION TO DENTAL IMPLANTS

The clinical reality is that implant restorations are continually subjected to joint-separating forces. These forces include:

Excursive contacts
Off-axis centric contacts
Angled abutments
Wide occlusal table
Interproximal contacts
Cantilever contacts
Nonpassive framework

MINIMIZE CLINICAL JOINT–SEPARATING FORCES

The joint-separating forces can be greatly influenced by the moment arm through which the force is applied. Excessive implant angles or prosthesis cantilevers can rapidly magnify the centric contacts not aligned with the long axis of the implant and may increase the joint-separating moment arm. Precision implant placement and treatment planning are the first crucial step in maintaining tight implant screws (Fig. 9–9).

Occlusion plays a primary role in keeping implant screws tight. Contacts in lateral excursions act as separating forces and should be avoided whenever possible. Remember, however, that light lateral forces below the threshold of the clamping force do not cause screw loosening. Therefore, minimal lateral guiding forces might be placed on *anterior* implant restorations without adverse consequences.

The most commonly overlooked separating forces are off-axis centric contacts. Normal centric contacts on molar cusp tips may exceed the clamping force threshold, especially if the general occlusal force generated by the patient is large (Fig. 9–10). This theory may explain the high incidence of screw loosening in single-implant molars. Molar implant screws should stay tight if the centric contacts can be directed in the long axis of the screw and excursive contacts eliminated. Heavy interproximal contacts may

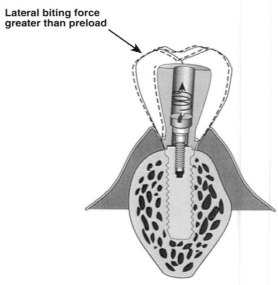

Lateral biting force greater than preload

Figure 9–9. If a lateral joint-separating force is applied to the crown that exceeds the preload, the screw will loosen.

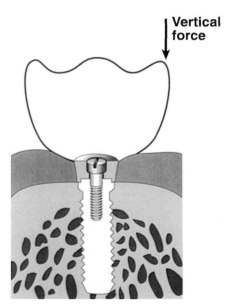

Figure 9–10. Centric contacts on a molar implant crown generate a large moment arm on implant screw.

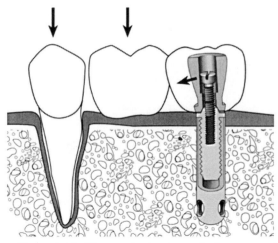

Figure 9–11. When an implant is attached to a natural tooth, the forces are concentrated on the implant screws.

also exert excessive lateral force on an implant crown, resulting in screw loosening.

Attaching implants to natural teeth with a fixed partial denture can commonly lead to loose screws in the implant abutment. The problem occurs because of mobility differences between the two types of abutments. The implant is immobile relative to the natural tooth, which can move within the limits of its periodontal ligament. Occlusal forces on the natural tooth can have a cantilever effect on the implant, generating a maximum resultant load up to two times the applied force. Much of this cantilever force is concentrated at the joint between the implant crown and its abutment screw (Fig. 9–11). It should not be surprising that screws loosen in this clinical situation.

Likewise, screw-loosening incidents increase if a nonpassive framework is forced to fit by tightening screws. The original framework applies joint-separating forces to the system because it attempts to return to its original position (Fig. 9–12). All nonpassive frameworks should be sectioned and soldered to ensure passive fit.

MAXIMIZE CLINICAL RESISTANCE TO JOINT SEPARATION

One possible advantage of the antirotational features used in dental implants is the resistance

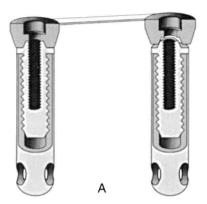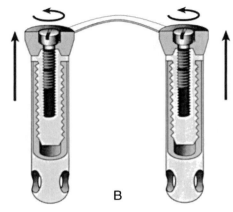

Figure 9–12. *A*, Implant framework with a nonpassive fit. *B*, If the screw is tightened to bend the framework, joint separating forces are applied, which may result in screw loosening.

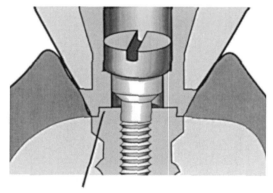

Figure 9–13. Cross-sectional view of the implant crown engaging the vertical walls of the hexagon.

they provide to joint-separating forces (Figs. 9–13 and 9–14). The possibility that vertical walls engage between the hexagon and the crown to resist applied force may explain the partial solution that these devices provide.[10] This occurrence would also explain why shorter hexes can allow some screws to loosen under heavy loads.

One of the simplest methods to ensure screw loosening is to make sure screws are tight.[2] The novice implant clinician often undertightens the implant component. One study suggests that the average torque placed with a screwdriver is only 11 Newton-cm (N-cm).[1] Most titanium components on the market can easily be tightened to twice that amount without consequences.[5] For torque levels greater than 20 N-cm, a torque wrench is usually required. In reality, the optimum torque values for many of the larger-diameter implant screws exceed the generally accepted limits of the bone-implant interface.[6] Although definitive torque removal values for the different implants have not been established in humans, animal studies suggest that no greater than 30 to

35 N-cm of torque should be applied to the bone-implant interface.[4, 8, 10] In fact, the safest method of applying higher torque values intraorally is to use a countertorque mechanism. If countertorque is applied to the abutment as the screw is tightened, the net force at the bone interface should be zero. Currently, torque levels in the 20- to 30-N-cm range are thought to provide significant preload without risk to the bone interface.

The major clinical procedures necessary for tight implant screws are summarized as follows:

1. Implants placed parallel to the forces of occlusion
2. Restorations designed to minimize cantilever lengths
3. Occlusion adjusted to direct forces in the long axis of the implant
4. Antirotational feature engaged for single teeth
5. Components tightened with 20–30 N-cm of torque (unless specified by manufacturer)

If screw loosening occurs, all potential contributing causes should be evaluated. The clinician should pay particular attention to occlusal forces oblique to the implant long axis. Interproximal contacts and framework fit should also be evaluated. Implant screws should not be maximally tightened until joint-separating forces are controlled.

Caution: We cannot focus only on eliminating loose screws; we must also eliminate the cause of screw loosening.

The danger for the patient lies in the fact that if the screws do not loosen, excessive forces may be directed to more deleterious locations in the system. Proper implant placement, framework fit, and occlusal adjustment become even more important as screw joints improve. If these fundamentals are not addressed, more stable screw connections could result in fractured implant bodies or crestal bone loss. Loose screws should be seen as a clinical symptom that may indicate that the forces are not appropriately balanced on a particular implant restoration.

References

1. Dellinges MA, Tebrock OC: A measurement of torque values obtained with hand-held drivers in a simulated clinical setting. J Prosthodont 2:212–214, 1993.
2. Griffith HT: Suggested tightening torques for structural

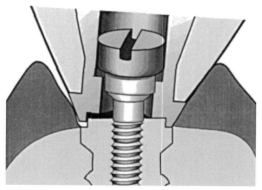

Figure 9–14. The antirotational hexagon may work by providing resistance form against joint-separating forces.

bolts. Fastener Technology/February 1987. *In* Torque Tensioning: A Ten Part Compilation. Fastener Technology, Stow, Ohio.

3. Jemt T, Lacey WR, Harris D, et al: Osseointegrated implants for single tooth replacement: A 1-year report from a multicenter prospective study. Int J Oral Maxillofac Impl 6:29, 1991.
4. Johansson C, Albrektsson T: Integration of screw implants in the rabbit. A 1-year follow-up of removal torque of titanium implants. Int J Oral Maxillofac Impl 2:69–75, 1987.
5. McGlumphy EA, Elfers CL, Mendel DA: Torsional ductile fracture of implant coronal screws. J Dent Res 71:114, 1992.
6. McGlumphy EA, Elfers CL, Mendel DA: Optimum torque values for implant abutment screws. J Dent Res 72:191, 1993.
7. Quirynen NI, van Streenberghe D, Darius P: A six year prosthodontic study of 509 consecutively inserted implants for the treatment of partial edentulism. J Prosthet Dent 67:236–245, 1992.
8. Sennerby L, Thomsen P, Ericson L: A morphometric and biomechanic comparison of titanium implants inserted in rabbit cortical and cancellous bone. Int J Oral Maxillofac Impl 7:62–71, 1992.
9. Sones AD: Complications with osseointegrated implants. J Prosthet Dent 62:581–585, 1989.
10. Tjellstrom A, Jacobsson M, Albrektsson T: Removal torque of osseointegrated craniofacial implants: A clinical study. Int J Oral Maxillofac Impl 3:287–289, 1988.
11. Trilling J: Torque data for socket-head cap screws. Fastener Technology Feb: 3–4, 1988.
12. Zarb G, Schmitt A: The longitudinal clinical effectiveness of osseointegrated dental implants: The Toronto Study: III: Problems and complications encountered. J Prosthet Dent 64:185–194, 1990.

Study Questions

1. List the advantages of screw-retained implant restorations.

2. Preload is determined by which factors?

3. Name the joint-separating forces on dental implants.

4. Which major clinical procedures are necessary for tight implant screws?

CHAPTER *10*

Implant Overdentures

Arturo J. Mendez
Luis R. Guerra
Revised by Luis R. Guerra

Tissue-Borne Overdentures
    Multiple Implants
    Splinting
Implant-Borne Overdentures
Attachments
Fabrication of Implant Overdentures
    Impression Techniques

Double Impression Technique
Single Impression Technique
    Jaw Relation Records
    Occlusion
References

More than 41% of senior citizens in the United States are edentulous.[10, 26] Among this large number of individuals, many wear complete dentures and rely on the soft and hard tissues of the residual alveolar ridge for support, retention, and stability of their prostheses. These patients face the inevitable prospect of further bone resorption with decreasing retention and stability of their dentures and consequential discomfort.

A treatment alternative that has been beneficial to patients who still preserve a small number of healthy natural teeth is an overdenture. Overdentures must meet all the requirements of complete dentures except that they rely on the remaining dental structures to provide additional support, stability, and retention.

Brewer and Morrow[7] have advocated the use of overdentures in patients with insufficient dentition to support either fixed or removable partial prostheses. It has been noted that overdentures can be fabricated over a single remaining tooth or a full complement of teeth.[7] The location and the condition of the remaining dentition are key in the final determination as to the selection of the type of overdenture fabricated. The advantages given for the use of overdentures over natural teeth include (1) retained proprioception by means of the periodontal ligament, (2) reduced loading of the endodontically treated tooth roots, (3) reduced loading of the residual alveolar ridge, (4) increase in the occlusal forces generated, (5) increased retention and stability of the prosthesis, (6) preservation of the residual alveolar bone, and (7) simplification of oral hygiene

procedures. Overdentures have been used successfully for a number of years.

Guerra et al[11] have pointed out that although new techniques and materials have aided greatly in the caring for edentulous patients with conventional complete dentures, these have not resulted in long-term preservation of the residual alveolar ridges or increased long-term retention and stability of the removable prostheses used. With the advent of dental implants, the benefits and advantages of using an overdenture have become a reality for edentulous patients. This significant new technique, with a reported overall success rate of greater than 97%,[24, 38] has been demonstrated to preserve the mandibular residual alveolar ridge[35] and to increase the retention and stability of the removable prosthesis.[16] Endosseous cylindrical implants have proved to be useful and effective for the rehabilitation of atrophic mandibles of 10 mm or less in anterior height.[33] The overall success rate of 94% on these functionally and aesthetically compromised patients makes this a viable treatment modality. Studies have shown that the chewing efficiency in subjects with implant overdentures improves significantly compared with the complete denture patients.[12] Bone loss around mandibular implants supporting overdentures has been reported to be minimal.[25] The change in marginal bone height does not seem to correlate with parameters such as the occlusion and articulation pattern, the presence or absence of a soft liner around the abutments, and the magnitude of the interabutment distance.[25]

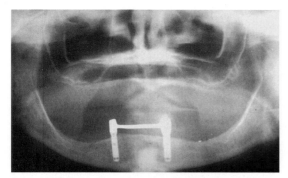

Figure 10–1. Radiograph of two IMZ endosseous implants in the mandible with bar assembly.

On the maxillary arch, however, the criteria for implant patient selection must be stringent. Studies indicate that compared with patients with more bone, patients with severely resorbed edentulous maxillae with overdentures supported by osseointegrated implants showed a lower success rate for the individual implants (84%) as well as for the prostheses (92.3%).[14] Patients who have suffered congenital or postsurgical defects can be helped functionally and aesthetically with overdentures supported by dental implants.[13]

There are basically two types of implant overdentures. The first type can be classified as being implant retained and tissue borne, the second type as being implant retained and implant borne.[1] An implant-retained, tissue-borne overdenture relies primarily on the residual alveolar ridge for support. The implants do provide support in the area of the arch in which they are placed, but this is generally limited by the number of implants used. An implant-retained, implant-supported overdenture does not rely on tissue support. Loading of the denture results in the implants bearing the full load of the occlusion. The periphery of the dentures must rest on soft tissue to prevent debris from accumulating beneath the denture. Retention is provided by the implants, and retention provided by negative air pressure is not required.

The use of implants to support overdentures has been advocated by many,[8, 9, 17, 31, 37] with the following advantages:[23] (1) higher patient acceptance of prosthesis, (2) less trauma to the underlying tissues by the prosthesis, (3) improved retention and stability of the dentures, (4) improved support of facial soft tissues and thus improved aesthetics, (5) preservation of the remaining alveolar bone, and (6) improved oral function (improved occlusion owing to the increased stability of the denture). The disadvantages of implant overdentures include (1) increased hygiene requirements to prevent peri-implantitis, (2) use of attachments to retain the denture to the implants, (3) increased cost, and (4) possible loss of the implants.

A well-founded rationale exists for recommending to the patient the use of implant overdentures.[19] The experience gained from the use of conventional overdentures includes the amount of support required, the location of the support structures in the arch, and the types of attachments that can be used. The difference between the attachment of a tooth to bone and an implant to bone explains the primary difference between conventional overdentures and implant overdentures. This difference influences the design of the support system. An example is the routine use of cantilever support for an implant overdenture versus a conventional overdenture. If this is kept in mind, it should facilitate the transition from the fabrication of conventional overdentures to implant overdentures.

A variety of implant systems have been used in supporting overdentures. These include endosseous (Figs. 10–1 and 10–2),[24] transosseous (Fig. 10–3),[3, 5, 27, 29, 30] and subperiosteal (Figs. 10–4 and 10–5)[4, 34, 39] implants. Root form endosseous implants are the type of implants most frequently used in implant overdentures at present, although there are indications for the use of the other types in specific cases. Modern endosseous implants offer the practitioner a predictable, simple, less costly alternative. In patients with pencil-thin mandibles, onlaying bone graft-

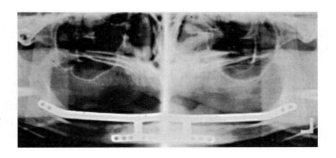

Figure 10–2. Panoramic radiograph of an endosseous ramus frame implant.

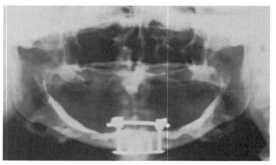

Figure 10–3. One of various designs of the staple implant that corresponds to the transosseous group of implants. This implant has been used to support a mandibular overdenture.

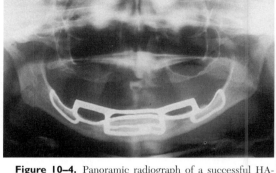

Figure 10–4. Panoramic radiograph of a successful HA-coated subperiosteal implant.

ing techniques have been used. In this situation, a screw form implant can be used to secure the graft to the underlying bone. A period of 6 to 9 months of healing is required as a minimum before denture fabrication. This delay may seem a contraindication to this type of treatment, but most patients accept this limitation if made aware of the long-term benefits.

In the severely resorbed mandible or maxilla, in which there is insufficient bone to support endosseous implants, the use of a subperiosteal or transosseous implant may be indicated with or without bone grafting to augment the bone present.

Considerations that enter into the selection of one type of implant overdenture over another include

1. The patient's desires
2. The availability, location, and quality of bone in the arch
3. The opposing occlusion
4. The amount of interarch distance
5. The patient's manual dexterity
6. The patient's ability to understand the benefits of the treatment
7. The financial resources available

TISSUE-BORNE OVERDENTURES

The tissue-borne overdenture is attached to implants generally placed in the anterior portion of the maxillary or mandibular arch. Two implants are the minimum number required for this type of restoration. In the mandible, a commonly used type of attachment is the bar and clip (Figs. 10–6 and 10–7). This attachment not only allows for support and retention of the den-

ture in the anterior area by the implants, but also allows for stress breaking when the posterior portion of the denture is loaded. For the bar and clip to provide the required stress breaking, the area of the bar to which the clip attaches must be located in the symphysis, be in a straight line so it is parallel to the mandibular hinge axis,[18, 24] and be perpendicular to the midsagittal plane. This is often impossible to accomplish owing to space limitations when more than two implants are used. A bar length of 12 to 15 mm is desirable in a mandibular tissue-borne overdenture to provide adequate retention and prevent distortion of the clip (Fig. 10–8). Care must be taken to avoid contact of the superstructure with the impression surface of the denture in any area other than the clip. A new axis of rotation between the denture and the superstructure occurs if the impression surface of the prosthesis contacts the superstructure distal to the clip. Should this occur, occlusal loading of the posterior dentition results in the clip being lifted from the bar. This constant lifting of the clip, which results in

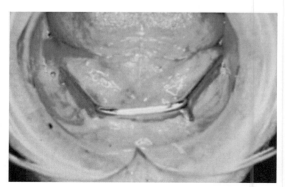

Figure 10–5. Clinical view of a subperiosteal implant. The overdenture made for this type of implant must be totally implant supported.

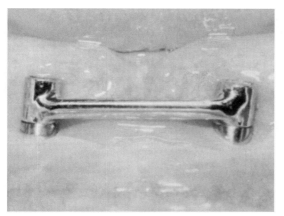

Figure 10–6. A high noble alloy bar and copings constitute the implant superstructure for a mandibular tissue–borne overdenture.

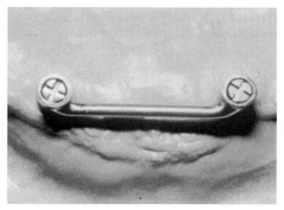

Figure 10–8. The length of the bar should be 12 to 15 mm to provide an adequate amount of retention. Note the bar placement over the crest of the residual alveolar ridge.

a rotational extraction force on the implants, must be avoided.

In the maxilla, bars and clips are not generally used in tissue-borne overdentures. These attachments, if used, prevent the denture from fully seating onto the tissues in the area where the implants are placed. This impedes the achievement of a seal around the periphery of the denture with resultant loss of retention of the denture.

Multiple Implants

Patients with a tapered mandibular arch are not considered good candidates for a two-implant bar and clip system[2] because the bar would encroach on the tongue space. In these patients, a

minimum of four implants is required if a connecting bar is to be used in combination with other types of attachments.

The use of more than two implants makes the selection of the type of attachment to be used more complex (Fig. 10–9). It must be kept in mind that although three, four, or more implants are being used, the prosthesis remains primarily a tissue-borne restoration. Therefore, stress breaking must be incorporated into the design, or overloading of the implants may result. The use of bar and clip types of attachments is generally contraindicated. Other types of attachments are available for use when more than two implants are placed. Should the implants be splinted together, the attachments are generally placed in an area distal to the implants. There are stress-breaking attachments of various designs (Table 10–1). The type of attachment se-

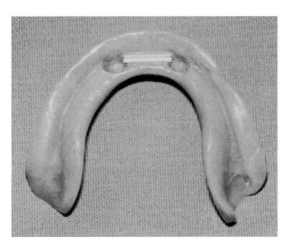

Figure 10–7. The retentive clip in the mandibular overdenture attaches to the bar illustrated in Figure 10–6.

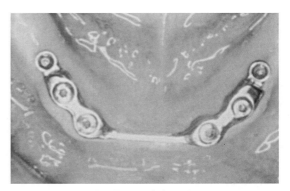

Figure 10–9. The design of this superstructure consists of a connecting bar and two ERA attachments on the distal ends. All four implants are splinted, but no retentive clip is used. The bar provides anterior support; the stress-breaking-type ERA attachments provide retention.

Table 10–1. Attachments for Tissue-Borne Implant Overdentures

Name	Characteristics	Distributor
Bar and Clip Systems		
Dolder Bar System	Elliptical gold bar/gold sleeve	Attachments Intl Inc (San Mateo, CA), APM-Sterngold (Attleboro, MA)
CM Bar and Rider	Round gold bar/gold rider	Attachments Intl Inc
CM Bar and Ackerman Clip	Round gold bar/gold rider	Attachments Intl Inc
Hader Bar System	Round with skirt plastic castable bar/plastic clip	Attachments Intl Inc, Lifecore Biomedical Inc (Chaska, MN), APM-Sterngold
EDS Bar System	Round with short skirt plastic castable bar/plastic clip	Attachments Intl Inc
CBS Bar and CM rider	I, oval, round, EDS plastic castable bar/gold rider	Attachments Intl Inc
UMA Bar System	Round, oval, EDS plastic castable bar/gold rider	Attachments Intl Inc
IMZ Bar and Clip	Round gold or plastic castable bar/plastic clip	Interpore Intl (Irvine, CA)
Machined Gold Clip System	Round precious bar/gold clip	Implant Innovations Inc (West Palm Beach, FL)
Plastic Castable System	Round or oval plastic castable bar/gold rider	Implant Innovations Inc
Hader Clip System	Round, oval, or round with skirt plastic castable bar/plastic clip	Implant innovations Inc
Overdenture Bar	Round gold plastic castable bar/ gold clip	Nobelpharma (Chicago, IL)
Round Bar and Rider	Round precious bar/metal rider	APM-Sterngold
Stud Attachments		
ERA Implant Abutment	Titanium female abutment/ plastic male	APM-Sterngold
ERA Overdenture	Plastic castable female/plastic male	APM-Sterngold
Ball Overdenture	Titanium spherical abutment	Calcitek Inc (Carlsbad, CA), Steri-Oss Inc (Anaheim, CA)
Nobelpharma Ball	Titanium male abutment/elastic ring female	Nobelpharma
Straight Ball Insert	Titanium male abutment/plastic female	Dentsply Intl Inc (York, PA)
O-Ring	Titanium male abutment/elastic ring female	Calcitek Inc, Steri-Oss Inc, Attachments Intl Inc, Implant Innovations Inc, Lifecore Biomedical Inc
O-Ring Castable and ORS-DE Plus	Plastic castable male/elastic ring female	Attachments Intl Inc, Implant Innovations, Lifecore Biomedical Inc
Dal-Ro	Titanium male abutment/metal female	Implant Innovations Inc
Dal-Ro Castable	Plastic castable male/metal female	Implant Innovations Inc
Dalla Bona Overdenture	Titanium male abutment/ titanium alloy or gold female	Lifecore Biomedical Inc, Attachments Intl Inc
Dalla Bona	Gold or plastic castable male/ gold, titanium, or plastic castable female	Attachments Int, APM-Sterngold
Swiss Anchor	Metal male/precious alloy and plastic female	Attachments Intl Inc
Dalbo	Gold female/high heat cast to ceramic alloy male	Attachments Intl Inc, APM-Sterngold
Plunger Type Attachments		
ASC-52	Stainless steel male/plantium iridium or plastic female	Attachments Intl Inc
Combination Bar Attachments		
Dolder Bar-ERA		
Dolder Bar-Swiss Anchor		
CBS Bar-O-Ring		
IMZ Bar-ERA		
IMA Bar-O-Ring		

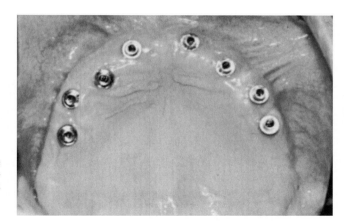

Figure 10–10. Eight maxillary implants have been strategically located to receive an implant-borne overdenture. Note the favorable distribution of the implants and interabutment distances.

lected depends on the location and number of implants used.

Splinting

Splinting of the implants deserves careful consideration. It has generally been believed[6, 32] that by splinting the implants, the lateral and torquing forces on the individual implants are reduced. Research indicates that attachments placed directly on the implant bodies without splinting to the adjacent implants may not place as much detrimental force on the implants as previously thought.[22] Although there is limited evidence to support either splinting or not splinting of the implants, it would seem prudent to join implants that are short (less than 10 mm) or implants placed in relatively poor bone (class III or IV).

IMPLANT-BORNE OVERDENTURES

This type of overdenture relies on the implants to bear the full occlusal loading. A properly de-signed implant-borne overdenture can satisfy the patient's needs in aesthetics, phonetics, and comfort and should facilitate oral hygiene measures. This prosthesis requires the use of a sufficient number of implants to accommodate the load placed on the prosthesis (Figs. 10–10 through 10–12). Because the implants carry all of the occlusal loading, the same rules are followed as in the fabrication of hybrid dentures (see Chapter 11). The minimum number of implants required is four in the mandible and six to eight in the maxilla. This minimum number reflects the differences in the quality and quantity of bone found in the two arches. It is important to avoid cantilevers on the maxillary arch. This can be accomplished by the symmetric placement of implants in the tuberosity, canine, and incisor regions. A removable denture supported by a precision milled bar completes the prosthetic design.[20]

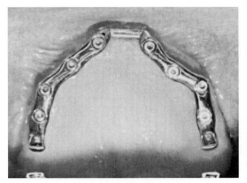

Figure 10–11. Maxillary slant-lock metal superstructure for an implant-borne overdenture.

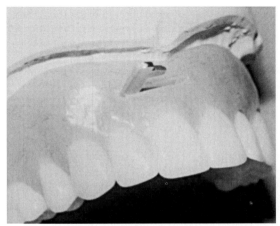

Figure 10–12. A small latch is part of the slant-lock–type overdenture. When closed, the latch engages underneath the anterior portion of the superstructure, providing excellent retention.

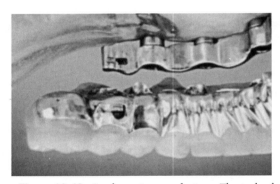

Figure 10–13. Spark erosion overdenture. The technology employed in fabrication of this type of prosthesis results in a precise fit of the components. This results in a rigid union between the denture and the superstructure. Small lingual latches in the denture engage the receptacles in the superstructure.

The firmer the connection of the prosthesis to the superstructure on the implants, the more precise the tooth contacts can be in centric and eccentric occlusion because the movement encountered in tissue-borne overdentures is not a factor. Bars and clips are the most popular methods of attaching the prosthesis to the implants. It is necessary, therefore, to space the implants to allow for the placement of clips of adequate length. Multiple clips of 5 to 6 mm are adequate to retain an implant-supported overdenture.

To provide a firm union of the prosthesis to the superstructure, a variety of attachments have been developed. Included in this group are the slant-lock, latch types, milled bars, and the spark erosion attachments (Fig. 10–13). Other attachments, such as the ERA, Swiss anchor, and O-ring attachments, that have been used do not provide the security or rigidity of the previously mentioned attachments. They rely on the attachment for retention and the resting of the prosthesis on the superstructure for support and stability.

Although the patient's desires are an important determinant in the consideration of the type of attachment to use for a particular case, an overriding consideration is the amount of interocclusal space available. The occlusal plane may be altered somewhat to accommodate an attachment, by increasing the distance between the crest of the ridge and the occlusal plane. If this results in an unaesthetic effect or a mechanical disharmony, however, it may be necessary to use an alternate attachment.

In general, the more firm the connection of the prosthesis to the superstructure, the more difficult the attachment is to manage by the patient. Therefore, careful consideration must be given to the patient's ability to manipulate the attachment chosen. Patients with debilitating diseases such as arthritides or who have suffered traumatic injuries to the hands must be evaluated as to their ability to engage and disengage the retentive devices used.

Although the cementing of superstructures to abutments may be appealing from a simplicity point of view, this is not recommended by the authors. A cementable-type superstructure can increase the difficulty of achieving the level of hygiene required for long-term maintenance. A superstructure that is retrievable can be removed for evaluation or treatment of the individual implants.

ATTACHMENTS

A variety of attachments are available for use with implant overdentures (see Table 10–1; Table 10–2). The selection of a specific attachment depend on various factors: (1) the type of overdenture to be fabricated, (2) the relative importance of stability and retention, (3) the condition of the residual alveolar ridges, (4) the length of the implants used, (5) the aesthetic requirements, (6) the dexterity of the patient in being able to insert and remove the prosthesis, (7) the psychosocial needs of the patient, and (8) the position of the implants within the ridge.

The characteristics of the attachments for a tissue-supported overdenture are quite different from those required for an implant-borne overdenture. The tissue-supported overdenture relies primarily on the residual alveolar ridge for support, although the implants do provide support when loading is directed over them. Therefore the prosthesis must be able to rotate around the

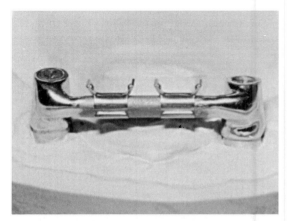

Figure 10–14. The attachment selected for a tissue-borne overdenture must allow for stress breaking. This bar assembly consists of a cast CBS bar and two CM riders, which can rotate around the bar.

Table 10–2. Attachments for Implant-Borne Overdentures

Name	Characteristics	Distributor
Bar and Clip Systems		
Dolder Bar System	Elliptical gold bar/gold sleeve	Attachments Int Inc (San Mateo, CA), APM-Sterngold (Attleboro, MA)
CM Bar and Rider	Round gold bar/gold rider	Attachments Intl Inc
CM Bar and Ackerman Clip	Round gold bar/gold rider	Attachments Intl Inc
Hader Bar System	Round with skirt plastic castable bar/plastic clip	Attachments Intl Inc, Lifecore Biomedical Inc (Chaska, MN), APM-Sterngold
EDS Bar System	Round with short skirt plastic castable bar/plastic clip	Attachments Intl Inc
CBS Bar and CM Rider	I, oval, round, EDS plastic castable bar/gold rider	Attachments Intl Inc
UMA Bar System	Round, oval, EDS plastic castable bar/gold rider	Attachments Intl Inc
Machined Gold Clip System	Round precious bar/gold clip	Implant Innovations Inc (West Palm Beach, FL)
Plastic Castable System	Round or oval plastic castable bar/gold rider	Implant Innovations Inc
Hader Clip System	Round, oval, or round with skirt plastic castable bar/plastic clip	Implant Innovations Inc
Overdenture Bar	Round gold or plastic castable bar/gold clip	Nobelpharma (Chicago, IL)
Round Bar and Rider	Round precious bar/metal rider	APM-Sterngold
Combination Bar Attachments		
Dolder Bar-ERA		
Dolder Bar-Swiss Anchor		
CBS Bar-O-Ring		
IMZ Bar-ERA		
IMA Bar-O-Ring		
Special Designs		
Slant-Lock	Metal connecting bars/metal latch	
Milled Bars	Metal precision type framework/ metal precision sleeves	
Spark-Erosion	Metal high precision type framework/metal latches	

implant attachment to settle onto the resilient tissues of the residual alveolar ridge. The bar and clip systems, which are probably the most widely used attachments for tissue-supported overdentures, provide a means of accomplishing this goal (Fig. 10–14). One must be careful to ensure that the bar is placed so the prosthesis can freely rotate in an anteroposterior direction. As explained earlier in this chapter, the bar must be placed so that it lies perpendicular to the midsagittal plane and parallel to the axis of rotation of the mandible.[18, 24] This ensures that there will be no torquing forces over the implants. The clips used depend on the cross-sectional shape of the bar. A round bar requires the use of a clip that is free to rotate around the bar. A Dolder bar, which is elliptic in cross section, must be used with the corresponding clip to accommodate the shape of the bar. The Dolder bar has the advantage of providing some direct-indirect retention by preventing the lifting of the distal portion of the prosthesis away from the tissues. This may

be minimal and is related to the length of the working portion of the bar. A bar and clip system should include a bar that is of sufficient length to provide the necessary retention and prevent distortion of the clip, as might occur when a denture with a short clip is seated over the bar.

Other attachments that can be used to control the torquing forces on the implants include plunger types of attachments such as the ASC-52 (Fig. 10–15). Stud attachments properly selected are also used. The Swiss anchor (Fig. 10–16) and O-ring (Fig. 10–17) attachments have been successfully used. Many of the implant systems provide abutments with stud-type attachments incorporated in their design (Figs. 10–18 through 10–21). These abutments are available with gingival cuffs of various lengths.

The requirements for attachments used for an implant-supported overdenture do not include the need for stress breaking. On this type of prosthesis, the purpose of the attachment is to fix the denture to the implants. This can be

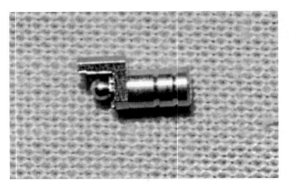

Figure 10–15. This ASC-52 attachment allows hinge rotation in every direction.

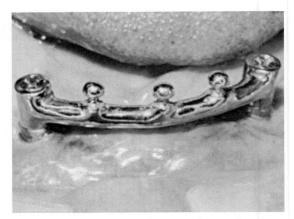

Figure 10–17. O-ring stud-type attachments have been cast with a round bar to serve as a means of retention for a mandibular tissue-borne overdenture.

accomplished with bar and clip types of attachments without regard to the shape of the bar. The ERA attachment is a versatile attachment for use with both tissue-borne and implant-borne overdentures (Figs. 10–22 and 10–23). More sophisticated attachments include the slant-lock and the spark erosion types of attachments.[28]

Generally the more complicated the attachment, the more difficult to repair and maintain. The patient's manual dexterity should also be a prime concern. As explained earlier, some patients with debilitating conditions may not be able to manage a more sophisticated attachment. Another consideration is the type of framework used with the attachment and its influence on the ability of the patient to maintain the health of the implants and the tissues surrounding them.

FABRICATION OF IMPLANT OVERDENTURES

The armamentarium needed to fabricate an implant overdenture varies, depending on the

implant system and the attachments used. In general, however, the equipment, instruments, and supplies required are few and simple.

Ten to fourteen days after the implants have been uncovered, the soft tissues are evaluated. If the tissues have healed normally, the healing cuffs are removed and the thickness of the soft tissues around the implant opening is measured with a plastic periodontal probe. These measurements are used for the abutment selection. The height of the abutment's cuff is selected based on the thickness of the soft tissue. The shoulder of the abutment must be slightly supragingival (0.5 to 1.0 mm).

Impression Techniques

Impression techniques for use in implant overdentures should be considered in light of the fact

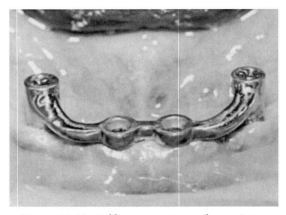

Figure 10–16. Gold superstructure with two Swiss-anchor female attachments.

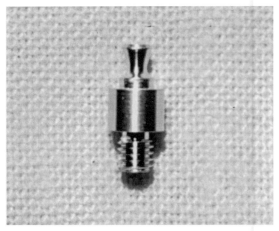

Figure 10–18. This abutment can be screwed directly into the implant body to engage an elastic O-ring in the overdenture.

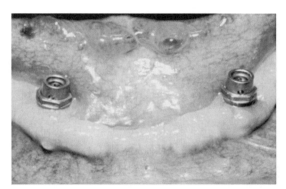

Figure 10–19. ERA female attachments secured to two osseointegrated implants.

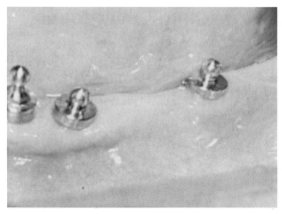

Figure 10–21. In a distal extension removable partial overdenture, two Dalla-bona attachments and one O-ring implant attachment are used. The Dalla-bona attachments provide retention and support, and the O-ring in a nonparallel implant provides complementary retention.

that the material must be accurate to reproduce the exact location of the implants or abutments and be of a viscosity that does not distort the soft tissues. Also the impression material should be one that is stiff enough to retain the implant or abutment analog during the pouring procedures. The use of a two-component impression material has proved beneficial in accomplishing this task. The heavy putty-like material provides the necessary stiffness, and the light-bodied material accurately reproduces the area around the transfer components and the soft tissues. The addition-type polysiloxane materials possess the qualities required. High-viscosity and low-viscosity polyether materials are also recommended.

DOUBLE IMPRESSION TECHNIQUE

There are several methods for making impressions to obtain a master cast for the fabrication

of overdentures. The same impression techniques can be used whether the final prosthesis will be a tissue-borne or implant-borne overdenture, but the extension of the tray is more critical on the former. The base of the tissue-borne overdenture should be as large as possible within the functional and anatomic limitations to optimize the distribution of occlusal forces.[37]

In one technique, the metal superstructure is first constructed and then secured in position intraorally and a final impression is made. The superstructure is reproduced in stone in the master cast. This requires two impressions: one that transfers the position of either the abutments or the implants to a working cast and a final impression for the fabrication of the prosthesis itself.

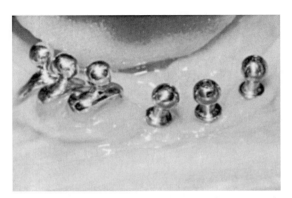

Figure 10–20. Three ball implant overdenture attachments are used on this patient in conjunction with three post and copings over natural teeth. Note the strategic location of the implants to provide optimum retention and stability to the prosthesis.

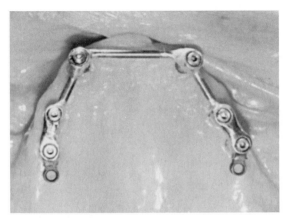

Figure 10–22. Two female ERA attachments have been incorporated on the distal end of the maxillary superstructure. The resiliency of the corresponding male attachments provides stress-breaking action.

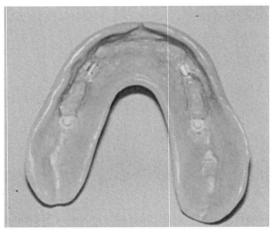

Figure 10–23. Maxillary overdenture with two small CM riders anteriorly and two ERA attachments posteriorly. Because rotation around the ERA attachments would cause lifting of the CM riders, they are not retentive but serve as anterior stops.

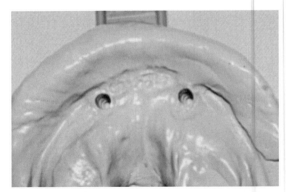

Figure 10–25. This impression exhibits intimate adaptation of the impression material to the transfer copings.

The first impression is obtained by placing transfer copings on the abutments or impression posts on the implants themselves (Fig. 10–24).

In the closed tray technique, the implant system provides for removal of the impression without removal of retaining screws and a conventional stock tray can be used. The impression material used is a vinyl polysiloxane, and both the low-viscosity and putty materials are utilized. The tray is loaded with the putty material that is lined with the light-bodied material; simultaneously, low-viscosity material is syringed around the transfer copings or impression posts. The materials are allowed to set, and the impression is removed from the mouth. The impression must have accurate border extensions, exhibit accurate reproduction of the tissues, and accu-

rately capture the transfer of the copings or posts (Fig. 10–25).

On approval of the impression, the transfer copings are removed and replaced with comfort caps. If impression posts were used, these are replaced with healing cuffs. The patient's old denture is relieved and relined with a temporary soft liner. The appropriate abutment analogs or implant body analogs are threaded to the respective transfer copings or impression posts, and these are carefully but completely seated onto the impression (Fig. 10–26). A small drop of cyanacrylate is placed where the analog meets the impression material.

The impression is poured in dental stone. The framework is waxed with the selected attachments, cast in a precious alloy with a minimum yield strength of 80,000 psi. The framework is then carefully finished and checked for fit on the working cast (Fig. 10–27). The bar assembly should be positioned over the crest of the ridge and as low as possible. This is to avoid excessive

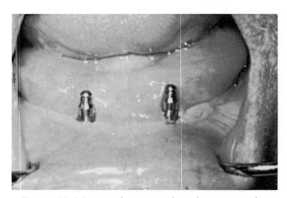

Figure 10–24. Transfer copings have been screwed over the implant abutments in preparation for the impression.

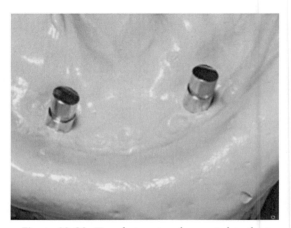

Figure 10–26. Two abutment analogs seated in the impression in preparation for the pouring procedure.

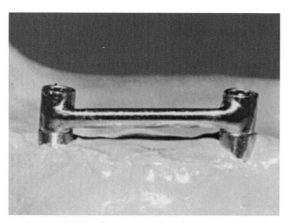

Figure 10–27. The copings that form part of the bar assembly must fit the abutment analogs on the master cast precisely.

bulk, which, in turn, would make the denture base thin, bulky, and fracture prone. Clearance of 1.5 to 2.0 mm beneath the bar, however, should be allowed to facilitate proper cleansing procedures. If the framework does not fit the working cast, it must be corrected. The framework is tried intraorally using a disclosing material to detect binding areas. The framework must have a passive fit over the abutments. Slight corrections can be made by selective grinding of the framework, but these should be kept to a minimum and not jeopardize the intimate fit of the framework over the abutments. Because there may be an error in the position of the implant or abutment analogs in the working cast, it is best to make the correction intraorally. If an error on the fit is detected, the framework is sectioned and reassembled by joining the segments with light-cured or autopolymerizing resin in the mouth. The framework is then removed, soldered, and carefully polished, preventing any distortion of the portions of the framework that contact the implants or abutments. The reassembled framework is again taken to the mouth and tried for fit. No attempt should be made to force the framework onto the implants or abutments. This ensures that the framework will not cause undue stress on the implants. Forceful seating causes stresses at the implant-bone interface and may produce microfractures, resulting in the initiation of a process that inevitably leads to implant loss.[15] Once the framework is seated, the final impression can be made.

With the framework secured to the abutments, a preliminary impression is made for the fabrication of a custom tray. The undercuts around the framework are blocked out. The framework is

then removed to allow the patient to use the interim or modified denture that has been utilized since the implants were exposed. On the resultant cast, a custom tray can be made after providing the proper relief over the stone reproduction of the framework. The flange areas are adjusted to allow for proper border molding during the making of the final impression.

At the final impression appointment, the framework is seated and screwed into position. The undercuts around the copings and bars are carefully blocked out with utility wax before making the impression. Border molding is completed, and the final impression is made with a resilient impression material in the same manner as the one used for the fabrication of a conventional complete denture.

Some implant systems require the transfer coping or impression post to be secured to the implant or abutment by means of auxiliary screws. In that case, a tray with an opening on the occlusal surface must be first prepared. After setting of the impression material, the open tray allows for the removal of the securing screws, which then allows for the removal of the transfer copings or impression posts in the impression (Figs. 10–28 and 10–29). The transfer copings or impression posts are secured to the appropriate abutment or implant analogs with the screws. The impression is poured in dental stone, and the fabrication of the framework and overdenture is completed as previously described.

At the time of delivery, the framework is placed on the abutments in the mouth and secured into place. The denture is then seated over the framework, and any adjustments to the impression surface and occlusion are accom-

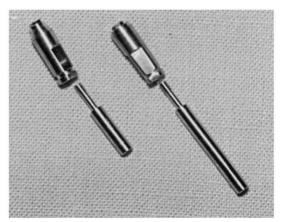

Figure 10–28. Impression posts with auxiliary screws of two different lengths. The use of these impression posts necessitates a tray with an opening on the occlusal surface.

plished. The retentive portion of the attachments can then be placed in the denture using auto-polymerizing acrylic resin with careful attention to blocking out all undercuts. The denture is then finished and instructions given to the patient concerning oral hygiene, denture care, and follow-up visits.

The advantages of the double impression technique are

1. Conventional and simplified processing of the final prosthesis
2. Eliminating the possibility of damaging the framework during processing of the denture

The disadvantages of this technique are

1. Necessity for the blocking out of the framework before making the final impression and placing the retentive portion of the attachments
2. The inability to use an index for the fabrication of the framework to ensure its fit within the confines of the denture
3. The inability to recognize compromises in aesthetics caused by the position of the implants in the wax-up stage before the fabrication of the framework
4. Extended chairside time at delivery to accomplish placement of the attachments

SINGLE IMPRESSION TECHNIQUE

This technique deals with the making of a single final impression both for the fabrication of the framework and the processing of the denture. After the implants are exposed and proper soft tissue healing has occurred, the temporary gingival cuffs are removed, and abutments of the proper length are placed. If a shouldered abutment is being used, the shoulder should be 0.5 to 1.0 mm above the gingival margin (Fig. 10–30). Comfort caps or similar parts are secured to the abutments. A preliminary impression is made in a stock tray to obtain a cast on which a custom tray is to be fabricated. Depending on the implant system used, either a conventional tray or an open tray is used. The custom tray is relieved over the comfort caps to accommodate the individual transfer copings or impression posts and

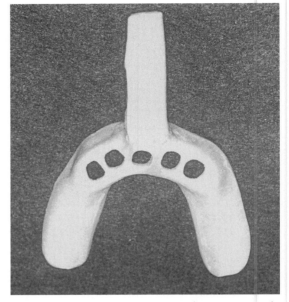

Figure 10–29. An impression tray with an opening on the occlusal surface allows for the removal of the securing screws, which then allows for the removal of the impression posts.

the flanges adjusted to allow for proper border molding.

At the final impression appointment, the comfort caps are replaced with impression copings, and the tray is inspected in the mouth to ensure proper clearance over the transfer copings, for the proper amount of impression material and proper flange extension. Alternatively, impression posts may be used to transfer the position of the implants to the master cast rather than the position of the abutments. This is particularly indicated when individual attachments are used, such as the stud-type abutments. The flanges of the tray are border molded in a conventional manner.

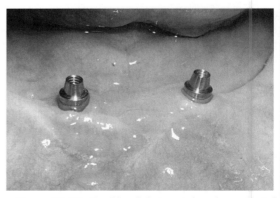

Figure 10–30. Shouldered abutments have been selected to have the shoulders 0.5 to 1.0 mm supragingivally.

The final impression is made in a two-component flexible material. A small amount of high-viscosity material is placed on the tray in each of the recesses over the individual implants, and the impression surface of the tray is loaded with low-viscosity material. A syringe is used to flow low-viscosity material around the transfer copings or impression posts. The impression is made in the same manner as an impression for a complete denture. After the impression material has set, the impression is removed, and the abutment or implant analogs are placed onto the impression attached to their respective impression copings or posts. The impression is poured in dental stone.

Bases and rims are fabricated, and the conventional procedures required in the fabrication of a complete denture are carried up to the stage of the wax try-in. After this is accomplished, the wax-up is returned to the laboratory, where an index is fabricated as described in Chapters 8 and 10. The denture wax-up is removed from the master cast, and the wax-up of the framework can be accomplished, ensuring that this will fit within the confines of the prosthesis (Figs. 10–31 and 10–32).

The framework is cast and finished and tried on the master cast and in the mouth. The framework is fitted as described earlier. The denture teeth are then modified as necessary to fit back in the original position. Usually the bulk of the framework makes it necessary to adjust the lingual and cervical aspects of the artificial teeth to place them back in position. The index can be used to accomplish this task rapidly.

A final wax try-in with the framework in position may be accomplished. This is a step that should not be ignored by the novice but may be omitted by the experienced practitioner working

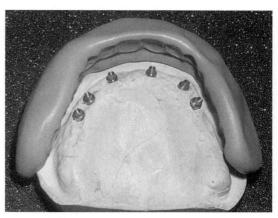

Figure 10–32. With the wax-up removed, the space available to fabricate the overdenture framework assembly to fit within the confines of the prosthesis is evident.

together with an experienced laboratory technician.

In processing the denture, it is necessary to block out all the undercuts around the framework as well as any part of the framework that may contact the impression surface of the denture in a manner to cause disruption of the correct functioning of the attachments. This can be accomplished with dental stone or vinyl polysiloxane putty impression material. The attachments, placed into position, are also blocked out to ensure that only the retentive portion comes into contact with the acrylic resin and is retained in the denture base. To ensure proper trial packing of the case, the split packing technique can be used. This consists of placing the bulk of the acrylic resin on the side of the flask that contains the teeth and a small amount around the attachments on the opposing side of the flask. During trial packing, a sheet of cellophane is placed between the two sides to prevent the attachments from being lifted out of place when the flask is opened.

Stud attachments are generally placed at the time of packing in the laboratory; however, they can also be placed at the delivery appointment intraorally with autopolymerizing acrylic resin.

The denture is completed in the conventional manner. Care should be taken during decasting to prevent damaging or distorting the framework.

At delivery, the framework is passively seated and secured to place. The denture is then placed in position, and the usual insertion inspections of occlusion, tissue fit, and flange extensions are accomplished. Oral hygiene, denture maintenance, and recall visits are also discussed with the patient.

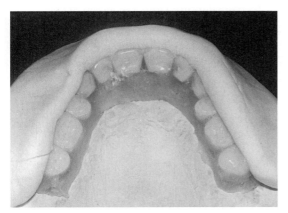

Figure 10–31. Index made with putty impression material around the diagnostic denture setup.

The advantages of this technique are

1. A single impression for the fabrication of the framework and the processing of the prosthesis
2. Decreased patient visits
3. The use of the wax-up and index to enhance aesthetics
4. The use of an index to ensure proper fit of framework within the prosthesis
5. Placement of the attachments in the laboratory instead of using valuable chair time.

The disadvantages of this technique are

1. Possible damage to the attachment and framework during the processing phase
2. More complex laboratory procedures during packing
3. Possible movement of the attachment during packing procedures.

There may be compelling reasons for the transfer of the implants rather than the abutments. In the case of malpositioned implants, the transferring of the implants rather than the abutments allows for versatility in the laboratory in selecting or modifying the appropriate implant abutments (Figs. 10–33 through 10–36).

Jaw Relation Records

For a tissue-supported overdenture, any of the conventional techniques that are acceptable for

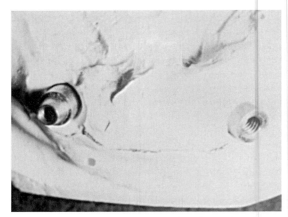

Figure 10–34. Master cast with shouldered abutment on the right side. Different abutments were tried directly on the implant analog (left side). The selection of a flat abutment allowed for draw of the superstructure.

use with complete dentures should suffice. For an implant-supported overdenture, one should consider the case as being more related to a fixed prosthetic restoration. The recording media should be accurate, stable, and easy to use. Although some have advocated the use of waxes, plaster, and other materials as the recording media, the more recently developed polysiloxane and polyether materials are preferred.[36, 40] The types of records obtained vary with the type of occlusion to be developed and the instrumentation used. In general, the use of a semiadjustable articulator and the obtaining of a centric relation-occlusion recorded along with either a protrusive or right and left lateral excursive records are indicated.

Occlusion

The occlusion developed for the tissue-supported overdenture can be selected according to

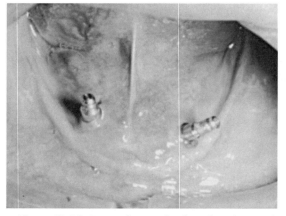

Figure 10–33. Intraoral view of malposed implants with transfer copings in place to emphasize the lack of parallelism. The transfer coping was removed from the divergent implant (left side) and an impression post screwed directly to the implant.

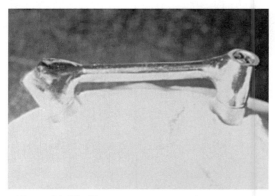

Figure 10–35. The superstructure on the master cast.

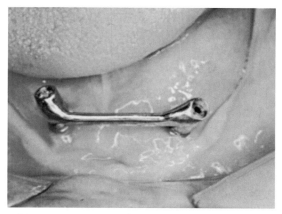

Figure 10–36. Intraoral view of the superstructure on the implants.

fossae and on the buccal and lingual inclines of the buccal and lingual cusps of the mandibular teeth. Some occlusal selective grinding is generally necessary to achieve a smooth movement. A lingualized occlusion can also be accomplished by the use of cusp teeth in the maxillary arch and zero degree teeth in the mandible. This requires extensive grinding of the mandibular teeth to achieve contact of the maxillary lingual cusps in eccentric movements. Special tooth forms marketed by several manufacturers such as the IPN Anatoline (Dentsply Intl Inc, York, PA) and the MLI (Myerson Tooth Division of Austenal, Chicago, IL) make the use of a lingualized occlusion much easier to achieve.[21]

the practitioner's preference for the occlusion for conventional complete dentures. Although the denture over the arch with the implants is more stable and retentive, it is still capable of movement owing to compressibility of the soft tissues and the lack of rigidity in the attachments used. Thus the overdenture functions more closely like a conventional denture than a fixed prosthesis.

The occlusion for the tissue-borne overdenture should include multiple bilateral, even contacts in centric relation and eccentric positions for proper distribution of force.[37] The types of occlusal schemes that can be used include the following types:

1. A full balance scheme of occlusion can be developed using any of the various types of cusp artificial teeth with a compensating curve. This is more easily accomplished with an implant overdenture versus a conventional complete denture owing to the greater stability and retention of the implant overdenture. This provides for greater ease in making occlusal and transfer records.
2. A flat plane type of occlusion can be developed. This is accomplished by the use of zero degree teeth in the opposing arches.
3. A lingualized occlusal scheme can be accomplished in various ways. A common approach is the use of dissimilar cusp teeth in the opposing arches. The teeth with the greater cusp degree are placed in the maxillary arch. This allows for the lingual cusps of the maxillary posterior teeth to glide from the central

The occlusion chosen for the implant-supported overdenture should be carefully considered. As already explained, the implant-borne overdenture is comparable to a fixed restoration. The restoration is stable and retentive and gains its support from the rigid implants and not the compressible, resilient tissues of the residual alveolar ridge. Therefore, in the edentulous patient, the arch with the implants becomes the dominant arch in terms of occlusion. An edentulous patient who previously complained of a loose, ill-fitting conventional mandibular denture and is fitted with an implant-borne overdenture will now feel that the maxillary complete denture is less secure. For these patients, it is highly recommended that a balanced type of occlusion be developed, which should provide balancing contacts on the working and balancing sides of the arch. Balanced occlusion ensures that there is no interference with jaw movements to eccentric positions.[37] A lingualized occlusion provides an excellent alternative to a full balanced occlusal scheme.

References

1. Adrian ED, Krantz WA, Ivanhoe JR: The use of processed silicone to retain the implant-supported tissue-borne overdenture. J Prosthet Dent 67:219-222, 1992.
2. Babbush CA: Dental Implants: Principles and Practice. Philadelphia, WB Saunders, 1991.
3. Barber HD, Fonseca RJ, Betts NJ: The transmandibular implant: Implant reconstruction and rehabilitation for the atrophic mandible. Implant Dent 1:297-301, 1992.
4. Bodine RL: Evaluation of 27 mandibular subperiosteal implant dentures after 15 to 22 years. J Prosthet Dent 32:188-197, 1974.

5. Bosker H, van Dijk L: The transmandibular implant: A 12-year follow-up study. J Oral Maxillofac Surg 47:442-450, 1989.
6. Brånemark P-I, Zarb GA, Albrektsson T: Tissue Integrated Prostheses. Osseointegration in Clinical Dentistry. London, Quintessence Publishing, 1985.
7. Brewer AA, Morrow RM: Overdentures, ed 2. St. Louis, CV Mosby, 1980.
8. DeBoer J: Edentulous implants: Overdenture versus fixed. J Prosthet Dent 69:386-390, 1993.
9. Finger IM, Guerra LR: The Integral implant system: Prosthetic considerations. Dent Clin North Am 36:189-206, 1992.
10. Gift HC, Newman JF: How older adults use oral health core services: Results of a national health interview survey. J Am Dent Assoc 124:89-93, 1993.
11. Guerra LR, Finger IM, Block MS: Tissue-supported implant overdentures. Impl Dent 1:69-77, 1992.
12. Haraldson T, Jemt T, Stålblad P-Å, Lekholm U: Oral function in subjects with overdentures supported by osseointegrated implants. Scand J Dent Res 96:235-242, 1988.
13. Hobo S, Ichida E, Garcia LT: Osseointegration and Occlusal Rehabilitation. London, Quintessence Publishing, 1990.
14. Jemt T, Book K, Linden B, Urde G: Failures and complications in 92 consecutively inserted overdentures supported by Brånemark implants in severely resorbed edentulous maxillae: A study from prosthetic treatment to first annual check-up. Int J Oral Maxillofac Impl 7:162-167, 1992.
15. Jemt T, Carlsson L, Boss A, Jorneus L: In vivo load measurements on osseointegrated implants supporting fixed or removable prostheses: A comparative pilot study. Int J Oral Maxillofac Impl 6:413-417, 1991.
16. Jemt T, Stålblad P-Å, Haraldson T: Functional evaluation of patients treated with overdentures in the mandible supported by osseointegrated fixtures; a one-year follow-up study. In van Steenberghe D (ed): Tissue Integration in Oral and Maxillofacial Reconstruction. Amsterdam, Excerpta Medica, 1986.
17. Johns RB, Jemt T, Heath MR, Hutton JE, McKenna S, McNamara DC, van Steenberghe D, Taylor R, Watson RM, Hermann I: A multicenter study of overdentures supported by Brånemark implants. Int J Oral Maxillofac Impl 7:513-522, 1992.
18. Kirsch A: Fünf Jahre I.M.Z.-Implantat-System. Grundlagen, Methodik, Erfahrungen. Symposium Der heutige Stand der Implantologie, herausgegeben von Prof Dr Dr J Franke, 1979. München, Carl Hanser Verlag, 1980.
19. Kopp CD: Overdentures and osseointegration. Dent Clin North Am 34:729-739, 1990.
20. Krämer A, Weber H, Benzing J: Implant and prosthetic treatment of the edentulous maxilla using a bar supported prosthesis. Int J Oral Maxillofac Impl 7:251-255, 1992.
21. Lang BR, Razzoog ME: Lingualized integration: Tooth molds and an occlusal scheme for edentulous implant patients. Impl Dent 1:204-211, 1992.
22. Mericske-Stern R: Clinical evaluation of overdenture restorations supported by osseointegrated titanium implants:
A retrospective study. Int J Oral Maxillofac Impl 5:375-383, 1990.
23. Misch CE: Prosthetic options in implant dentistry. Int J Oral Implantol 7:17-21, 1991.
24. Naert I, DeClercq M, Theuniers G, Schepers E: Overdentures supported by osseointegrated fixtures for the edentulous mandible: A 2.5-year report. Int J Oral Maxillofac Impl 3:191-196, 1988.
25. Naert I, Quirynen M, Theuniers G, van Steenberghe D: Prosthetic aspects of osseointegrated fixtures supporting overdentures. A 4-year report. J Prosthet Dent 65:671-680, 1991.
26. National Survey of Oral Health in U.S. Employed Adults and Seniors: Oral Health of United States Adults. National Findings. U.S. Department of Health and Human Services. Bethesda, Public Health Service National Institutes of Health, 1985-1986.
27. Powers MP, Maxson BB, Scott RF, et al: The transmandibular implant: A 2-year prospective study. J Oral Maxillofac Surg 47:679-683, 1989.
28. Salinas TJ, Finger IM, Thaler JJ, Clark RS: Spark erosion implant-supported overdentures: Clinical and laboratory techniques. Implant Dent 1:246-251, 1992.
29. Small IA, Chalmers J: Lyons memorial lecture: Metal implants and the mandibular staple bone plate. J Oral Surg 33:571-585, 1975.
30. Small IA, Metz H, Kobernick S: The mandibular staple implant for the atrophic mandible. J Biomed Mater Res 8 (4 Pt 2):365-371, 1974.
31. Smedberg J-I, Lothigius E, Bodin I, Frykholm A, Nilner K: A clinical and radiological two-year follow-up study of maxillary overdentures on osseointegrated implants. Clin Oral Impl Res 4:39-46, 1993.
32. Smedberg J-I, Lothigius E, Nilner K, DeBuck V: A new design for a hybrid prosthesis supported by osseointegrated implants: Part 2. Preliminary clinical aspects. Int J Oral Maxillofac Impl 6:154-159, 1991.
33. Triplett RG, Mason ME, Alfonso WF, McAnear JT: Endosseous cylinder implants in severely atrophic mandibles. Int J Oral Maxillofac Impl 6:264-269, 1991.
34. Truitt HP: The application of high technology in contour replication of jaw bones (abstract). 32nd Annual Meeting of American Academy of Implant Dentists, Washington, DC, 1983.
35. von Wowern N, Harder F, Hjirting-Hansen E, Gotfredsen K: ITI implants with overdentures: A prevention of bone loss in edentulous mandibles? Int J Oral Maxillofac Impl 5:135-139, 1990.
36. Winkler S: Essentials of Complete Denture Prosthodontics, ed 2. Littleton, MA, PSG Publishing, 1988.
37. Winkler S, Mahosky GE: The edentulous mandible opposing maxillary natural teeth: Treatment considerations utilizing implant overdentures. Impl Dent 2:44-47, 1993.
38. Wismeijer D, Vermeeren JIJH, van Waas MAJ: Patient satisfaction with overdentures supported by one-stage TPS implants. Int J Oral Maxillofac Impl 7:51-55, 1992.
39. Young L, Michel JD, Moore DJ: A twenty-year evaluation of subperiosteal implants. J Prosthet Dent 49:690-694, 1983.
40. Zarb GA, Bolender CL, Hickey JC, Carlsson GE: Boucher's Prosthodontic Treatment for Edentulous Patients, ed 10. St Louis, CV Mosby, 1990.

Study Questions

1. Describe the advantages of a tissue-borne, implant-retained overdenture as compared with a conventional complete denture.

2. Describe an implant-borne overdenture.

3. Describe the selection process for choosing a specific attachment.

4. Outline the steps in the impression-making procedure for implant-retained, tissue-supported overdentures.

5. Discuss the occlusal schemes desirable in a patient with implant-retained overdentures.

CHAPTER 11

Hybrid Dentures

Luis R. Guerra
Harold S. Cardash
Revised by Luis R. Guerra

Factors Affecting Hybrid Denture
   Construction
Diagnostic Dentures Method
Stent Fabrication
Implant Exposure

Impression
Design of the Superstructure
Placement of the Prosthesis
References

A hybrid prosthesis is fabricated over a metal framework and retained by screws threaded into the implant abutments (Fig. 11–1). This is more commonly used in the mandible than in the maxilla. The prosthesis can be secured to implants placed in the anterior portion of the mandible, while the posterior part of a prosthesis is cantilevered from the implants. In the maxilla, every effort is made to maximize the number of implants used, spacing them evenly throughout the arch and avoiding the use of cantilevers.

Screws allow the prosthesis to be rigidly attached to the implant abutments and facilitate removal. Removal of the prosthesis may be necessary owing to implant failure, the need for further prosthodontic service, or soft tissue alteration. Unless aesthetic reasons dictate otherwise, it is preferable to have no contact between the prosthesis and the soft tissue of the residual alveolar ridge.

The most common indications for implant placement are patients who are edentulous in one or both arches and whose dentures lack support, retention, and stability. In the United States a national survey[15] in 1988 revealed a 10% incidence in one-arch edentulism in adults aged 50 years, rising to 15% in seniors over age 65. Total edentulism reached 50% in seniors 80 years of age.

Complete removable dentures are often poorly tolerated by the oral tissues, especially in geriatric patients. Continual ridge resorption is a problem faced by denture wearers,[3, 12, 20] necessitating constant adjustments, replacements of dentures, and eventually reduced ability to retain and control the prosthesis. Loss of bone from the buccal and lingual surfaces and the crest of the ridge leads to a variety of ridge forms.[2] Knife edge and depressed arch forms, sharp mylohyoid ridges, and high muscle attachments are all unfavorable to successful complete denture wearing.

Patients with implant-borne dentures are free of the injuries and problems associated with tissue-borne dentures. Chewing efficiency, known to be reduced in complete denture wearers,[10] has been shown to be comparable to that of dentate patients when an implant-borne prosthesis is utilized.[9] Thus the implant-borne prosthesis provides the patient with the best substitute for the natural dentition available at present.

In this section, we describe the general principles that must be applied to fabricate hybrid implant-borne prostheses for the edentulous jaw.

FACTORS AFFECTING HYBRID DENTURE CONSTRUCTION

Patient selection, diagnosis, treatment planning, and an explanation of the expected results to the patient are keys to successful implant prosthodontic rehabilitation. The medical history should elicit whether the patient is a medical risk for implant surgery and reveal any systemic disease that might compromise the survival of the implants. Unless the underlying factors are corrected, patients with orally manifested health problems (e.g., xerostomia, burning mouth syndrome, nutritional or hormonal problems) may not be free of symptoms on completion of treatment, even though the implant-borne prosthesis

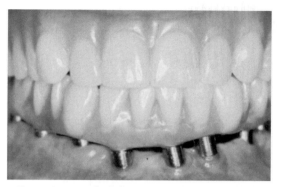

Figure 11–1. Hybrid denture resembles a complete denture and is screw retained.

may be much more comfortable to wear than a tissue-borne denture.

A careful examination of the soft tissue at the potential implant site avoids undesirable gingivae sequelae following insertion of the implants. Less than a 2 mm collar of attached gingiva around the implant may be insufficient to maintain the health of the peri-implant tissue and places the marginal integrity of the epithelium in jeopardy. Good oral and denture hygiene is a prerequisite for the implant patient. Lack of commitment by the patient to a supervised maintenance program may lead to eventual loss of the implants.

Diagnostic casts mounted on a semiadjustable articulator are indispensable to treatment planning. Assessment of the size and shape of the alveolar ridges aids in revealing any limitation in placement of the implants. Evaluation of the interarch distance and interarch relationship ensures that adequate space exists for the prosthesis and that the implant abutment does not encroach on tooth space. A minimum of 7 mm between the implant site and the opposing dentition or occlusal plane is considered adequate for tooth and abutment.

When a normal jaw relationship exists between moderately resorbed edentulous arches, the residual alveolar ridges are approximately opposite each other in frontal and sagittal planes at the correct vertical dimension of occlusion. This enables teeth to be set in a bilateral balanced occlusion centralizing the forces of occlusal function over the alveolar ridges. In addition, implants may be set in an almost vertical position, allowing occlusal forces to be directed along the long axis of the implants.

With increasing resorption, changes occur in the vertical and horizontal relationship of the residual ridges. The maxillary residual alveolar ridge resorbs superiorly and palatally, and the mandibular residual alveolar ridge resorbs inferiorly and laterally. This resorptive pattern tends to place the arches in a relatively prognathic jaw relationship.

The prognathic (Cl III) jaw relationship may require inclination or lingual placement of the implants in the anterior portion of the mandible to avoid the screw access holes being located on the labial surface of the teeth. This would also minimize excessive force to the anterior region of the denture-bearing edentulous maxilla, reducing the potential for bony resorption and subsequent loss of stability of the maxillary denture.[5] Inclination greater than 20 degrees from the vertical, however, probably contraindicates a hybrid prosthesis.

A retrognathic (Cl II) jaw relationship often requires labial positioning of the mandibular incisors to achieve satisfactory aesthetics. Therefore, implants should be angled slightly labial to the residual alveolar ridge to avoid an excessive labiolingual dimension of the anterior portion of the restoration. This allows normal tongue function and speech and easier cleaning of the prosthesis. Excessive inclination of implants should be avoided when possible so as not to subject them to nonaxial forces.

Less flexibility is available in positioning the artificial teeth and consequently the implants where the prosthesis is opposed by natural teeth. Every effort should be made to restore the opposing teeth to an acceptable plane of occlusion.

Mandibular implant-borne overdentures generally require four to six implants placed anterior to the mental foramina. This obviates encroachment on the inferior alveolar nerve. Occlusion can be provided to the first molar area by using a distal cantilever of 15 mm or less. When implants are placed bilaterally distal to the mental foramina, potential flexure of the mandible in function may loosen the prosthesis or the implants. In such cases it is advisable to construct a metal superstructure that is split at the midline and joined by the acrylic resin of the prosthesis.

In the maxilla the most common area for implant placement is the cuspid area limited by the medial wall of the maxillary sinus posteriorly and the nasal cavity anteriorly. Minimally six to eight implants are considered necessary to retain a complete maxillary prosthesis (Fig. 11–2).

The length and mobility of the upper lip are important factors in designing the maxillary prosthesis. A high smile line exposes a broad expanse of gingiva, and the implant abutments are visible between the tissue surface of the prosthesis and the crest of the residual alveolar ridge (Fig. 11–3). In this situation, it would be preferable to

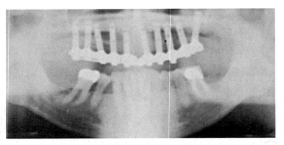

Figure 11–2. Radiograph of prosthesis in place.

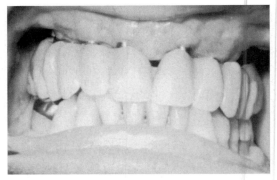

Figure 11–3. Long tooth with a high smile line leaves poor aesthetic result.

place the implants in the canine and first and second bicuspid sites if sufficient bone exists in that region.

The space recommended for hygiene beneath a fixed prosthesis may also cause significant phonetic discrepancies even in patients with a long upper lip. Normal tooth length and gingiva are displayed if a pink removable facade is added to cover the gingival margins (Fig. 11–4). Alternatively a removable prosthesis with a labial flange should be considered, especially if lip support is also required.

Severe bony resorption may also require teeth of abnormal length to satisfy aesthetics. This may lead to an unfavorable crown-to-implant ratio, placing excessive torque on the implant, especially in protrusive movements of the mandible. In such cases a removable prosthesis is preferred.

The final choice between an operator-removable and a patient-removable prosthesis rests with the patient. When a good dentist-patient relationship exists, however, the patient is guided by the dentist. The three main factors to be discussed between them are the amount of bone available, aesthetic factors, and hygienic considerations.

DIAGNOSTIC DENTURES METHOD

Before surgical placement of the implants, it is important that the patient be satisfied with the aesthetics of the new prosthesis. Diagnostic dentures are constructed up to the trial stage using conventional methods. Anterior tooth position, arrangement, and lip support are finalized to meet the aesthetic and phonetic requirements of the patient.

The diagnostic denture is used to ensure that implants are correctly positioned to ensure that the superstructure is contained within the contours of the denture. Screw-retentive elements should not exit in an area that may compromise

aesthetics or function. A surgical stent aids in proper placement of the implants.

STENT FABRICATION

In the maxilla, the central part of the palate of the maxillary denture wax-up is removed and the flanges reduced to the cervical portion of the teeth. A silicone putty or irreversible hydrocolloid impression is made of the denture wax-up on the cast and the impression poured. A vacuum-formed or clear acrylic transitional stent is made on the new cast, including the palate. The clear transitional stent is trimmed and transferred to the original cast without the waxed diagnostic denture. Guide holes are drilled through the transitional stent into the cast in the desired implant locations. Lastly the final surgical stent is fabricated in clear acrylic resin on the scored original master cast. Holes are drilled through the surgical stent corresponding to the holes in the master cast. The surgical stent is retained after implant insertion and used as an aid in

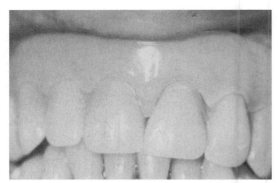

Figure 11–4. Removable acrylic resin facade to correct poor aesthetic result shown in Figure 11–3.

relocating the implants at the second surgical stage (see Chapter 8).

IMPLANT EXPOSURE

During the period the implants are integrating, the patients may use their present dentures, or transitional dentures may be fabricated. These are inserted approximately 2 weeks after implant placement to allow for tissue healing. They are lined with a tissue-conditioning material.

Approximately 12 to 16 weeks are allowed to elapse before implants placed in the mandible are uncovered. Because the maxilla generally has somewhat less dense bone, implant exposure is delayed until 16 to 24 weeks to allow osseointegration of the implants to take place.[14] The adaptation of bone to the implant continues to improve at least up to 18 months, so a longer healing time is advised if bone is less dense or if anatomic limitations have necessitated the use of short implants.

On exposure of the implant, the healing cap or screw is removed, and the appropriate abutment or transmucosal sleeve is attached while ensuring that no soft tissue interposes between the implant and the abutment. The denture is relined with a tissue conditioner to act as a bandage over the tissues surrounding the implants. The liner is changed as necessary.

A meticulous oral hygiene program is instituted at this point even though the tissues may be inflamed. The tissues are massaged with a toothbrush and the abutment heads kept clean with an end-tufted brush, proxy brush, pipe cleaners, gauze strips, or dental floss, together with twice-daily rinses of chlorhexidine gluconate.

IMPRESSION

The object of the impression is to transfer the implant positions to a master working cast. Attention to detail is essential to obtain an exact replica of the implant, abutments, and adjacent soft tissues.

The healing cap or transmucosal sleeves are removed and the abutments inspected for cleanliness, screwed into the implants, and checked for tightness. It is desirable that the shoulder of the abutment be located a minimum of 1 mm supragingivally (Fig. 11–5).

Transfer copings used to locate the abutment analogs in the impression are threaded into the

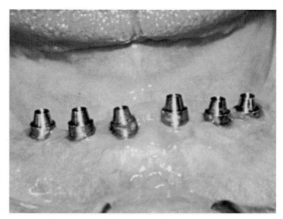

Figure 11–5. Shoulders of abutments must be placed 1 to 2 mm supragingivally.

abutments. Preliminary impressions are made with irreversible hydrocolloid impression material and a custom tray constructed with autopolymerized or light-cured resin. Although the final impression may be made in a stock tray, a custom tray is preferred to record more accurately the sulci and the retromolar pad area, which are useful guides in determining the occlusal plane. The optimum height of the posterior occlusal plane is considered to be two-thirds the height of the retromolar pad.[11]

The custom tray is border molded with modeling compound or high-viscosity elastomeric impression material compatible with the material to be used for the final impression. The final impression is made with medium or heavy body addition-type silicones or polyether, these materials being among the stiffest of the available elastomers.[17] A material that is rigid and not too elastic is preferred. This facilitates accurate relocation of the transfer copings into the impression. The abutment with the transfer coping in place is dried and impression material injected with a syringe, taking care not to incorporate air bubbles into the material. The loaded impression tray is then seated. On removal from the mouth, the impression is carefully inspected. The transfer copings are unscrewed from the abutments. Abutment analogs are threaded into the transfer copings, which are, in turn, relocated into the impression (Figs. 11–6 and 11–7). Some systems use impression posts splinted with acrylic resin, which remain in the impression material when it is withdrawn from the mouth.

Inaccuracies in the master cast arise from improper threading of the abutment head into the implant and the transfer coping onto the abutment head, lack of attention in removing these

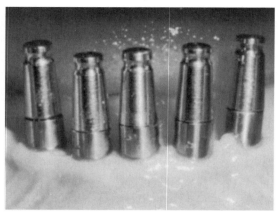

Figure 11–6. Transfer copings placed over fixture abutments in preparation for impression.

and then relocating the transfer coping into the impression, and distortion of the autopolymerizing acrylic when it is used to splint impression posts together. This distortion occurs during removal of the posts from the implant, which allows release of the stresses set up during polymerization.[19]

Incorporation of these errors in the impression leads to fabrication of an ill-fitting implant superstructure, which imparts stress to the implant or screwed-in abutment when seated.

In evaluating impression techniques, Spector et al[19] found no significant difference in accuracy whether or not posts were splinted together or when different elastomeric impression materials were used.

The impressions are poured in improved stone, record bases are constructed, and a centric relation record is made at the proper vertical dimension of occlusion. The maxillary cast is positioned on a semiadjustable articulator using a facebow transfer record and the maxillary and

mandibular casts articulated. Teeth are selected and set in bilateral balanced occlusion. Because the appearance of the diagnostic dentures has already been approved by the patient, they may be used as a guide to selecting and setting the teeth.

The vertical dimension of occlusion, centric relation, and aesthetics are verified at the next clinical try-in appointment and a protrusive record taken with a recording medium of choice. The condylar inclinations are set according to the protrusive record.

It is essential that the contours of the metal framework of the denture be contained within the volume of the denture and be compatible with the position of the teeth. This is accomplished by recording the position of the teeth with indices and using the indices as a guide during fabrication of the framework. The waxed-up denture is replaced on the cast. The exterior base of the cast is keyed, and silicone putty or plaster indices are made of the labial-buccal and lingual surfaces of the waxed-up denture (Fig. 11–8). The waxed denture is removed from the cast, the indices are replaced on the cast, and the space available for the metal superstructure can be visualized (Fig. 11–9).

DESIGN OF THE SUPERSTRUCTURE

Because anatomic considerations generally necessitate the implants being placed in the anterior segment of the arch, the posterior section of the framework is cantilevered posteriorly from the distal abutment. To provide a sufficiently long masticatory area and to achieve a bilateral balanced occlusion, it is desirable to extend the

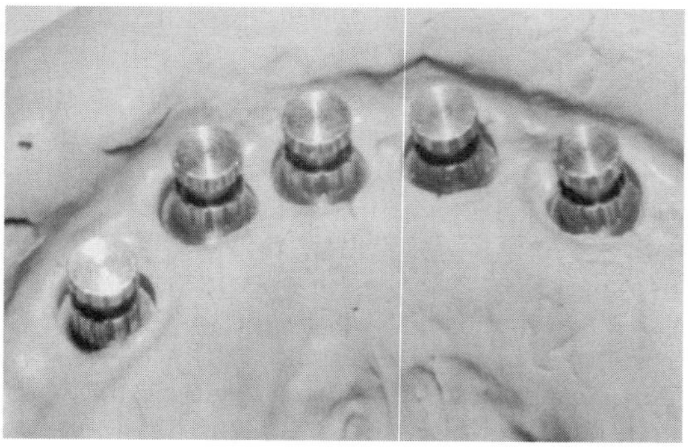

Figure 11–7 Laboratory analogs screwed to transfer copings placed into the impression.

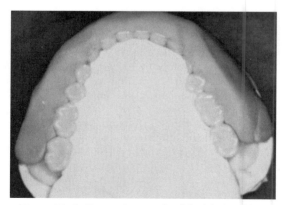

Figure 11–8. Putty indices made of the labial and lingual surfaces of the waxed-up denture on the master cast.

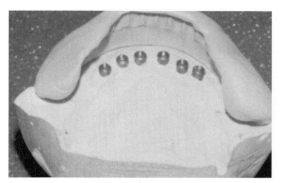

Figure 11–9. Denture wax-up removed from cast and the space available for the hybrid superstructure is visualized.

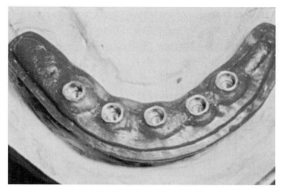

Figure 11–11. Final wax-up of framework with finish line developed. Cantilevers are short and wide.

cantilever to the first molar region. In the mandibular prosthesis, the cantilever should not exceed 15 mm when five abutments are used or 12 mm when using four abutments (Fig. 11–10).[22]

The volume of bone available and its density are generally less in the maxilla than in the mandible.[1] It has been suggested that the maximum cantilever length in the maxillary arch be 10 to 12 mm.[22] This provides room for one premolar tooth distal to the most posterior implant. Depending on the position of the distal implant, this might pose a problem by creating an edentulous space in the buccal corridor during smiling or speech. In addition, the lack of molar teeth in the maxilla may not provide sufficient occlusal contact for a full complement of mandibular teeth. Therefore, for aesthetic or functional reasons, it may be necessary to restore the maxillary arch with a removable overdenture prosthesis retained by implants anteriorly and tissue supported posteriorly.

The dimensions of the cantilever are most important in reducing deformation of the restoration and hence stress on the implants. No precise equations exist for describing functional defor-

mations of cantilevered pontics; however, deformation is minimized when the modulus of elasticity is high and when the height and width of the bar are increased.[7] A width of 4.5 mm and thickness of 5 mm are considered adequate (Figs. 11–11 and 11–12).[21] Short, thick cantilevers are preferred. Added bulk is necessary at the junction of the cantilever and the distal abutment because this is a site of potential increased stress and is susceptible to fracture. A cross section of the pattern shows a shape that provides rigidity and strength in the framework with minimum bulk and weight.[4] This shape aids in retention of acrylic and allows polished metal to be adjacent to the tissue in the final prosthesis (Table 11–1).

To facilitate oral hygiene and avoid food impaction, a space of approximately 2 to 3 mm should exist between the residual ridge and the framework (Fig. 11–13). In the maxilla, too great a space, however, may lead to difficulty with phonetics owing to escape of air. An overly wide buccolingual dimension may give rise to difficulties in cleaning the undersurface of the prosthesis. Similarly a convex contour of the tissue surface is more amenable to cleaning.

The importance of the framework fitting accu-

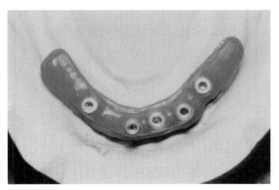

Figure 11–10. Wax-up of framework around gold copings with cantilever 15 mm distal to the first implant.

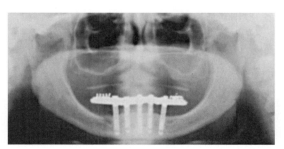

Figure 11–12. Metal framework tried in the mouth. Note the thickness of the framework at the cantilever sites. The thickness in this area should be no less than 5 mm.

Table 11–1. Hybrid Framework Characteristics

Well-planned screw access "chimney" holes
Precious or semiprecious alloy
Convex tissue surface
Highly polished tissue surface
Framework
    Minimum 3 mm thick
    Minimum 4 mm wide
Cantilever 15 mm or less
Retention for resin
Hygiene consideration

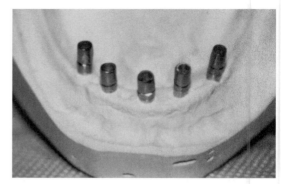

Figure 11–14. Metal copings secured to the abutment analogs on the cast in preparation for construction of a verification framework.

rately and passively over the abutments cannot be overemphasized. Any malalignment of the superstructure to the osseointegrated implants results in internal stresses in the prosthesis, the implants, and the bone. Such stresses cannot be detected usually, but may substantially reduce the load required to cause failure.[18] Forced tightening of the screws against the ill-fitting superstructure may lead to microfractures of bone or a vertical loss of marginal bone.[1]

It is therefore advisable to verify the accuracy of the master cast by trying in a verification framework made with autopolymerizing acrylic resin before the wax-up of the framework is completed. The framework base is constructed in acrylic resin, on gold cylinders or plastic sleeves, which seat accurately on the abutments (Figs. 11–14 and 11–15). The acrylic framework is left to stand on the cast overnight to minimize distortion. Should the plastic framework not fit, a new impression must be made.

Various metals have been used to cast the framework. A metal alloy of yield strength 300

MPa and modulus of elasticity 80,000 MPa withstands occlusal forces sufficiently to prevent deformation and breakage of the cantilevers.[16] Type IV gold, silver/palladium, and chrome/cobalt have been used.[4, 23] The gold alloys are, however, expensive. Silver/palladium has a tendency to tarnish, and chrome/cobalt is difficult to solder. An alloy of platinum/palladium is recommended.

The casting process may be a source of error in the ultimate fit of the superstructure. The larger the casting, the greater the inaccuracy.[6] An alternative to a one-piece casting is to cast the superstructure in sections and solder it together after trial insertions in the mouth.[13] Other techniques include light-cured resin and laser welding to join the components.

When the superstructure is cast, it is retried in the mouth for a passive and accurate fit. The framework is held by one screw in the middle positioned abutment, while the contact with the other abutments is checked. The stability of the framework on the abutments is inspected, and the screws should easily thread into the abut-

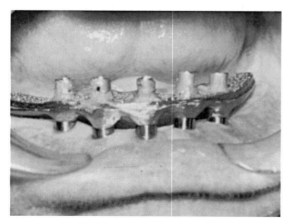

Figure 11–13. The framework of the hybrid prosthesis should be designed with spaces of 3 to 4 mm between the residual ridge and the framework.

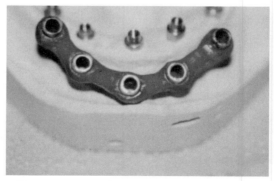

Figure 11–15. Verification framework in acrylic resin.

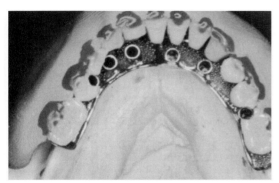

Figure 11–16. The index has been used to wax the artificial teeth to the superstructure.

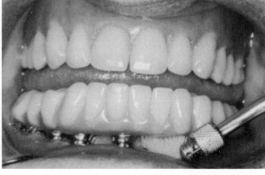

Figure 11–18. A nylon-coated interproximal brush to clean the impression surface of the prosthesis and abutments.

ments without binding. It has been reported that a discrepancy of fit of more than 30 μm on more than 10% of the interface circumference is unacceptable.[13] Goll[8] notes that 25% of metal frameworks for full arch restorations do not fit accurately despite meticulous attention to detail.

If the seating of the framework is judged unacceptable, the framework is sectioned, rescrewed to the abutments, joined with acrylic resin, and soldered together. On obtaining a satisfactory seat, the framework is tested by applying occlusal forces to the cantilevers. As the distal end of the cantilever is approached, pain may be elicited around the most distal abutment. The point on the cantilever where pain is first noted is marked and the cantilever shortened.[16]

The acrylic teeth are set on the superstructure and retried in the mouth (Fig. 11–16). The prosthesis is then processed and polished using conventional techniques.

A problem occasionally noted with hybrid restorations is the dark shadow of metal seen through the thin translucent resin. The metal framework can be opaqued with a heat-cured pink opaque veneer that bonds chemically with polymethyl methacrylate resin; the final thickness of resin and metal is expected to be 2 mm or less.[22]

PLACEMENT OF THE PROSTHESIS

At the delivery appointment, the prosthesis is screwed firmly into place on the abutments. An interocclusal record is made and the prosthesis remounted on an articulator to correct occlusal discrepancies arising from polymerization.

After insertion of the prosthesis, the screws are tightened and covered with gutta-percha. Panoramic and intraoral radiographs are taken to verify the fit of the abutments (Fig. 11–17).

The implant-borne prosthesis is placed temporarily for a short period to determine if the patient is comfortable and to assist him or her in oral hygiene techniques.

Oral hygiene instructions are given, including care of the prosthesis and the abutments. The

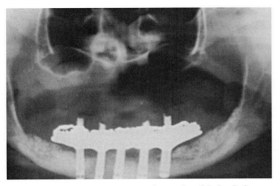

Figure 11–17. Panoramic radiograph of hybrid denture in place. It is important to verify correct seating of the prosthesis on the abutments.

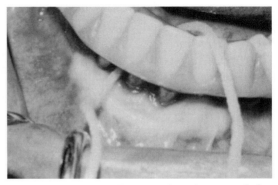

Figure 11–19. Superfloss is used to clean around abutments.

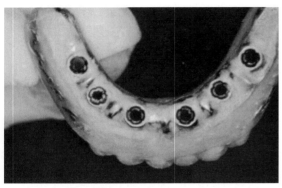

Figure 11–20. It is important to remove the prosthesis periodically at the recall appointments to evaluate the peri-implant tissues and to clean the denture. Note accumulation of plaque on the impression surface of the prosthesis. Ultrasonic cleaners are used to clean the denture and implant components thoroughly.

major part of the prosthesis can be cleaned with a toothbrush. The impression surfaces of the prosthesis and abutments, however, require special attention. The lip is retracted and the visible areas of the tissue surface of the prosthesis cleaned with a proxy brush, pipe cleaner, or Superfloss (Fig. 11–18). Proxy brushes with metal stems coated with nylon are preferred to avoid scratching the abutments or implants. The lingual areas and abutments are cleaned with an end-tufted brush. Superfloss or "shoelaces" are threaded under the prosthesis and around each abutment in turn (Fig. 11–19).

The patient is seen after 24 hours. Minor adjustments of denture flanges may be necessary at this postinsertion visit, and plaque control is evaluated.

After 1 month when the patient has demonstrated the necessary ability to maintain satisfactory oral hygiene, the gutta-percha is removed over the screw holes. The screws are tightened, gutta-percha is placed in the slots or hex hole of the screws. The remaining void is filled with light-cured composite resin. The patient is placed on a 3-month recall schedule (Fig. 11–20).

References

1. Adell R, Lekholm U, Rockler B, Brånemark P-I: A 15 year study of osseointegrated implants in the treatment of the edentulous jaw. Int J Oral Surg 6:387–416, 1981.
2. Atwood D: Reduction of residual ridges: A major oral disease entity. J Prosthet Dent 26:266–279, 1971.
3. Campbell R: A comparative study of the resorption of the alveolar ridges in denture wearers and non-denture wearers. J Am Dent Assoc 60:143–153, 1960.
4. Cox J, Zarb G: Alternative prosthodontic superstructure designs. Swed Dent J 28(suppl):71–75, 1985.
5. Desjardins RP: Tissue-integrated prostheses for edentulous patients with normal and abnormal jaw relationships. J Prosthet Dent 59:180–187, 1988.
6. Fusayama T, Wakumoto S, Hosada H: Accuracy of fixed partial dentures made by various soldering techniques and one piece casting. J Prosthet Dent 14:334–342, 1964.
7. Glantz PO: Aspects of prosthodontic design. In Brånemark P-I, Zarb G, Albrektsson T (eds): Tissue Integrated Prostheses. Osseointegration in Clinical Dentistry. Chicago, Quintessence Publishing, 1985, pp 329–332.
8. Goll GE: Production of accurately fitting full-arch implant frameworks: 1. Clinical procedures. J Prosthet Dent 66:377–384, 1991.
9. Haroldson T, Carlsson GE: Chewing efficiency in patients with osseointegrated oral implant bridges. Swed Dent J 3:183–191, 1979.
10. Haroldson T, Karlsson V, Carlsson GE: Bite force and oral function in complete denture wearers. J Oral Rehab 6:41–48, 1979.
11. Hickey JC, Zarb GA, Bolender CL: Boucher's Prosthodontic Treatment for Edentulous Patient, ed 9. St. Louis, CV Mosby, 1985.
12. Jozefowicz W: The influence of wearing dentures on the residual ridge: A comparative study. J Prosthet Dent 24:137–144, 1970.
13. Klineberg IJ, Murray GM: Design of superstructures for osseointegrated fixtures. Swed Dent J 28(suppl):63–69, 1985.
14. Lundqvis S, Carlsson GE: Maxillary fixed prostheses in osseointegrated dental implants. J Prosthet Dent 50:262–270, 1983.
15. Meskin LH, Jackson BL: Prevalence and patterns of tooth loss in U.S. employed adult and senior populations 1985–86. J Dent Educ 52:686–691, 1988.
16. Minsley GE, Koth DL: Prosthodontic procedures for dental implants. In Fagan MJ (ed): Implant Prosthodontics. Surgical and Prosthetic Techniques for Dental Implants. Chicago, Year Book Medical Publishers, 1990, p 211.
17. Schelb E, Norliny BK: Impression materials and techniques. In Malone WPK, Koth DL (eds): Tylman's Theory and Practice of Fixed Prosthetics, ed 8. St. Louis, Ishiyaka Euroamerica, 1989.
18. Skalak R: Biomechanical considerations in osseointegrated prostheses. J Prosthet Dent 49:843–848, 1983.
19. Spector MR, Donovan TE, Nicholls JI: An evaluation of impression techniques for osseointegrated implants. J Prosthet Dent 63:444–447, 1990.
20. Tallgren A: The continuing reduction of the residual alveolar ridges in complete denture wearers: A mixed longitudinal study covering 25 years. J Prosthet Dent 27:120–132, 1972.
21. Taylor R, Bergman G: Laboratory Techniques for the Brånemark System. Chicago, Quintessence Publishing, 1990.
22. Taylor TD: Fixed implant rehabilitation on the edentulous maxilla. Int J Oral Maxillofac Impl 6:329–337, 1991.
23. Zarb GN, Symington JM: Osseointegrated dental implants: Preliminary report on a replication study. J Prosthet Dent 50:271–276, 1983.

Study Questions

1. Define the term hybrid denture.

2. Discuss the factors affecting the fabrication of a hybrid denture for a patient.

3. List the characteristics of a hybrid denture framework.

4. Describe the steps required at the delivery appointment of a hybrid denture.

CHAPTER 12

Fixed Prosthodontics

Israel M. Finger
Luis R. Guerra
Neil Boner
Revised by Luis R. Guerra

Clinical and Biomechanical Considerations
    Hard Tissue Factors
    Soft Tissue Factors
    Spacing of Implants
    Number of Implants
    Connection to Teeth
    Crown-to-Root Ratio
    Implant Orientation
Retrievable or Cementable Restoration
Provisional or Temporary Restorations
Fabrication of Restorations
    Impressions
    Transfer Systems

Laboratory Considerations
    Infection Control Procedures
    General Considerations
    Abutment Head Selection
    Metal Framework Considerations
    Aesthetic Considerations
    Loading Forces
Single-Tooth Restorations
    Treatment Planning
    Posterior Restoration
    Anterior Restoration
    Retention
References

Patients who present for implant prosthodontic restorations will require three types of restorations as it relates to the support provided by the implants: implant to implant, implant to tooth, and single implants (Fig. 12–1). Although there are general principles that apply to all of these patients, the patient requiring a single-implant restoration has unique conditions and is addressed separately at the end of this chapter.

CLINICAL AND BIOMECHANICAL CONSIDERAIONS

Hard Tissue Factors

The type of bone available determines the quality of support available. Maxillary and mandibular bone density and type have been classified by various authors[30] and include the following classification:

1. The entire jaw is composed of homogeneous compact bone.
2. A thick layer of compact bone surrounds a core of dense trabecular bone.
3. A thin layer of cortical bone surrounds a core of dense trabecular bone of favorable strength.
4. A thin layer of cortical bone surrounds a core of low-density trabecular bone.

Based on this classification, the most dense and favorable bone is generally found in the symphysis of the mandible. The posterior mandible and anterior and posterior maxilla generally have less favorable bone. The bone in these areas is generally composed of various combinations of cortical bone.[36] Therefore, alternative treatment plans should be considered that may change the site and number of implants used. An example of this is finding less desirable bone at the time of implant placement and increasing the number of implants to reduce the load on the individual implants.[42]

There are sophisticated radiologic methods for

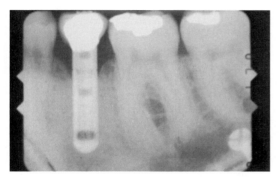

Figure 12–1. Periapical radiograph demonstrating single-implant restoration.

determining the density of bone.[1, 21, 27, 29, 37, 40, 49, 50, 57] In addition, a valuable method of determining the quality of the bone density is the visual assessment made at the time of drilling the bone for implant placement. Unfortunately this assessment is done after the treatment plan has been finalized. It is possible, however, to alter the treatment plan based on this assessment if close communication exists between the surgeon and restorative dentist.

The support of facial structures is also of major concern. Although this may not be a problem in the partially edentulous patient who has remaining anterior teeth, it may present a problem for those patients who have been edentulous in the maxillary anterior zone for some time. In these individuals, the resorptive process is advanced, so the implant is placed much more superiorly and palatally than the original dentition. This leads to a poor aesthetic result from lack of lip support. It may be necessary to graft the deficit area to place the implant in a more desirable position not only to improve the support of facial tissues, but also to bring the residual alveolar ridge to a more normal appearance and enhance the aesthetic result.[60]

Soft Tissue Factors

The quality and quantity of soft tissue at the site of implant placement must be evaluated. The soft tissue must be capable of withstanding the techniques used in completing the prosthesis and the rigors of maintaining the oral hygiene around the implants. Keratinized, fixed gingival tissues are the most desirable.[8] It is desirable to have a minimum of 1 mm of keratinized tissue around natural dentition. Around implants, however, there should be a minimum of 2 mm of keratinized tissue.[2] Long-standing edentulous

spaces may not have adequate quality or quantity of soft tissue. In these cases, it may be necessary to graft more desirable soft tissue to the area. This is particularly true in the posterior mandible, where movable mucosal tissue is often present.

The quantity of tissue at the implant site also deserves close attention. If implants are placed in thick soft tissue, excessive pockets may result around the abutments. This leads to the patient having increased difficulty in complying with hygiene measures. The tissues should be thinned at the time of implant exposure and the placement of the temporary healing cuffs.

The smile line is thought of in terms of anterior maxillary restorations (Fig. 12–2). It may play a role in restorations completed on the mandible as well. It is well to think of the aesthetic zone as encompassing the dentition from the first premolar on one side to the first premolar on the opposite side of the same arch. This ensures that aesthetic requirements can be more easily achieved and provide a wider range for developing proper tooth shape and size to establish an aesthetic result.[34]

Spacing of Implants

The main goal in spacing the implants is to place the greatest number of implants that can be accommodated into the edentulous area without compromising the viability of the remaining bone (Fig. 12–3). The implants should be spaced so that they emerge through the central fossa of posterior teeth and not through the embrasures of the restoration (Fig. 12–4). This is often difficult to accomplish. A diagnostic wax-up can be

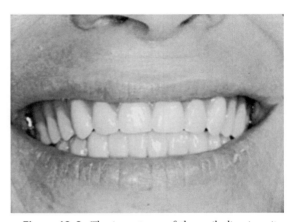

Figure 12–2. The importance of the smile line is quite evident in this illustration.

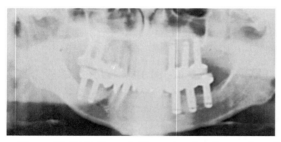

Figure 12–3. Radiograph illustrating that the number of implants varies depending on the site of placement and bone available.

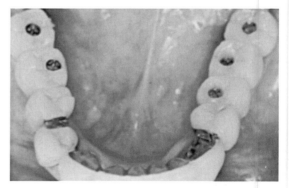

Figure 12–5. Three-unit restoration supported by two implants and attached to a natural tooth on the left. Four-unit restoration supported by three implants and attached to natural tooth on the right.

invaluable in disclosing this problem and the compromise in aesthetics that can result.

Number of Implants

The number of implants required for a fixed restoration depends on the length of the span, the location of the span in the arch, and whether the implants are to be placed in the maxilla or mandible.[24] In general, the following rules can be used to determine the number of implants required: Two implants can support a three-unit freestanding restoration in the mandible. One implant attached to a sound natural tooth can support a two-unit restoration in the mandible.[41] Multiples of these different types of support can be used for larger restorations (Fig. 12–5). In the maxilla, every effort should be made to maximize the number of implants because of variances of the density of bone at different sites. A minimum of six implants should be used in the edentulous maxilla to support a totally implant-borne restoration.

Connection to Teeth

As a result of the differences in which implants and teeth are anchored to bone, a great deal of

controversy exists whether implants should be attached to teeth. It has been stated that because of the immobility of the implant, it may cause disuse atrophy of the periodontal ligament when an implant is rigidly attached to a tooth.[53] To avoid this problem, mobile elements have been incorporated into some implant systems to allow the tooth to move within its periodontal ligament when rigidly attached to an implant. These have taken the form of resilient intramobile elements, flexible gold screws, and semiprecision attachments. Unfortunately the use of attachments has led to reports of intrusion of the tooth attached to an implant.

There is little research to guide the clinician in resolving this problem. Some basic concepts can be distilled from the knowledge that is known. It is best not to attach implant-supported prostheses to the natural dentition.[44] When possible, the number of implants placed should be increased to make the restoration completely implant borne. When sufficient implants cannot be

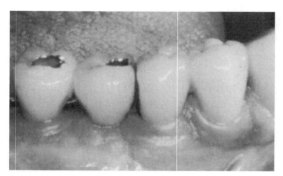

Figure 12–4. Emergence of screws through central fossae of posterior teeth restoration.

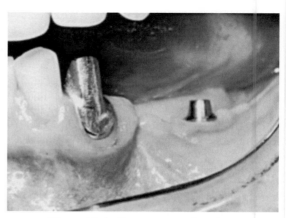

Figure 12–6. Coping cemented in place.

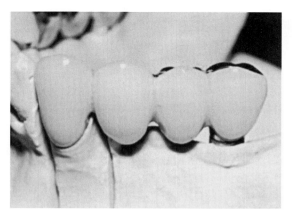

Figure 12–7. A retrievable restoration supported by one implant and a natural tooth restored with a coping and a telescopic crown.

Table 12–1. Surface Area of Implants

Implant (Cylinder)	Implant Length (mm)	Surface Area (mm²)
3.25 mm	8	88.4
	10	109.7
	13	140.0
	15	160.6
	18	192.2
4.0 mm	8	112.9
	10	138.1
	13	174.8
	15	200.0
	18	238.7

Calcitek Technical Product Manual. Calcitek, Inc, Carlsbad, CA. (Copyright material reprinted courtesy of Calcitek.]

placed and the prosthesis must be attached to the natural dentition, it is best to use a rigid, precision attachment to avoid rotational and uneven forces. Alternatively, copings can be cemented to the natural tooth. A prosthesis retained by screws to the implant and with a telescopic crown cemented to the coping can be fabricated (Figs. 12–6 and 12–7).

Crown-to-Root Ratio

Guidelines have been developed to determine the loading that can be placed on the natural dentition when supporting fixed restorations. Attempts have been made to correlate the surface area in contact with bone in implants and natural teeth (Tables 12–1 and 12–2). These have been imprecise owing to the various morphologic designs used in the implant systems. It is also difficult to evaluate the differences in the manner in which bone "attaches" to the various surfaces used on implants.

Shorter implants have a higher rate of loss than longer ones of the same type.[5, 48] The diameter of the implant seems to play a lesser role than the length of the implant in assessing the implant's ability to sustain the added load of a fixed restoration. Therefore the use of the longest implant possible should be the goal in selecting an implant (Fig. 12–8). Restorations supported by multiple implants fare better than those supported by fewer implants.

Implant Orientation

The orientation of the implants in the edentulous space plays an important role in controlling the forces placed on the implant-bone interface. Optimum orientation provides for the forces on the implant to be directed along its long axis. Any deviation from this optimum orientation results in a variety of unfavorable sequelae. Lateral forces are increased, resulting in a tilting force

Table 12–2. Root Surface Area of Teeth

Tooth	Maxillary Surface Area (mm²)	Ranking	Mandibular Surface Area (mm²)	Ranking
Central	204	6	154	7
Lateral	179	7	168	6
Canine	273	3	268	3
First premolar	234	4	180	5
Second premolar	220	5	207	4
First molar	433	1	431	1
Second molar	431	2	426	2

From Jepsen A: Root surface measurement and a method for x-ray determination of root surface area. Acta Odont Scand 21:35–46, 1963. By permission of Scandinavian University Press.

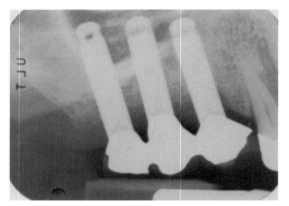

Figure 12–8. Bone grafting to the sinus allows for the use of the longest implant possible to improve the crown-to-root ratio.

on the implants. Decentralizing of the occlusal loading leads to mesial or distal forces, particularly when a cantilever design is used.

To minimize the problems associated with implant orientation, it is recommended that the occlusal table be narrowed. This eliminates or minimizes the length of the lever arm of lateral force. Implants should not be placed in a straight line. Implants should be placed to maximize a tripodal support for the restoration.[13] Excessively long implant crowns should be avoided, and splinting of these should be considered if long crown length cannot be avoided. The number of implants should be maximized to reduce the per unit load of the individual implants.

RETRIEVABLE OR CEMENTABLE RESTORATION

The restorative dentist must decide whether a retrievable or nonretrievable restoration is to be

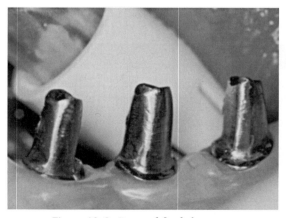

Figure 12–9. Prepared fixed abutments.

fabricated (Figs. 12–9, 12–10, 12–11). There are advantages and disadvantages to either selection.

The disadvantages of a retrievable restoration include the following:

1. There is an increase in the number of components required to fabricate the restoration.
2. The restoration is more complex to fabricate and therefore more costly.
3. It is often more bulky and therefore may interfere with the aesthetic results.
4. The opening for the retentive screw may also interfere with the aesthetic result.
5. Owing to the bulk required for attachments and other components, it may also compromise the contours of the crowns and pontics.
6. Compromised contours of the restoration may hinder the ability to have open embrasures to allow easy access for cleaning.
7. Extra components are required for temporization.
8. Loosening of the retentive screw may result in loss of components and damage to the implants.

The advantages of the retrievable restoration are primarily those of convenience and include:

1. The components can be easily replaced if they fail.
2. The evaluation of the soft tissue around the implants can be done more easily if the prosthesis is removable.
3. The evaluation of the implants is accomplished more accurately if the restoration is removable. The implants can be evaluated as freestanding units rather than as ones that are splinted to a tooth or other implant.
4. Repair or modification of the restoration can be easily accomplished.
5. Cleaning of the restoration can be done on a periodic basis.

The cemented restoration has the following advantages:

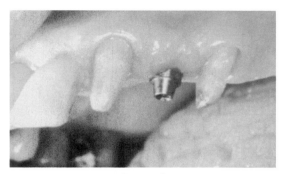

Figure 12–10. Use of an implant as a pier pontic in a retrievable four-unit restoration.

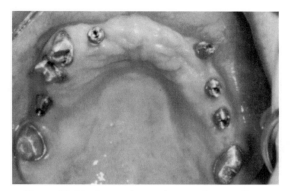

Figure 12–11. Intraoral view showing the use of copings on natural teeth combined with implants to support a retrievable restoration.

1. Fewer components are required.
2. It is a familiar type of procedure for both the dentist and the laboratory technician.
3. Because the bulk can be more favorably managed, it is easier to accomplish aesthetic restorations.
4. Minor divergences of the implants are easily corrected in preparation of the abutments.
5. The restoration can be made retrievable by the use of temporary cement.
6. Temporization can be accomplished in a traditional manner.

The disadvantages to cemented restorations include the following:

1. Grinding of a metal abutment is necessary to obtain a proper preparation.
2. The prepared abutments are generally small and difficult to transfer in the form of a cast.
3. Gingival retraction is required to reproduce accurately the subgingival margins of the preparation.
4. It is not possible to evaluate the implants as freestanding units.
5. Temporary cements may wash out, leading to a foul taste or smell.
6. Temporary cements have been unpredictable in terms of longevity.

The restorative dentist must carefully weigh the advantages and disadvantages of the different methods of retaining a restoration. The considerations listed here must be evaluated based on the patient's needs and the ability to fabricate an aesthetic and functional prosthesis. Improvements in the prosthetic components add greatly

in the restorative dentist's ability to deliver this type of restoration. An example of this is the improvement in the machining of components, which has lessened the loosening of restorations retained by screws.

PROVISIONAL OR TEMPORARY RESTORATIONS

Before fabrication of the final restoration, it is well to consider the fabrication of the provisional or temporary restoration.[11, 13, 59, 61] Provisional restorations allow a period to finalize the definitive prosthesis (Figs. 12–12 and 12–13). An additional advantage is the ability to refine aesthetics and the final form of the restoration. Transitional restorations fabricated of acrylic resin are easily modified to address the factors encountered in aesthetics, occlusion, and cleansability. To gain the patient's cooperation, it is important that the patient understand the rationale for the use of

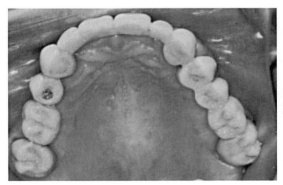

Figure 12–12. Occlusal view of completed provisional restoration.

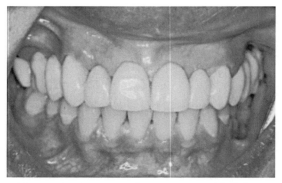

Figure 12–13. Provisional restoration modified for aesthetics and tissue health.

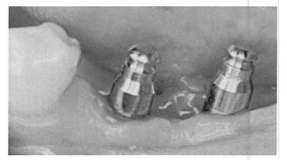

Figure 12–14. Transfer copings screwed to implant abutment heads.

provisional restorations in achieving the best definitive restoration possible.

Transitional loading[35] and *provisional loading*[7] are both used in the dental literature to describe the placement of an increasing load on the implants before final placement of the definitive prosthesis. Transitional loading has been advocated as a means of allowing the implant to achieve osseointegration and maturation of the bone around the implant without undue trauma during early bone adaptation to the implant. There seem to be advantages to this viewpoint despite the fact that there is little research on the role of progressive loading as it affects the long-term survival of the implants.[14, 47]

FABRICATION OF RESTORATIONS

Impressions

A primary concern when dealing with implant restorations is the accurate transfer of the relationship of the implants and/or any remaining dentition to a master cast. Several options exist when dealing with impressions in implant prosthodontics. The implant analogs or the abutment analogs may be transferred to the master cast. An impression may be made of the prepared implant abutments and these are reproduced in the master cast. Each of these options requires careful consideration in the choice of the impression material and the technique used.

The transfer of components requires the use of an impression material that is resilient enough to spring out of the undercuts encountered and stiff enough to allow for the accurate seating of the components into the impression. The material should also prevent any dislodging of the

components during the pouring of the impression. The replication of the prepared abutments in the master cast requires a material that is of sufficient flexibility to spring over the delicate prepared abutments. The smallness of the prepared abutments may also require the use of alternate materials in pouring the master cast to avoid fracture of the stone.

The addition-type of polysiloxanes, polyethers, and rubber base impression materials have all been used successfully. In general, the impression materials that use a putty-like heavy body component and a less viscous wash material are preferred. This allows for the less viscous material to be injected around the abutments without incorporating air bubbles and allows for the seating of the heavy body material to give added rigidity to the impression to receive the transfer components.

Transfer Systems

There are two transfer systems that are used in implant dentistry. The first transfers an abutment head analog, and the second transfers an implant analog to the master cast. Each implant system

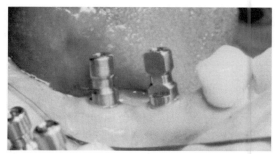

Figure 12–15. Impression posts screwed directly to implants.

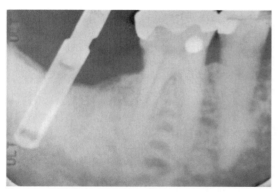

Figure 12–16. Radiograph illustrating proper seating of the impression post on an implant.

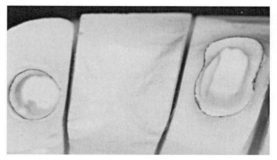

Figure 12–18. Stone cast of prepared abutment and crown preparation.

has its own method of accomplishing these transfers (Figs. 12–14 and 12–15).

All implant systems, however, require that the transfer be accomplished in the most accurate method to ensure an accurate fit of the prosthesis to the implants. Earlier systems used copings resting on abutment heads to accomplish this transfer. Because the impression techniques involved blindly seating the impression tray with impression material, it was possible that the transfer copings could be disturbed, producing an inaccurate impression. Newer systems rely on threaded transfer copings that screw onto the appropriate abutment head or impression posts that screw directly to the implant. Some systems use a coping or impression post without threads, but use a screw to fasten these to the abutment heads or implant body. A flush fit between the transfer component and the abutment head or implant is necessary in either method (Fig. 12–16). The same transfer component is then placed over an abutment head analog or implant analog, and this is securely seated into the impression.

The different transfer systems do require their own special impression techniques.[3, 12, 20, 52]

The threaded transfer copings use an impression of the transfer coping on the abutment head (see Fig. 12–14). The transfer coping is then removed from the abutment head and threaded onto the abutment head analog. The analog-transfer coping complex is then firmly seated into the impression and the cast poured. The transfer copings that are retained with separate screws require the use of an open window in the impression tray to allow for removal of the retaining screw, allowing the transfer coping that is incorporated into the impression to be removed from the mouth.

Abutment heads that are used for prostheses that will be cemented into place can also be transferred if they are not altered in any way. If the abutment heads are altered, they are managed as a prepared tooth abutment. These are reproduced in stone or other suitable material on the master cast (Figs. 12–17 to 12–19).

Most of the systems provide for an alternative method of developing an accurate master cast. In this method, the position of the implants rather than the abutment heads is transferred to the master cast. An impression post is used for

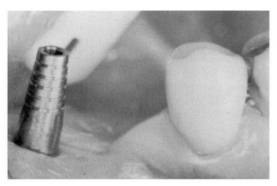

Figure 12–17. Abutment head screwed to place. An impression is made and the abutment head prepared in the laboratory.

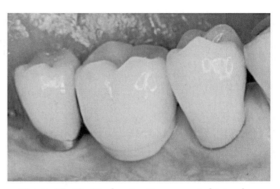

Figure 12–19. Final restoration cemented into place.

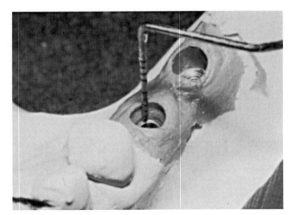

Figure 12–20. Master cast with gingival tissues reproduced in resilient material allowing for proper abutment head selection.

this purpose. Instead of attaching to the abutment head, the impression post is secured to the body of the implant itself. After making the impression, the impression post is removed from the implant intraorally and secured to an implant body analog. This implant body analog–impression post complex is then securely seated in the impression and a cast poured in dental stone. These impression posts must allow for the same orientation of the implant-abutment orally and on the master cast.

Techniques have been described that allow the soft tissue aspects of the cast around the implants to be reproduced in a resilient material (Fig. 12–20). This allows for better managing of the aesthetic requirements because the areas of the cast can accommodate the placement of the abutment heads in the laboratory without having to remove the stone in this area. This is a particularly useful system when there is any doubt about the final selection of the abutment heads to be used. It also allows selection of the abutment heads in the laboratory phase. This method is also required when abutment heads are to be prepared or modified. The preparation should *not* be done with the abutment heads attached to the implants in the mouth. There is danger of heat buildup, which can damage the implant-bone interface. The drill may also cause undue vibrations, which may lead to damage at the bone-implant interface.

LABORATORY CONSIDERATIONS
Infection Control Procedures

Infection control requires the restorative dentist to be knowledgeable concerning these proce-

dures and what effect they may have on the dental materials used. The laboratory technician must also comply with the standards in using different chemical agents not only to protect the laboratory personnel, but also to avoid damage to the impression materials.[17, 38]

General Considerations

Before pouring the impression the technician must verify that the implant components are properly seated in the impression. The impression is then boxed and poured in a suitable material. It has been previously discussed that the choice of material depends on the individual requirements of the restorative dentist The material most frequently chosen is improved dental stone. Alternate materials include resilient material used to replicate the gingival tissues around the implant–abutment head complex or the epoxy resin used in replication of prepared abutments with the remaining cast reproduced in dental stone.

The restorative dentist must understand the laboratory procedures involved in fabricating an implant prosthesis, and the laboratory technician must understand the needs of the restorative dentist and the patient. Although many dentists generally use only a limited number of implant systems in their practice, the laboratory technician is faced with a wider spectrum of systems to satisfy the needs of dentists. Unless the laboratory consists of several individuals, it is impossible for a single technician to have in-depth knowledge of all systems in use today. It is incumbent on the restorative dentist to select the laboratory with expertise in the system that is being used.

Abutment Head Selection

Examination of the mounted master cast in the laboratory may reveal that a suitable restoration cannot be fabricated owing to malalignment of the abutment heads or insufficient interocclusal space. If the master cast reproduces the abutment heads or prepared abutments, the only solution is to change the abutments intraorally or reprepare the abutments and make a new impression. If the cast reproduces the implants in the form of implant analogs, however, the abutments can be changed in the laboratory to correct for discrepancies (Fig. 12–21).

The use of angled abutments is particularly helpful in correcting implants that are mal-

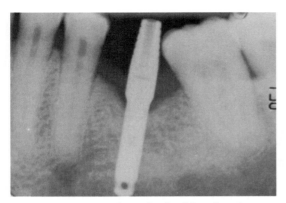

Figure 12–21. Radiograph of malaligned implant.

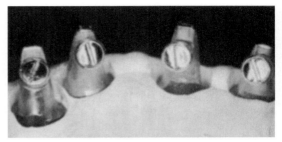

Figure 12–23. Customized preangled abutments with lingual accessory screw holes.

aligned.[16] Additionally the angled abutments lead to a restoration that can be designed to ensure optimum hygiene maintenance, prevent screw emergence in undesirable areas of the restoration, and provide for proper tooth form and improved aesthetics (Fig. 12–22).

If the implant system components cannot correct the problem, consideration must be given to custom abutments. These include modification of components by grinding, customized preangled abutments, or mesiostructures. The retention of the restoration can be obtained by the use of accessory screws or temporary cement (Figs. 12–23 and 12–24).

Although every effort should be made to restore the implants that are in place, it must be emphasized that the use of the described alternate abutments may lead to increased loading of the implants. The forces are not directed along the long axis of the implants, and lateral forces are increased.

Metal Framework Considerations

The major consideration in the laboratory is the fabrication of an accurately fitting metal superstructure. This may be a structure to support an overdenture, hybrid prosthesis, or a fixed restoration. The metal structure must have a passive fit over the abutment analogs.[58] This means that the framework must not depend on excessive force to allow for full seating. Excessive forces exerted either by screws in a retrievable prosthesis or by biting forces in the case of cementing procedure place the implants in a continual stress-bearing situation. If this stress is beyond the ability of the bone to react to stress, failure results. Because this force is extremely difficult to measure in a clinical setting, it is important that passive seating be achieved.

The framework for a fixed restoration should provide open embrasures to allow access to the gingival margin for cleaning of the area (Fig. 12–25). The connections, whether solder joints or attachments, must be kept as close to the occlusal table as possible to allow easy access for maintenance of the gingival tissues. Although this is more easily accomplished in the posterior quadrants, it becomes more difficult in the aesthetic zone, where emergent profile of the restoration is important in meeting cosmetic demands. In this area, the use of impressions where the implant position is transferred to the master cast by the use of implant analogs can be most

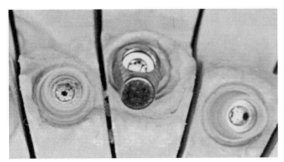

Figure 12–22. Angled abutment head. This can be screwed directly to an implant to correct for malalignment of the implant.

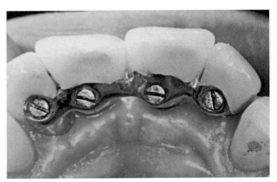

Figure 12–24. Restoration screwed to position with lingual screws.

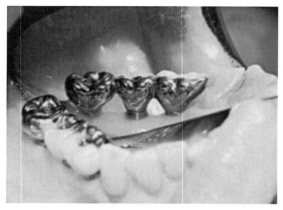

Figure 12–25. Restoration in place demonstrating easy access to implant–soft tissue interface.

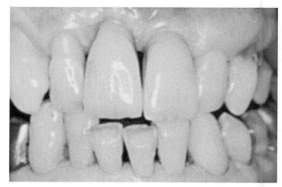

Figure 12–27. Clinical view of completed restoration demonstrated in Figure 12–26.

useful. This allows for more options in selecting the most suitable type of abutment head or other restorative components.

Aesthetic Considerations

Components are available that allow the restoration to connect directly to the implant body itself rather than to an abutment. This means that the technician can better control emergent profile because the restoration can be shaped from the implant, which is generally subgingivally, rather than from the abutment head, which may prevent proper contouring and gingival adaptation (Figs. 12–26 to 12–28).

In the posterior quadrants, experience has shown that it is best to place the margins of the restoration supragingivally and design the prostheses to allow for cleansability at the gingival area. This must be done with great care so as not to interfere with aesthetics along the buccal corridor. It is generally easier to comply with aesthetic requirements if this accessibility to the gingival area is accomplished on the lingual of mandibular restorations and on the palatal of maxillary restorations.

Loading Forces

It is a misconception to perceive the implant buried in a solid medium with 100% contact between the implant and the bone. Block et al[9] and others[18, 46, 51] have demonstrated varied amounts of bone contact depending on the site, shape, surface characteristics, and time the implant has been in place. Therefore the occlusion must be developed as described in Chapter 13.

SINGLE-TOOTH RESTORATIONS

Treatment Planning

Single-tooth restorations are often required in patients with congenitally missing teeth or those

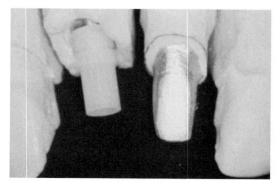

Figure 12–26. Direct connection of restoration to implant does allow an improved emergent profile.

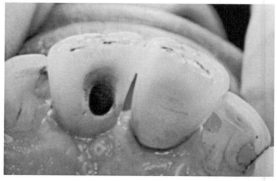

Figure 12–28. Emergent profile of restoration in place.

patients who have lost a tooth owing to trauma or dental disease.[50] The primary concern in these patients is the condition of the hard and soft tissues.[22, 55, 56]

The bone height, width, and form must be evaluated. These determine the direction of the long axis of the implant. The residual alveolar ridges have been classified as to bone width and height (Table 12–3).[5]

The long axis of the implant must be directed toward the cingulum area of an anterior tooth and the central fossa of a posterior tooth. This prevents weakening the incisal edge of the restoration and avoids overcontours of the crown (Fig. 12–28).

In the anterior area when viewed from the frontal plane, there must be at least 1 mm of bone between the implant and the adjacent teeth. The long axis of the implant must be placed in harmony with the long axis of the roots of the remaining teeth to achieve the proper long axis orientation in this plane.

In the horizontal plane, sufficient soft tissue must exist to achieve a natural-appearing emergent profile. This generall requires a depth of 2 to 4 mm of soft tissue over the implant. A close look at the cementoenamel junction of the adjacent teeth as well as the gingival margin of the adjacent teeth is a guide that can be used to determine the depth of soft tissue required.

In patients with congenitally missing teeth, the bone is often inadequate. If the defect is significant as a result of a congenital defect or trauma, the restoration will be more difficult to fabricate. The dimensions of the alveolar bone are affected, and the placement of the implant is compromised unless grafting to the area is done first. Scarring of the soft tissues can be a significant finding after repairs of congenital defects (cleft palate), thus affecting the aesthetic result owing to improper soft tissue contours and depth resulting in a less than desirable emergent profile of the restoration.

It is important to accomplish the grafting of bone, alloplastic materials, and/or soft tissues before the placement of the implant. This allows the restorative dentist the opportunity to deal with the conditions as they exist, rather than

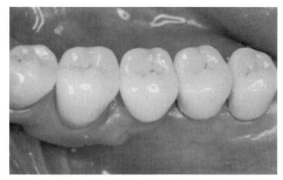

Figure 12–29. Narrowing of occlusal surface on implant-borne restoration to diminish lateral forces on the implants.

trying to improve conditions after implant placement. A complete treatment plan and work-up must be accomplished to establish whether a single implant can support the intended prosthesis.

Posterior Restoration

In cases of a single-tooth restoration replacing a posterior tooth, it is difficult to control the occlusal morphology because it must conform to the adjacent teeth (Fig. 12–29). This may result in a single implant being placed in an edentulous space measuring more than 12 mm in length and can lead to overloading the single-tooth restoration (Fig. 12–30).[23, 25] If the implant is not placed in the center of the edentulous space, cantilever forces can be generated, resulting in increased loading of the implant. Another factor that affects long-term success is the use of short (less than 10 mm) implants. This is particularly encountered more frequently in the posterior maxilla,

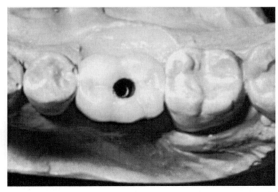

Figure 12–30. Single-tooth posterior restoration. The occlusal anatomy corresponds to the adjacent natural dentition.

Table 12–3. Bone Quantity		
Type of Ridge	**Width**	**Height**
1	>5 mm	>10 mm
2	>4–5 mm	8–10 mm
3	<4 mm	<8 mm

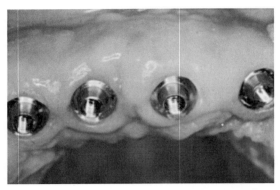

Figure 12–31. The width of the edentulous space determines the number of implants that can be placed.

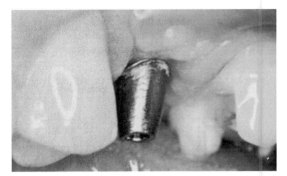

Figure 12–33. Prepared abutment head.

where the floor of the maxillary sinus may encroach on the residual alveolar ridge.

The single posterior implant restoration should rely on the adjacent posterior natural dentition to prevent excessive loading.[4, 6, 15, 19, 43, 45] After careful study it may be found that the space is long enough for the placement of two implants rather than a single implant. Although the occlusal morphology may be compromised, the added support enhances the long-term success. When large restorations have been placed on single implants, fracture of the implant or abutment components has been observed.

Anterior Restoration

The smile line is a consideration that must not be ignored. This determines the amount of tooth structure that will be exposed. It plays a dominant role in the gingival area of a restoration. Although a person with a high smile line demands greater efforts in achieving the proper emergent profile and contouring of the gingival

portion of the restoration, the person with a low smile line must not be denied the best efforts possible. Patients may not always view their dentition under what may be considered normal conditions.

In the anterior aesthetic zone, the width of the space influences the final aesthetic result (Figs. 12–31 and 12–32).[39] It is common to see the adjacent teeth move into the space, making it impossible to achieve the proper dimensions to the restorations. Orthodontic therapy may have to be considered before implant placement. The same is true for spaces that may be of excessive width. Attempting to place a restoration in a large space results in a restoration that is wide and not in harmony with the adjacent or paired tooth.

The following observations can aid in determining the mesiodistal dimensions required for anterior tooth replacement. If a 4-mm diameter implant is used and the separation from the adjacent teeth is maintained at 1.5 mm on either side, it is evident that a 7-mm space must exist for implant placement. If a smaller diameter im-

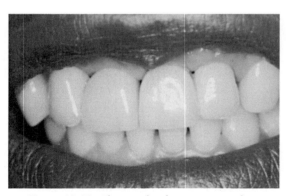

Figure 12–32. The completed restoration in place.

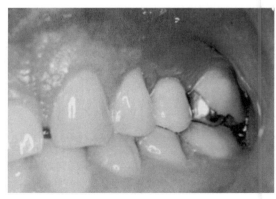

Figure 12–34. Restoration in place on implant in second bicuspid position.

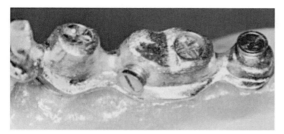

Figure 12–35. Mesiostructure attached to abutments on malplaced implants allowing for placement of retaining screws for the restoration in proper position. Note lingual screw in first molar position.

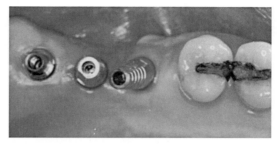

Figure 12–37. Occlusal view demonstrating malaligned implants.

plant is used, such as 3.15 mm, a 6.25-mm space is required.

To improve the aesthetic and functional results, several options are available to replace the conventional abutment heads. The fabrication of crowns on components that are retained directly to the implant rather than an abutment head enables the laboratory technician to achieve a more normal-appearing emergent profile.[31, 32] These have taken the form of castable plastic components as well as machined metal copings and sintered ceramic abutments. The fit of machined metal parts is more accurate than that of cast parts. This may be a critical concern in single-tooth restorations owing to the requirement of a nonrotational restoration. The nonrotational design varies among the different implant systems, but is generally achieved by the use of an opposing male and female geometric design in the implant and the joined component.

These components allow the contour of the crown to begin within the gingival sulcus and not supragingivally as might occur with a conventional abutment head. The use of porcelain abutments to which porcelain can be directly added has also led to improved aesthetic restorations.

Retention

There are basically two methods of retaining the single-tooth restoration to the implants (Figs. 12–33 and 12–34). The restorations either can be made retrievable[33] or cemented onto the implant. Each has advantages and disadvantages as already discussed. In the aesthetic zone it means that the placement of the implant must be carefully controlled. An implant just a millimeter or two out of the planned alignment may prevent realizing the desired result. The angulation of the implant is also important. A malaligned implant may prevent placement of a retrievable prosthesis owing to the location of the retaining screw. Although several options are available to correct for the misplacement of the implants,[26, 39, 54] a careful assessment by both the surgeon and the prosthodontist before placement of the implants diminishes the need for these improvisations. The positioning of implants in other than ideal conditions may be accepted, but this should be determined before placement of the implants (Figs. 12–35 through 12–39). This information can be imparted to the patient, and the anticipated aesthetic result can be demonstrated.

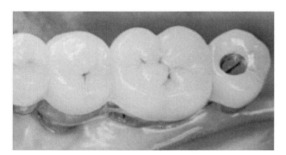

Figure 12–36. Restoration seated over mesiostructure shown in Figure 12–35.

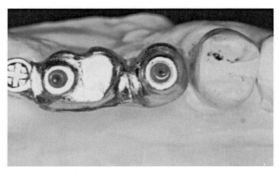

Figure 12–38. Restoration framework seated over mesiostructure.

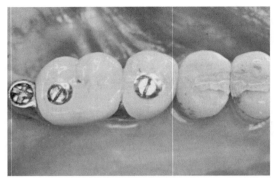

Figure 12–39. Occlusal view of completed restoration in place.

References

1. Abrahams JJ: The role of diagnostic imaging in dental implantology. Radiol Clin North Am 31:163–180, 1993.
2. Artzi Z, Tal H, Moses O, Kozlovsky A: Mucosal considerations for osseointegrated implants. J Prosthet Dent 70: 427–432, 1993.
3. Assif D, Fenton A, Zarb G, Schmitt A: Comparative accuracy of implant impression procedures. Int J Periodont Restor Dent 12:113–121, 1992.
4. Astrand P, et al: Combination of natural teeth and osseointegrated implants as prosthesis abutments: A 2-year longitudinal study. Int J Oral Maxillofac Impl 6:305–312, 1991.
5. Bahat O: Treatment planning and placement of implants in the posterior maxillae: Report of 732 consecutive Nobelpharma implants. Int J Oral Maxillofac Impl 8:151–161, 1993.
6. Balshi TJ: Preventing and resolving complications with osseointegrated implants. Dent Clin North Am 33:821–867, 1989.
7. Binon P, Sullivan D: Provisional fixed restorations technique for osseointegrated implants. CDA J 18:28–30, 1990.
8. Block MS, Kent JN: Factors associated with soft- and hard-tissue compromise endosseous implants. J Oral Maxillofac Surg 48:1153–1160, 1990.
9. Block MS, Kent JN, Kay JF: Evaluation of HA-coated titanium dental implants. J Oral Maxillofac Surg 45:601–607, 1987.
10. Brunski JB, Skalak R: Biomechanical considerations. In Worthington P, Brånemark P-I (eds): Advanced Osseointegration Surgery. London, Quintessence Publishing, 1992, pp 15–39.
11. Callan DP, Strong SM: Immediate aesthetic provisionalization for the dental implant patient. Pract Periodont Aesthet Dent 3:17–21, 1991.
12. Carr AB: A comparison of impression techniques for a five implant mandibular model. Int J Oral Maxillofac Impl 6:448–455, 1991.
13. Chiche GJ, Pinault A, Weaver C, Finger I: Adapting fixed prosthodontics principles to screw-retained restorations. Int J Prosthodont 2:317–322, 1989.
14. Currey JD: The Mechanical Adaptations of Bones. Princeton, Princeton University Press, 1984.
15. Ericsson I, et al: A clinical evaluation of fixed-bridge restorations supported by the combination of teeth and osseointegrated titanium implants. J Ging Periodontol 13:307–312, 1986.
16. Gelb DA, Lazzara RJ: Hierarchy of objectives in implant placement to maximize esthetics: Use of pre-angulated abutments. Int J Periodont Restor Dent 13:277–287, 1993.
17. Giblin J, Podesta R, White J: Dimensional stability of impression materials immersed in an iodophor disinfectant. Int J Prosthodont 3:72–77, 1990.
18. Gottlander M, Albrektsson T: Histomorphometric studies of hydroxylapatite-coated and uncoated CP titanium threaded implants in bone. Int J Oral Maxillofac Impl 6:399–404, 1991.
19. Gunne J, Astrand P, Ahlen K, Borg K, Olsson M: Implants in partially edentulous patients. A longitudinal study of bridges supported by both implants and natural teeth. Clin Oral Impl Res 3:49–56, 1992.
20. Inturregui JA, et al: Evaluation of three impression techniques for osseointegrated implants. J Prosthet Dent 69:503–509, 1993.
21. Jeffcoat MK: Digital radiology for implant treatment planning and evaluation. Dentomaxillofac Radiol 21:203–207, 1992.
22. Jemt T, Lekholm U, Adell R: Osseointegrated implants in the treatment of partially edentulous patients: A preliminary study on 876 consecutively placed fixtures. Int J Oral Maxillofac Impl 4:211–217, 1989.
23. Jemt T, et al: Osseointegrated implants for single tooth replacement: A 1-year report from a multicenter prospective study. Int J Oral Maxillofac Impl 6:29–36, 1991.
24. Jensen O: The classification of the osseointegrated implant. J Prosthet Dent 61:228–234, 1989.
25. Jorneus L, Jemt T, Carlsson L: Loads and designs of screw joints for single crowns supported by osseointegrated implants. Int J Oral Maxillofac Impl 7:353–359, 1992.
26. Kallas T, et al: Clinical evaluation of angulated abutments for the Brånemark system: A pilot study. Int J Oral Maxillofac Impl 5:39–45, 1990.
27. Kattapuram SV, Lodwick GS, Chandler H, Khurana JS, Ehara S, Rosenthal DI: Porous-coated anatomic total hip prostheses: Radiographic analysis and clinical correlation. Radiology 174 (Pt 1):861–864, 1990.
28. Keller EE, Tolman DE, Brånemark P-I: Surgical reconstruction of advanced maxillary resorption with composite grafts. In Worthington P, Brånemark P-I: Advanced Osseointegration Surgery. Chicago, Quintessence, 1992, pp 146–161.
29. Kraut RA: Utilization of 3D/Dental software for precise implant site selection: clinical reports. Implant Dent 1:134–139, 1992.
30. Lekholm V, Zarb GA: Patient selection and preparation. In Brånemark P-I, Zarb G, Albrektsson TA (eds): Tissue Integrated Prostheses. Chicago, Quintessence, 1985, pp 199–209.
31. Lewis S: An esthetic titanium abutment: Report of a technique. Int J Oral Maxillofac Impl 6:195–201, 1991.
32. Lewis S, et al: The "UCLA" abutment. Int J Oral Maxillofac Impl 3:183–189, 1988.
33. Lewis SG, et al: Single tooth implant supported restorations. Int J Oral Maxillofac Impl 3:25–30, 1988.
34. Miller CJ: The smile line as a guide to anterior esthetics. Dent Clin North Am 33:157–164, 1989.
35. Misch CE: Density of bone: Effect on treatment plans, surgical approach, healing, and progressive bone loading. Int J Oral Implantol 6:23–31, 1990.
36. Misch CE: Contemporary Implant Dentistry. St. Louis, CV Mosby, 1993.
37. Nasr HF, Meffert RM: A proposed radiographic index for assessment of the current status of osseointegration. Int J Oral Maxillofac Impl 8:323–328, 1993.

38. Owen CP, Goolam R: Disinfection of impression materials to prevent viral cross contamination: A review and a protocol. Int J Prosthodont 6: 480–494, 1993.
39. Parel SM, Sullivan DY: Esthetics and Osseointegration. Dallas, Taylor Publishing, 1989.
40. Pharoah MJ: Imaging techniques and their clinical significance. Int J Prosthodont 6:176–179, 1993.
41. Rangert B, Gunne J, Sullivan DY: Mechanical aspects of a Brånemark implant connected to a natural tooth: An in vitro study. Int J Oral Maxillofac Impl 6:177–186, 1991.
42. Rangert B, Jemt T, Jörneus L: Forces and moments on Brånemark implants. Int J Oral Maxillofac Impl 4:241–247, 1989.
43. Rangert B, Gunne J, Sullivan DY: Mechanical aspects of a Brånemark implant connected to a natural tooth: An in vitro study. Int J Oral Maxillofac Impl 6:177–186, 1991.
44. Rieder C, Parel S: A survey of natural tooth abutment intrusion with implant-connected fixed partial dentures. Int J Periodont Restor Dent 13:334–347, 1983.
45. Rigdon TF: Retrievable/fixed prosthetics for implant and natural dentitions. Int J Oral Implantol 8:59–62, 1991.
46. Roberts WE, Garetto LP, DeCastro RA: Remodeling of devitalized bone threatens periosteal margin integrity of endosseous titanium implants with threaded or smooth surfaces: Indications for provisional loading and axially directed occlusion. J Indiana Dent Assoc 68:19–24, 1989.
47. Roberts WE, Smith RK, Zilberman Y, Mozsary PG, Smith RS: Osseous adaptation to continuous loading of rigid endosseous implants. Am J Orthodont 86:95–111, 1984.
48. Saadoun AP, LeGall ML: Clinical results and guidelines on Steri-oss endosseous implants. Int J Periodont Restor Dent 12: 486–495, 1992.
49. Serman NJ: Pitfalls of panoramic radiology in implant surgery. Ann Dent 48:13–16, 1989.
50. Shimura M, et al: Pre-surgical evaluation for dental implant reconstruction: Using computed tomography with a reformatted program. In Babbush CA (ed): Dental Implants: Principles and Practice. Philadelphia, WB Saunders, 1991, pp 43–65.
51. Smith DE: Review of endosseous implants for partially edentulous patients. Int J Prosthodont 11:12–19, 1990.
52. Spector M, Donovan TE, Nicholls JI: An evaluation of impression techniques for osseointegrated implants. J Prosthet Dent 63:444–447, 1990.
53. Takayama H: Biomechanical considerations on osseointegrated implants. In Hobo S, Ichida E, Garcia LT (eds): Osseointegration and Occlusal Rehabilitation. Tokyo, Quintessence, 1990, pp 265–280.
54. ten Bruggenkate CM, Sutter F, Oosterbeek HS, Schroeder A: Indications for angled implants. J Prosthet Dent 67:85–93, 1992.
55. van Steenberghe D: A retrospective multicenter evaluation of the survival rate of osseointegrated fixtures supporting fixed partial prostheses in the treatment of partial edentulism. J Prosthet Dent 61:217–223, 1989.
56. van Steenberghe D et al: The applicability of osseointegrated oral implants in the rehabilitation of partial edentulism: A prospective multicenter study on 558 fixtures. Int J Oral Maxillofac Impl 5:272–281, 1990.
57. Weber HP, Buser D, Fiorellini JP, Williams RC: Radiographic evaluation of crestal bone levels adjacent to nonsubmerged titanium implants. Clin Oral Impl Res 3:181–188, 1992.
58. White GE: Osseointegrated Dental Technology. London, Quintessence Publishing, 1993.
59. White GE: Provisional prostheses. In White GE (ed): Osseointegrated Dental Technology. London, Quintessence Publishing, 1993, pp 47–58.
60. Wilson TG, Weber HP: Classification of and therapy for areas of deficient bony housing prior to dental implant placement. Int J Periodont Restor Dent 13:451–459, 1993.
61. Zarb GA, Harle T, DeGrandmont P, Caro S, Zarb FL: Use of provisional prostheses with osseointegration. Dent Clin North Am 33:323–333, 1989.

Study Questions

1. Classify the bone density and type for the maxilla and the mandible.

2. The number of implants for a patient requiring a fixed prosthesis is determined by which factors?

3. Discuss the advantages and disadvantages of fixed and retrievable fixed restorations.

4. Provisional or temporary restorations are utilized to accomplish what purposes?

5. Discuss single tooth restorations for the anterior maxilla.

6. Discuss single tooth restorations for the posterior mandible and posterior maxilla.

CHAPTER *13*

Development of the Occlusal Scheme in Implant Prosthodontics

Israel M. Finger
Luis R. Guerra
Revised by Luis R. Guerra

Impact Load and Stress Load Transfer
Arch Form
Interarch Distance and Jaw Relationship
Soft Tissue Attachments
Orientation of the Occlusal Plane
Abnormal Mandibular Movements
Condylar Guide Angle and Incisal Guide
    Angle
Phonetics
Rationale for Choice of Occlusal Schemes
Bone Support and Occlusion
Implant Occlusion in the Partially Edentulous
    Patient
Implant Occlusion in the Edentulous Patient
References

The goal of any restorative procedure must include the development of a functional occlusion.[28] Without occlusion receiving the attention required, the restoration may be subjected to abnormal forces and may eventually fail or cause problems with the supporting structures. This is particularly true in implant-supported prostheses.

Occlusion is one of the many factors that affects the long-term prognosis of a dental implant. The literature is replete with successful surgical techniques, including much discussion about implant surface characteristics, bone adaptation to implants, and soft tissue management.[1] Unfortunately the subject of implant-prosthetic occlusion has not received the same amount of research and study.

Levinson[21] has stressed requirements for optimum occlusal form. His primary considerations are (1) stability of the occlusion—to enhance jaw position, (2) distribution of occlusal force along the long axis of the tooth, and (3) freedom in lateral excursions. These observations concur with those of Ismail et al,[17] who added that the width of occlusal table should be narrowed and cusp heights minimized. This decreases lateral stresses to the implant.

There are meaningful differences between

support provided by the periodontal ligament of natural teeth and support provided by ankylosed implants. Not the least of these differences is the lack of proprioception that is normally found around natural teeth. It has been stated that the patient with an implant-supported prosthesis does feel pressure to a varying degree whether it is directed occlusally or laterally. There is not the sense of discrimination, however, as exists in the natural dentition between normal contact and harmful overloading.[18, 23, 27, 33]

IMPACT LOAD AND STRESS LOAD TRANSFER

The disparity between the amount of movement of an implant integrated in bone as compared to a natural tooth suspended in its periodontal ligament is noteworthy.[11] This disparity in the movement between an implant and a natural tooth has led to the development of the concept of stress breaking when attaching an implant to a natural tooth. This lack of mobility of an implant, however, is not absolute. The implant does, in fact, move. The movement depends on the elasticity of the bone in which it rests, and consequently it may well be that implants display varying amounts of mobility.[3] The various degrees of alveolar bone and cancellous bone elasticities may have a profound long-term effect on the survival of root-form implants.

The connection between bone and the integrated implant is relatively stiff, and it has been theorized that overloading of prostheses over implants can cause bony microfractures.[7] Several restorative techniques and materials have been proposed to reduce load on dental implants. Using finite element analysis,[10] the issue of shock absorption has been examined. It has been shown that under impact conditions, which is analogous to the clinical situation of hard objects being inadvertently encountered during mastication, the use of acrylic resin reduces the stress being transmitted to the implant. In 1991, in an in vitro study,[13] it was concluded that a 1.5-mm resin layer reduced the impact force by 57% and 53%, respectively, when compared with an equivalent thickness of porcelain and metal ceramic alloy.

The IMZ implant system uses an intramobile element in the restoration of implants.[19] Although the primary reason for this design was to compensate for the movement of the natural teeth when attached to an implant, it may act as a shock absorber to reduce forces acting on the implant-bone interface. Lacking the proprioception found in the periodontal ligament, it has been suggested that occlusal forces are controlled through neuromuscular mechanisms of the muscles of mastication in patients with implant-borne restorations. There may not be any appreciable difference, however, between maximum occlusal forces exerted in patients with natural dentition and those with implant-borne prostheses.

Occlusal forces in patients with natural dentition have been measured,[14] and these measurements can be used as an indicator of masticatory function.[8, 12] Patients can discern between different biting levels of force. Biting forces in edentulous patients increase when osseointegrated implants are used to support prostheses as compared with complete tissue-borne prostheses. An increase in loading forces has been noted in implant-borne cantilevered prostheses when compared with cantilevered prostheses supported by natural teeth.[22] The proprioceptive periodontal ligament around natural teeth limits destructive forces to the supporting tissues of the natural teeth. What limits destructive forces to the implant-bone interface around implants without this proprioception has yet to be determined or defined.

Attention to the mechanical loading over implants, transmission of the loading to the bone-implant interface tissues, and biologic reactions of interfacial tissue to transmitted loadings must be carefully monitored.[4, 5, 6] The effects of occlusal forces on the anterior mandibular osseointegrated implants have demonstrated that occlusal overloading appears to be the main cause of bone loss around mandibular implants.[24] Computerized models[26, 31] that are able to predict vertical and horizontal forces applied to implant-supported restorations have been developed. These models, however, do not admit to the many variables we see in daily clinical practice, such as bridge design, number of implants at various positions, and the actual in vivo loading of implants.

Various authors[9, 15, 16, 30] have given their guidelines for occlusion over dental implants. Although all appear to agree on a stable posterior occlusion with simultaneous contacts in the centric relation occlusion position, there are no clinical experimental data to substantiate these assumptions. Similar to many authors, they rely on the literature pertaining to the development of occlusion for natural tooth-borne restorations and transpose these principles to develop the occlusion for implant-borne prostheses.

There is insufficient research to support one occlusal concept over another for osseointegrated prostheses. Many of the cited goals, however, are similar: to reduce interfering occlusal contacts and reduce lateral stresses as a means of reducing implant-to-bone stresses. Regardless of the various views on restoration design, materials used, implant systems utilized, or the requirement for aesthetic results, there is agreement on the need for a stable nontraumatic occlusion. Stability is exemplified by centric cusp-to-fossa relationships that do not slide on inclined planes, whereas nontraumatic refers to either a nonoverloaded implant or a natural tooth prosthesis that allows for lateral excursions with an emphasis on the vertical placement of normal occlusal forces.

The development of a satisfactory occlusal scheme depends on many factors. Each person has unique circumstances, and the occlusal scheme developed must meet that individual's requirements. These differences must also be reflected in the final restoration. The needs of each patient are not always obvious and may require a great deal of study before a final occlusal scheme is developed.

ARCH FORM

Arch form describes the configuration of the arch when viewed from the occlusal aspect. It is

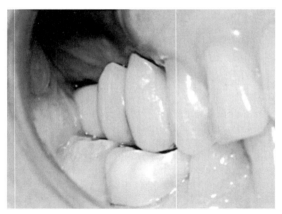

Figure 13–1. Resorption of the posterior maxillary alveolar ridge has required the placement of the implants in a palatal position, resulting in the development of a crossbite relationship.

the geometric shape of the dental arch (e.g., square, tapering, ovoid). The differences in arch form, varying from square to V-shaped, affect the positions in which the implants can be placed. The resulting occlusion is affected by the opposing arch form.

The visibility and resultant tooth arrangements are more pronounced in the anterior aspects of the arch than in the posterior areas. For example, in a narrow maxillary V-shaped arch, the amount of available room for the mesiodistal placement of implants is considerably less than in a broad square-shaped arch. For such a situation, the position of the implants in relation to the superimposed teeth may represent a compromise position in that ideal incisal guidance is precluded because of the vertical overjet configuration. Additionally the placement of the implants also has a bearing on the anteroposterior position of the teeth, which also influences the incisal guidance owing to the amount of horizontal overjet.

In the posterior areas a discrepancy between the maxillary and mandibular ridges may prevent the formulation of an ideal occlusion, and a crossbite type of occlusion may have to be developed. Crossbites are not unusual when posterior maxillary or mandibular areas have had excessive resorption. Although crossbites may present a challenge to the clinician and laboratory technician in developing a satisfactory scheme, this type of occlusion should be considered as indicated (Fig. 13–1).

INTERARCH DISTANCE AND JAW RELATIONSHIP

Interarch or inter-ridge distance may prevent the development of an acceptable occlusal

scheme. This space may be diminished owing to overeruption of the teeth into an opposing edentulous space or malplaced implants, or the space may be exaggerated because of the excessive resorption of the maxillary or mandibular bone before the placement of implants. In some instances, orthognathic surgical procedures must be instituted before restoration of the patient with implants. Decrease in the amount of space available may influence the type of tooth form used. This tooth form then dictates the type of occlusion developed. An increase in the interarch space requires close attention to the lateral forces acting on the implants owing to the increased length of the lever arm that results. Significance that has been given to crown-to-root ratio of natural teeth may be as important in projecting an implant-to-crown ratio. In attempting to reduce the lateral forces on implants, modifications to the occlusal scheme must be made. Maintaining the correct interarch distance in establishing the vertical dimension of occlusion and allowing for a distinct rest position are essential.

The horizontal or transverse relationship of the maxillary arch to the mandibular arch is important. Discrepancies between arch form may be due to the manner and direction in which the resorption process occurs in each arch (Fig. 13–2). When posterior alveolar bone resorbs in the mandible, the remaining basal bone is in a more lateral position to the remaining maxillary bone, requiring a crossbite relationship of the teeth in this area. In the anterior part of the mandible, resorption results in the remaining basal bone being more anterior to the maxillary basal bone. This discrepancy can be further aggravated by the placement of mandibular implants in the symphysis, which forces the setting of the artificial mandibular dentition in a further labial posi-

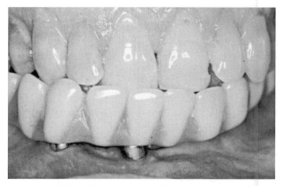

Figure 13–2. The resorption of the anterior mandibular arch has resulted in a pseudo-class III relationship. The placement of implants and the overlying prosthesis results in an anterior crossbite.

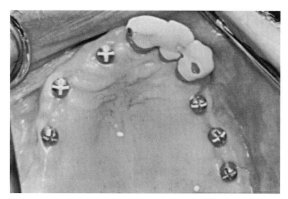

Figure 13–3. Implants placed in a palatal position in relationship to the remaining dentition.

tion. This anterior placement also influences the development of the anterior guidance and affects the occlusal scheme.

Similar resorptive processes occur, albeit not as noticeably, in partially edentulous patients. In the maxilla, for instance, the architecture resulting from these patterns of resorption may result in implants being placed palatally to achieve anchorage of the implants in solid bone (Figs. 13–3 and 13–4). This positioning of the implants has a bearing on the type of occlusion developed for the individual patient as well as on tongue placement and phonetics.

SOFT TISSUE ATTACHMENTS

The health of the soft tissue is influenced by the occlusal scheme that is developed. The main-

tenance of the soft tissue around the supporting structures of a prosthesis has always occupied a central position in the restorative procedures. Unless the soft tissues can be maintained, long-term survival of the implants is in jeopardy.[2] When one considers that the average implant is 4 mm in diameter and that it must support a reasonable replication of a natural tooth, the discrepancy between the diameter of the implant to the size of the artificial tooth must be considered. All these point to developing an occlusion that is nontraumatic to the soft tissues by designing an occlusal form that reduces the loading on the implants, is complemented by proper contours to avoid traumatizing the surrounding soft tissues, and ensures open embrasures to facilitate maintenance of the soft tissues by the patient while adhering to strict aesthetic requirements (Fig. 13–5).

An important aesthetic consideration in the anterior arch is the emergence profile of the restoration. The challenge in this area is to fabricate an aesthetic restoration that is acceptable in size, shape, and contours and capable of being maintained by the patient and that does not place adverse stresses on the underlying implants.

ORIENTATION OF THE OCCLUSAL PLANE

The partially edentulous patient has a defined occlusal plane, which may be altered by odontoplasties or crown reconstructions. Modificatons are possible, and these are often based on the condition of the remaining teeth, the amount of treatment desired by the patient, and not infrequently by the financial resources available to the patient.

In the totally edentulous patient there is more latitude in the development of the occlusal plane. The orientation of the occlusal plane depends on

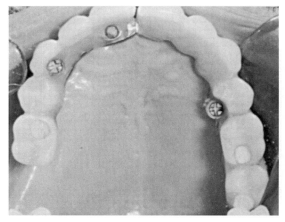

Figure 13–4. Restoration in place on patient shown in Figure 13–3. Note the elimination of the lingual cusp on the first bicuspid on the right owing to implant placement.

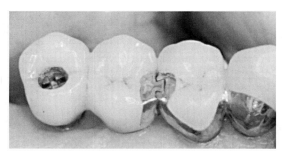

Figure 13–5. Properly placed implants result in a prosthesis that displays proper occlusal design, open embrasures, and well-shaped contours.

anterior placement of teeth to ensure proper incisal guidance. Placement of posterior teeth is done to ensure proper mastication. For the patient with implants, however, the amount of resorption of the residual alveolar ridges, the location of the available bone for implant placement, aesthetic considerations, and biomechanical considerations influence the development of an acceptable occlusal plane. It should always be kept in mind that the arch in which implants are placed usually becomes the dominant arch. That is, the opposing edentulous arch now becomes the weaker arch and the subject of patient complaints as to the inadequacy of stability, retention, and support of the prosthesis resting on this arch. The plane of occlusion must then be developed to take this heretofore nonissue into consideration when the opposing arch has received an implant-supported prosthesis. The arch without implants subsequently becomes the arch that may have to be favored with fine-tuned, noninterfering occlusal patterns.

ABNORMAL MANDIBULAR MOVEMENTS

Movements of the mandible that are out of the norm also influence the development of the occlusal scheme. Although the mandibular movements of patients who have undergone radical surgery are obvious, there are other patients who exhibit subtle deviations that have a bearing on final results.

Depending on the patient's individual needs, existing dental condition, and records obtained, group function or cuspid disclusion may be used to achieve the goal of lateral force dissipation.

CONDYLAR GUIDE ANGLE AND INCISAL GUIDE ANGLE

The condylar angles may be recorded by various techniques, including a functionally generated path, and transferred to the articulator. Regardless of which occlusal philosophy is followed, these angles should be recorded so that the occlusion developed is in harmony with the angles. The incisal guide, which is controlled by the clinician, plays a key role in the proper placement of the anterior dentition. Cusp height, cusp angulations, and compensating curves are affected by these determinants and affect the final aesthetic result.

PHONETICS

Phonetics, an area often neglected in prosthodontics, is important in implant dentistry. The position of the teeth and the contour of the palate relate to nonintrusive placement of implants. In proper articulation the tongue must contact these structures correctly to achieve favorable speech. Individual patients vary in the articulation required to produce certain sounds. These variations must be considered when the occlusal scheme is being developed.

The area that presents the greatest difficulty is the maxillary arch. As stated previously, the relative narrowing of the maxillary arch owing to bony resorption usually results in the implants being placed in a palatal position in relation to the natural dentition. This may result in crowding of the tongue and improper articulation. The contour of the palate may be adversely affected by implants placed in the resorbed anterior maxilla. This results in the implants being placed distally in relation to the position of the natural dentition (Fig. 13–6). This situation is further aggravated by the placement of structures over the implants to retain the maxillary prosthesis. This steepens the anterior palatal curve, crowding the tip of the tongue, and prevents proper tongue placement during articulation.

Implant maintenance in a fixed implant-borne prosthesis requires that a space of varying dimensions be provided between the prosthesis or superstructure and the crest of the ridge (Fig. 13–7). This space in the maxillary arch presents a unique problem in phonetics. It is not unusual to find speech problems in patients fitted with fixed prostheses because this space disrupts the normal articulation.

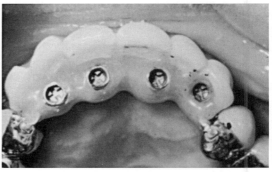

Figure 13–6. Implants placed palatally result in a bulky prosthesis when the anterior dentition is placed to optimize the aesthetics. This can affect speech by crowding the tongue.

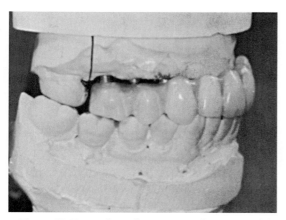

Figure 13–7. Prosthesis demonstrating the position of the anterior teeth in relation to the residual alveolar ridge.

RATIONALE FOR CHOICE OF OCCLUSAL SCHEMES

There are essentially two schools of thought in developing occlusal schemes for the patient with teeth. Stuart and Stallard[32] hold that an occlusal scheme that allows disclusion of the posterior teeth in eccentric occlusion eliminates or reduces lateral stress on the dentition. The disclusion is accomplished by the mandibular cuspid riding on the lingual slope of the maxillary cuspid.

In group function occlusion, lateral pressures are distributed to all working side teeth, in contrast to cuspid disclusion, in which lateral pressures are directed only to the working side canine. The elimination of reduction of the lateral stresses on the dentition is accomplished by having the dentition function as a group and thus distributing the lateral stress along the entire arch in eccentric movements of the mandible.

Although these seemingly divergent philosophies would seem to be mutually exclusive, there are some common points to both. The position of the cusp-to-fossa relationship in centric occlusion can be accomplished the same for both views. Therefore a sound centric occlusion is a requirement regardless of the types of contacts established in eccentric movement. Other points that are shared include the relationship of the restoration to the supporting structures (the crown-to-root ratio), the proper contouring of the individual restorations and pontics, and the need for fabricating a cleansable prothesis.

In attempting to develop an occlusal scheme for implant-supported prostheses, both philosophies have been helpful. This has been particularly true in development of occlusal schemes for long span restorations. In many of these cases

the implants have not been placed in the same position as the teeth that were lost. This has meant that the forces acting on the implant are not directed as they were on the natural tooth. The resultant vector of forces has required thoughtful modification and adaptation of these time-tested philosophies.

BONE SUPPORT AND OCCLUSION

Misch[25] has defined four main bone density groups that vary clinically in the amount of cortical and trabecular bone. The treatment at the uncovering stage and the loading of implants are varied, according to Misch, and depend on the site in which the implants are placed. Success in the various anatomic regions relates not only to bone density and implant size, but also to the time and length of time of loading of the implant. He suggests that each step of the progressive loading process be allowed sufficient time for bone to respond to the increased stimulation of loading.[25] Because of continued maturation of bone and changes observed around implants, it has been proposed by Misch that the progressive loading concept be used when restoring root-form dental implants. Misch's observations indicate that with the differing qualities of bone within the various mandibular and maxillary sites, loading sequences of implants differ. Each restoration is unique, and the provisional restoration suggested by Binon and Sullivan[4] allows the final form of the restoration to be developed while maintaining the concept of progressive loading (Fig. 13–8).

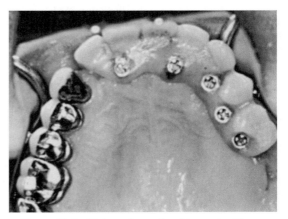

Figure 13–8. With implants placed into palatal bone, an acrylic resin temporary restoration is made. This aids in defining the occlusion before construction of the definitive prosthesis.

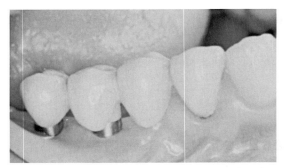

Figure 13–9. Temporary restoration allows the final form to be developed for occlusion and aesthetics.

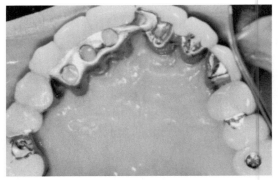

Figure 13–11. Implant-supported restoration replacing the cuspid and incisors.

In developing harmonious occlusions and providing for provisional restorations and provisional loading, a temporary retrievable acrylic resin restoration can be attached to the dental implant by means of either screws or cement (Fig. 13–9). The temporary restoration can be modified to meet aesthetic and functional needs. In the maxilla the patient uses this temporary restoration for 2 to 3 months. The final restoration can be developed using the transitional restorations to verify requirements of aesthetics, speech, and occlusion.

IMPLANT OCCLUSION IN THE PARTIALLY EDENTULOUS PATIENT

It is important to differentiate between anterior restorations over implants that replace the cuspid and those that do not. If the cuspid is not involved, forces on the anterior teeth can be controlled by the use of either cuspid disclusion or group function of the posterior teeth (Fig. 13–10). If the cuspid is involved in an implant restoration, great care must be exercised in de-

veloping the occlusion to avoid undue lateral stresses on the implants. In such an instance a group function type of occlusion must be developed. This group function involves the posterior teeth (Figs. 13–11 and 13–12). The chief concern is to spread the load and not have all the load on any single implant. The condylar and incisal guide angles have a bearing in the development of this occlusion to eliminate lateral and rotational forces on the occlusal and incisal surfaces of the restorations over implants.

Because the mandibular cuspid is generally the last tooth to be lost, most of the recorded experience with implant restorations that involve the cuspid teeth has generally been in the maxillary arch. In those individuals who have an edentulous mandible opposing a partially edentulous maxilla, however, implants have afforded an opportunity to provide fixed-type restorations in the edentulous mandible. Although the bone type in this area is generally more favorable than in the anterior maxilla, management of the occlusion is carried out in the same manner: that is, using group function to distribute the load to the implant-supported restoration as well as to the re-

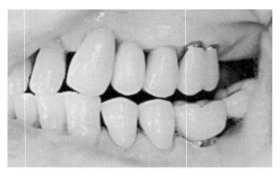

Figure 13–10. Anterior teeth are present with a posterior implant bridge. Cuspid disclusion avoids lateral stresses on the implants.

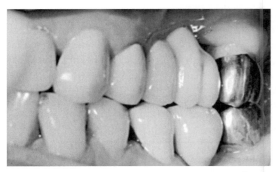

Figure 13–12. Same patient as in Figure 13–11 demonstrating the use of group function in eccentric movement. This dissipates lateral forces.

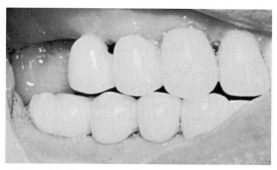

Figure 13–13. Owing to the quality and quantity of bone, only two implants are placed in the maxillary arch. A cantilever is required to meet aesthetic demands.

maining natural teeth. A great deal of care must be taken in creating free end cantilever designs into this type of prosthesis. These cantilevers should be kept to a minimum length (Figs. 13–13 and 13–14).

The advantage of having occlusal stops with natural teeth is obvious. The remaining teeth have great influence in the development of a harmonious occlusion. Undue lateral forces must still be avoided on the implant-supported restoration. Every attempt is made to bring the implant-supported restoration immediately out of occlusion in lateral and protrusive movements. In a posterior fixed-implant prosthesis, cuspid disclusion is recommended in lateral and protrusive movements. If this is not practical, group function is used.

Single-tooth restorations have been placed in both the anterior and the posterior region of the mandibular and maxillary arch. In the anterior region the cuspid and central incisor positions present the greatest challenge in controlling the forces to the implant-bone interface. In restoring a single-tooth implant in the posterior segment of the arch, every effort is made to achieve a reduction or elimination of lateral forces by the

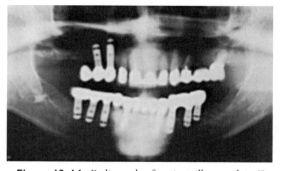

Figure 13–14. Radiograph of patient illustrated in Figure 13–13.

use of cuspid disclusion. This results in the disclusion of the single implant–supported restoration. When the patient has a mutually supported type of occlusion in eccentric movements, this type of function is maintained.

IMPLANT OCCLUSION IN THE EDENTULOUS PATIENT

Balanced occlusion in complete dentures can be defined as stable simultaneous contact of the opposing maxillary and mandibular teeth in the centric relation occlusion position and a continuous smooth bilateral gliding from this position to any eccentric position within the normal range of mandibular function. Balance in natural dentition is not needed because each tooth is supported independently by its periodontal ligament. The necessity of bilateral balanced occlusion in complete denture prosthodontics is not universally subscribed to by dentists, but few have raised objections to it.

The occlusal schemes described in the literature for the edentulous patient are numerous. In 1982, Parr and Loft[29] reviewed the various occlusal schemes, which ranged from full anatomic balance to neutrocentric occlusion. It should be remembered, however, that these different occlusal schemes were developed to function on unstable denture bases. Even the denture base fabricated in the most precise manner moves owing to the looseness and compressibility of the soft tissue on which the denture base rests. Although it would appear that the development of an occlusal scheme for the edentulous patient would be a relatively simple procedure because the implants provide for a stable denture base, it is quite the contrary. In many edentulous patients, the type of prosthesis and position of implants are the chief determining factors. Tissue-supported overdentures, implant-borne overdentures, and hybrid prostheses are options available in restoring the edentulous patient. Each of these options presents conditions for developing a harmonious occlusion. An additional consideration is the amount of resorption that has occurred on the residual ridge. The more resorption that has occurred, the greater the lever arm acting on the implants themselves. The occlusion then depends on the type of prosthesis to be fabricated, the number of implants used, the type of superstructure placed over the implants, and the type of attachment used to retain the prosthesis to the implants or superstructure.

Bilateral occlusal balance is present when there is equilibrium on both sides of the arches owing to simultaneous contact of the artificial teeth in centric and eccentric occlusion. It requires a minimum of three contacts for establishing a plane of equilibrium. This type of balance depends on the interaction of the incisal guidance, plane of occlusion, angulation of the teeth (tilt and inclination), cusp angulation (height), compensating curve, and inclination of the condylar path.

In the edentulous patient there is more leeway in control of the incisal guidance. The role of condylar guidance also varies with the type of occlusion developed. If a balanced occlusion is desired, a three-point contact balance between the working and balancing sides is achieved. This simplifies achieving the desired results because only three points of contact are involved. No attempt should be made to obtain a full balanced occlusion. To eliminate or reduce lateral stress, the use of a lingualized type of occlusion is preferred.[20] This eliminates contacting of the maxillary buccal cusp on the working side, thus (it is hoped) lingualizing or centralizing the forces on the prosthesis. It might be argued that this reduction of the horizontal lever arm is insignificant, but any reduction in the lateral stresses generated should be considered.

It should be carefully noted that regardless of the scheme of occlusion used when implants are placed in one arch, there is always the possibility of rendering an opposing complete denture unstable. Therefore the occlusion must be carefully developed to provide support, stability, and retention to the soft tissue–supported opposing prosthesis. It is recommended that in the edentulous patient, the type of occlusion used should follow the precepts of a balanced or a lingualized occlusion.

When a totally implant-borne prosthesis opposes an arch with natural dentition, it is usually neither possible nor desirable to use a balance-type occlusion. Instead, a group function–supported type of occlusion developed from carefully generated records is used.

References

1. Albrektsson T, Zarb GE: The Brånemark Osseointegrated Implant. Chicago, Quintessence Publishing, 1989.
2. Artzi Z, Tal H, Moses O, Kozlovsky A: Mucosal considerations for osseointegrated implants. J Prosthet Dent 70:427–432, 1993.
3. Bidez MW, Misch CE: Force transfer in implant dentistry: Basic concepts and principles. J Oral Implantol 18:264–274, 1992.
4. Binon P, Sullivan D: Provisional fixed restorations technique for osseointegrated implants. J Calif Dent Assoc 18:28–30, 1990.
5. Brunski JB: Biomaterials and biomechanics in dental implant design. Int J Oral Maxillofac Imp 3:85–97, 1988.
6. Brunski JB: Biomechanics of oral implants: Future research direction. J Dent Educ 52:775–787, 1988.
7. Brunski JB: Avoid pitfalls of overloading and micromotion of intraosseous implants. Dent Impl Update 4:77–81, 1993.
8. Carr AB, Laney WR: Maximum occlusal force levels in patients with osseointegrated oral implant prostheses and patients with complete dentures. Int J Oral Maxillofac Impl 2:101–108, 1987.
9. Chapman R: Principles of occlusion for implant prostheses: Guidelines for position, timing and force of occlusal contacts. Quint Int 20:473–480, 1989.
10. Davis DM, Rimrott R, Zarb GA: Studies on frameworks for osseointegrated prostheses: 2. The effect of adding acrylic resin or porcelain to form the occlusal superstructure. Int J Oral Maxillofac Impl 3:275–280, 1988.
11. English CE: Root intrusion in tooth-implant combination cases. Impl Dent 2:79–85, 1993.
12. Falk H: On occlusal forces in dentitions with implant-supported fixed cantilever prostheses. Swed Dent J 69 (suppl):1–40, 1990.
13. Gracis SE, Nicholls JI, Chalupnik JD, Yuodelis RA: Shock-absorbing behavior of five restorative materials used on implants. Int J Prosthodont 4:282–291, 1991.
14. Haraldson T, Carlsson GE: Bite force and oral function in patients with osseointegrated oral implants. Scand J Dent Restor 85:200–208, 1977.
15. Hobo S: Occlusion for the osseointegrated prosthesis. J Gnathol 10:9–17, 1991.
16. Ingber A: The osseointegration implant system and its influence upon occlusal design. Alpha Omegan 78:73–78, 1985.
17. Ismail Y, Kukunas S, Pipho D, Ibiary W: Comparative study of various occlusal materials for implant prosthodontics (abstract). J Dent Res 68 (spec iss):962, 1989.
18. Jacobs R, van Steenberghe D: Comparative evaluation of the oral tactile function by means of teeth or implant-supported prostheses. Clin Oral Impl Res 2:75–80, 1991.
19. Kirsch A, Ackerman K-L: The IMZ osseointegrated implants system. Dent Clin North Am 33:733–761, 1989.
20. Lang BR, Razzoog ME: Lingualized integration: Tooth molds and an occlusal scheme for edentulous implant patients. Impl Dent 1:204–211, 1992.
21. Levinson E: Requirements for ideal restorative posterior tooth occlusal anatomy—a working clinical hypothesis. Alpha Omegan 78:82–86, 1985.
22. Lundgren D, Laurell L, Falk H, Bergendal T: Occlusal force pattern during mastication in dentitions with mandibular fixed partial dentures supported on osseointegrated implants. J Prosthet Dent 58:197–204, 1987.
23. Lundqvist S, Haraldson T: Occlusal perception of thickness in patients with bridges on osseointegrated oral implants. Scand J Dent Res 92:88–92, 1993.
24. Lindqvist LW, et al: Bone resorption around fixtures in edentulous patients treated with mandibular fixed integrated prostheses. J Prosthet Dent 59:59–63, 1988.
25. Misch CE: Contemporary Implant Dentistry. St Louis, CV Mosby, 1993.
26. Monteith B: Minimizing biomechanical overload in implant prostheses: A computerized aid to design. J Prosthet Dent 69:495–502, 1993.
27. Muhlbradt L, Ulrich R, Mohmann HH, Schmid H:

Mechanoperception of natural teeth versus endosseous implants revealed by magnitude estimation. Int J Oral Maxillofac Impl 4:125–130, 1989.

28. Parker MW: The significance of occlusion in restorative dentistry. Dent Clin North Am 37:341–351, 1993.

29. Parr GR, Loft GH: The occlusal spectrum and complete dentures. Comp Contin Educ 3:241, 1982.

30. Schulte JK, Peterson TA: Occlusal and prosthetic considerations. J Calif Dent Assoc 15:64–72, 1987.

31. Skalak R: Biomechanical considerations in osseointegrated prostheses. J Prosthet Dent 49:843–848, 1983.

32. Stuart CE, Stallard H: Principles involved in restoring occlusion to natural teeth. J Prosthet Dent 10:308–310, 1960.

33. Trulsson M, Johansson RS, Olsson KA: Directional sensitivity of human periodontal mechanoreceptive afferents to forces applied to the teeth. J Physiol 447:373–389, 1992.

Study Questions

1. Discuss the movement of an implant in bone as compared to a natural tooth.

2. Discuss the factors that influence the occlusion in a fixed implant prosthetic restoration.

3. Discuss the role of the cuspids in development of the occlusal scheme in the partially endentulous patient.

4. Discuss the occlusion developed for the edentulous patient utilizing implant restorations.

SECTION 3

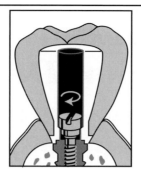

Surgical Considerations

CHAPTER 14

Anesthesia, Incision Design, Surgical Principles, Exposure Techniques

Michael S. Block

Anesthesia
Incision Design
   Anterior Mandible
   Posterior Mandible
   Maxillary Incisions

Exposure Techniques
   Exposure Techniques for Aesthetic
      Restorations
References

ANESTHESIA

Most endosseous implant operations can be performed using local anesthesia with or without conscious sedation. A careful review of the patient's medical history may reveal medical problems that limit the amount of local anesthesia or epinephrine that can be administered or indicate that the patient's condition must be monitored by a clinician trained in anesthesia, such as an anesthesiologist or an oral and maxillofacial surgeon. Patients with a compromised cardiovascular status with unstable angina or patients requesting implant surgery after a recent myocardial infarction need treatment delayed to improve their medical status before administration of a local anesthetic and the stress of surgery.

Routine inferior alveolar nerve blocks and maxillary infiltration anesthesia provide satisfactory local anesthesia for the implant patient. Local anesthesia infiltrated directly into the planned incision line reduces bleeding and simultaneously performs a hydropic dissection. This eases the development of a subperiosteal dissection during development of a full-thickness mucoperiosteal flap.

The specific local anesthetic is chosen by operator preference. Lidocaine 1% or 2% (Xylocaine) with 1:100,000 or 1:200,000 epinephrine or a similar anesthetic is most commonly used. Longer-acting anesthetics can also be used if the

clinician and patient desire anesthesia time for 6 to 8 hours.

Intravenous conscious sedation is useful for the anxious patient or for the patient who is undergoing a lengthy procedure. One disadvantage with sedation is the lack of the patient's ability to close the mouth gently during the procedure. Often when placing implants, the surgeon asks the patient to close the mouth gently to confirm the implant angulation using paralleling pins. This shows the expected retaining screw emergence. With intravenous sedation, the patient may clamp down harshly on the pins, or the patient may resist rotation of the mandible to check implant placement. The deeper the plane of general anesthesia or conscious sedation, the more difficult it is to rely on patient cooperation during surgery. General anesthesia is rarely necessary except for patients with extreme dental phobia or those requiring bone graft harvesting from the iliac crest, cranium, or multiple intraoral sites.

INCISION DESIGN

Anterior Mandible

The two most popular incisions for placement of implants into the anterior mandible are crestal and vestibular incisions (Figs. 14–1 and 14–2). The crestal incision is useful when the mandible

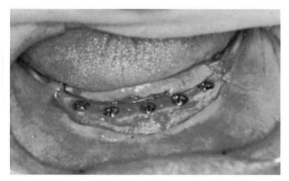

Figure 14–1. Crestal incisions can be used to place anterior mandibular implants. Note this incision bisecting the keratinized gingiva with small vertical release incisions posteriorly. The full-thickness mucoperiosteal flaps have been elevated to expose the labial and lingual cortices.

has sufficient height and the mentalis and lip musculature insert below the alveolar crest. For the patient with an adequate (at least 4 mm) band of attached gingiva, a crestal incision bisecting the keratinized gingiva provides excellent access to both the labial and the lingual regions for visualization during implant placement. A full-thickness mucoperiosteal flap is raised, exposing the facial and lingual aspects of the mandible. The reflection should be sufficient to allow for access to the bone without placing excessive retraction forces on the tissue, preventing tearing of the edges of the incision. Adequate reflection also allows one to visualize directly the slope of the bone and its quality.

For the patient without an adequate band of attached tissue or for the patient whose mentalis muscle inserts close to the crest, a vestibular incision is recommended[2] (Fig. 14–2). High muscle attachments result with mobile tissue against the labial portion of the implant's abutment, and

thus simultaneous vestibuloplasty or presurgical soft tissue grafting is recommended when lip musculature with its mobile tissue is present along the crest at the implant site (Fig. 14–2).

The incision is made in the lip mucosa and a lingual-based, mucosa-only flap developed superficial to the mentalis musculature. Once the crest of the mandible is reached, a periosteal incision is made, and the periosteum is reflected labially, exposing the labial cortical bone. A full-thickness periosteal reflection (lingual based) is then made to expose the lingual cortical bone. The implant sites are prepared following manufacturer's recommendations. After implant placement, the mucosa flap is sutured to the depth of the vestibule with the periosteum reflected labially, "switching" their positions. This lip-switch procedure provides nonmobile tissue labial to the implant.[4] The partially denuded lip tissue is allowed to heal by re-epithelialization. In the extremely atrophic mandible (less than 12 mm in vertical height), one must be careful to avoid stripping the mentalis muscle from the symphysis. In general, 10 mm of mentalis muscle should be left attached to the mandible to avoid chin laxity, otherwise known as a witch's chin.

Posterior Mandible

In the edentulous posterior mandible the residual band of keratinized gingiva tissue may only be 2 mm wide. It is important to preserve this thin band of keratinized tissue and plan on repositioning it along the labial aspect of the implants at the time of exposure of the implant and abutment placement. (Figs. 14–3 and 14–4). Vertical releasing incisions with flap reflection allow excellent access and direct visualization of the mental foramen.

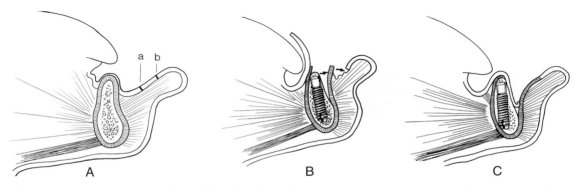

Figure 14–2. *A*, Cross section of mandible with high muscle attachments; *a* denotes incision used to increase vestibular depth conservatively for implants, whereas *b* indicates location of incision for more extensive vestibular deepening. *B*, A lingual-based, mucosa-only flap is raised, superficial to the orbicularis muscle. The periosteum is incised on the crest and reflected labially; the implant is then placed. *C*, After implant placement, the periosteum is sutured to the lip, and the mucosa is sutured to the depth of the vestibule, "switching" the tissues' positions. By gently rolling the edge of the mucosa deep in the vestibule, less scarring results.

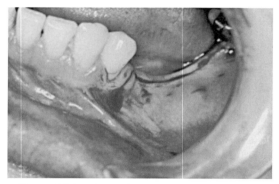

Figure 14–3. A crestal incision is recommended for placement of implants into the posterior mandible. The crestal incision bisecting the thin band of keratinized gingiva is shown, with vertical release incisions to allow for reflection of the flaps facially and lingually. Note how the attached gingiva adjacent to the natural tooth is not raised with the flap.

A crestal incision is also useful when using membranes and guided tissue regeneration techniques for alveolar ridge. After the mucosa is reflected the membrane is placed along with the graft material, and the incision is closed without tension along the crest. Horizontal scoring of the periosteal membrane is required, combined with a supraperiosteal dissection to allow for a tension-free closure.

Incision breakdown can be avoided by preventing the patient from chewing on the incision and by avoidance of wearing removable prostheses during the first 2 to 4 weeks of healing following implant placement. The patient's removable partial denture should be relined with a soft liner for optimal tissue conditioning during the healing period until the implants are exposed.

Maxillary Incisions

The most commonly used incision is slightly palatal to the alveolar crest (Fig. 14–5). This incision is placed into fixed, keratinized gingiva. By placing the incision slightly palatal to the crest, the surgeon can easily visualize palatal bone contours without the aid of additional retractors. For full arch maxillary implant placement, the anterior portion of the incision should trace around the incisive foramen to avoid cutting through its accompanying structures.

EXPOSURE TECHNIQUES

After placement of the implant into bone and suturing of the gingiva everting the incision, time

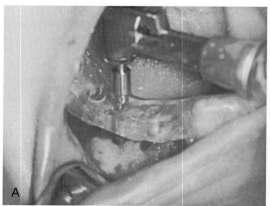

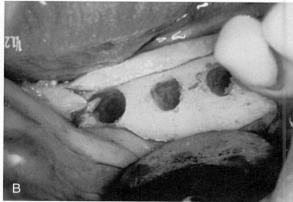

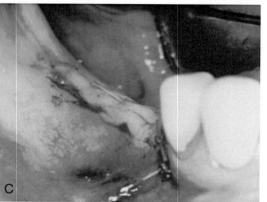

Figure 14–4. *A,* A vertical releasing incision allows for lateral reflection of the flap. The template is then placed and the implant site prepared. Here one sees the drill entering the bone. This allows the surgeon confirmation of placing the implants properly into adequate bone. *B,* After final preparation, the implant sites should be clean and precise. *C,* The posterior mandibular crestal incisions are closed with a horizontal mattress suture technique. This suturing technique everts the incision margin, preserving the kertatinized gingiva and providing a band of tissue at the time of exposure.

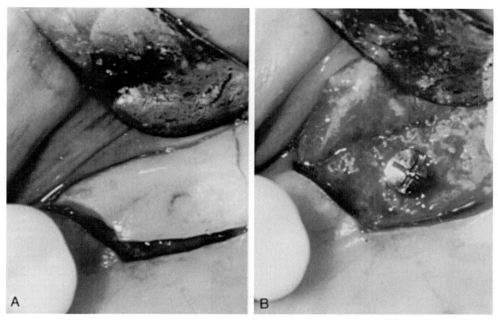

Figure 14–5. *A*, For implants placed in the posterior maxilla, an incision is made slightly palatal to the crest, with vertical release incisions to allow for reflection of a full-thickness mucoperiosteal flap. *B*, The implant is placed, countersinking it 1 to 2 mm apical to the alveolar crest, anticipating bone resorption during the healing period.

is allowed for healing and integration to occur. Depending on the manufacturer's recommendations, 4 to 6 months are generally allowed until exposure (stage 2) surgery. Before exposing the implants the surgeon confers with the restorative dentist, and the proper abutments or temporary gingival abutments are chosen. For some patients, gingival grafting is performed prior to implant exposure to ensure that an adequate band of keratinized gingiva is present. It is customary for the patient to see the restorative dentist after the surgeon exposes the implants for adjustments to the patient's removable prostheses or fabrication of temporary prostheses.

Local infiltration or field blocks can be given. After a satisfactory plane of anesthesia has been reached, an incision is made bisecting and thus preserving all of the keratinized gingiva through the periosteum to bone. Gentle reflection allows for visualization of the implants (Fig. 14–6). Once the implant is identified, small, vertical releasing incisions can be made conservatively avoiding the papilla, and the gingiva reflected to expose the implants. A tissue punch should be used only when a broad band (10 mm) of keratinized gingiva is present; otherwise it should be used with caution because it removes keratinized gingiva.

After the implant is exposed, a curet is used to remove soft and hard tissue that may be present over the top of the healing screw in the implant. Once the top of the healing screw is

clean, it is removed and the internal portion of the implant irrigated with sterile saline. The transgingival component is then placed with direct visualization, avoiding trapping soft tissue between the abutment and the implant.

The keratinized gingiva is then apposed to the labial or facial surface of the implant. Sutures are used along the mesial and distal aspects of the implants. Tight suturing is avoided to prevent trauma and damage to the interdental papilla. This preserves all of the keratinized gingiva and also transposes it along the labial surface of the abutment, protecting the implant from irritation from mobile, unattached mucosa (Fig. 14–7).

When one is exposing implants in the edentulous maxilla, the gingiva is often greater than 3 mm in thickness. For this area, it is advisable to thin the gingival thickness by removing the subcutaneous tissues, leaving the keratinized tissue. Once the thickness of the maxillary gingiva has been reduced, the remaining keratinized gingiva needs to be trimmed to remove excess.

Exposure Techniques for Aesthetic Restorations

One must be extremely careful when exposing implants placed into the partially edentulous anterior maxilla. Considerations include preservation of papilla, creation of soft tissue bulk for a convex and esthetic ridge form, and creation of

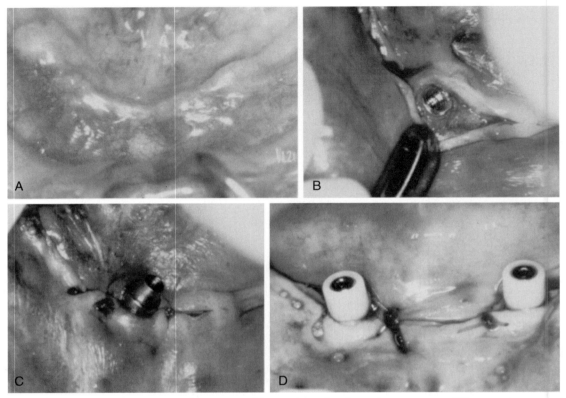

Figure 14–6. *A,* This patient returns for exposure of her implants placed into the anterior mandible 4 months previously through a crestal incision. *B,* The ridge is palpated, and the approximate location of the implant is identified by radiographs or the templates. A crestal incision is made bisecting the keratinized gingiva, with a small vertical release if necessary. The healing screw is removed from the implant body. The top of the implant is cleaned to avoid trapping soft tissue. The inside of the implant is irrigated with sterile saline. *C,* An abutment is placed. Either the abutment for the restoration can be placed, or a temporary gingival abutment can be placed. Sutures are then placed approximating the keratinized gingiva. This method preserves and places keratinized gingiva along the labial surface of the abutment. *D,* Comfort caps can be placed over the abutments to avoid sharp edges of the abutments lacerating the tongue and soft tissues of the floor of the mouth. The denture is then relined over these abutments.

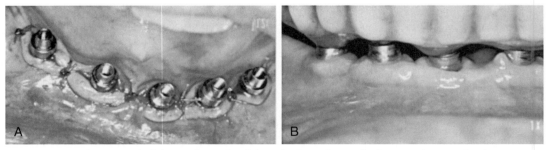

Figure 14–7. *A,* This patient had five implants placed for a fixed prosthesis. The keratinized gingiva has been preserved and placed labial to the abutments. *B,* The 4-year follow-up demonstrates excellent gingival health despite the patient's poor efforts to maintain oral hygiene.

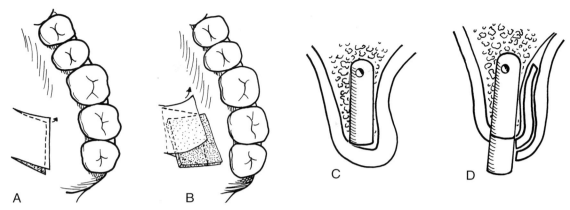

Figure 14–8. *A,* To harvest a piece of connective tissue, incisions are made and the palatal mucosa reflected. *B,* A thickness of connective tissue is harvested. The palatal flap is then reapproximated. *C,* This cross section of an anterior maxillary site demonstrates sufficient bone thickness for the implant but a concave labial profile. *D,* After gingival reflection, the connective tissue graft is placed plumping out the labial portion of the ridge providing convex ridge form.

keratinized gingiva along the labial aspect of the crown.

To preserve papillae and to avoid their loss, incisions should avoid the papillae and be made palatal to the crest to allow for transposition of gingiva labially. Upon crown delivery, the soft tissue can be carved to form an aesthetic soft tissue "socket." When palatal tissue is transposed labially it creates a bulk of tissue facially, which can then be carved after initial healing to form an aesthetic sulcus. This creates excellent soft tissue form over the implant crown.

For most anterior maxillary aesthetic restora-

tions, it is often necessary to augment the soft tissue thickness, creating a convex ridge form to enhance the aesthetic restoration. Soft tissue augmentation can be easily obtained by performing a subepithelial connective tissue graft harvested from the palate or by using a palatal roll-in procedure.[5–7]

The subepithelial connective tissue graft is harvested by removing a sheet of connective tissue from the palate. This sheet of tissue is then interposed within the facial gingiva to augment the ridge. The subepithelial connective tissue graft was designed and described by Langer and

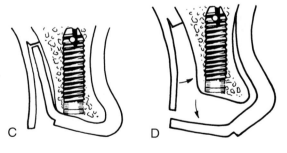

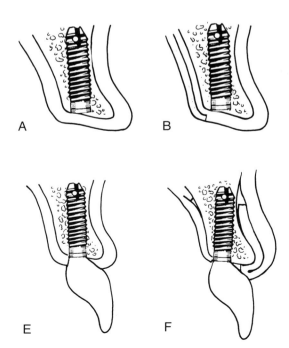

Figure 14–9. *A,* Cross section of an implant in a maxillary incisor location. Note the concave labial ridge form. *B,* An incision is made to allow development of a partial-thickness flap with a palatal base. *C,* The palatal flap is reflected, and the palatal base is incised then raised toward the facial aspect. *D,* The de-epithelialized portion of the palatal tissue is reflected to allow reapproximation of the palatal mucosa. *E,* This cross section shows what a crown and concave labial ridge would look like if no augmentation procedure were performed. *F,* The cross section shows the de-epithelialized palatal tissue rolled under the labial gingiva to create increased ridge width and a convex ridge form.

Langer[8] to minimize palatal de-epithelialization (Fig. 14–8).

The palatal roll-in procedure is also useful because it can be performed as part of the dissection to expose the implant[1, 11] (Fig. 14–9). An incision is made through mucosa only just palatal to the implant. The horizontal incision, which defines the border of keratinized gingiva, can be made further toward the palate when gingival height also needs to be augmented. Two vertical incisions are made and a palatally based flap created, leaving the underlying subepithelial tissue bed intact. A releasing incision is made under the base of the palatal flap, connecting with vertical periosteal incisions through periosteum toward the crest and over the labial surface. The subepithelial tissue is elevated toward the crest over the implant and coronally along the labial aspect of the ridge. The subepithelial tissue is then "rolled in" under the labial gingiva, plumping out the ridge to create a convex ridge form. Sutures are placed to hold the flap in place. This procedure creates a ridge form necessary for an aesthetic anterior restoration. The palatal flap is then approximated to the facial flap.

Creation of keratinized gingiva is easily accomplished by performing a split-thickness free palatal graft.[3, 9, 10] Mobile alveolar mucosa is incised and reflected in a supraperiosteal plane. This dissection should leave the host bed covered with periosteum to receive the palatal graft. The reflected alveolar mucosa is sutured in a reflected position with periosteal sutures. The graft is then trimmed to fit the defect and sutured in place. Four to six weeks are required for healing before implant exposure and completion of the restoration. Often this graft procedure is performed 1 month before second-stage surgery to create the ideal tissue for the final restoration. If necessary, other procedures then can be performed to touch up the gingival contours.

References

1. Abrams L: Augmentation of the deformed residual edentulous ridge for fixed prosthesis. Compend Contin Educ Dent 1:205, 1980.
2. Adell R, Lekholm U, Brånemark P-I: Surgical procedures. In Brånemark P-I, Zarb GA, Albrektsson T (eds): Tissue Integrated Prostheses: Osseointegration in Clinical Dentistry. Chicago, Quintessence Publishing, 1985, pp 214–232.
3. Huybers TJM, Stoelinga PJ, deKoomen HA, Tideman H: Mandibular vestibuloplasty using a free mucosal graft (2–7 year evaluation). Int J Oral Surg 14:11–15, 1985.
4. Kethley JL, Gamble JW: The lipswitch: A modification of Kazanjian's labial vestibuloplasty. J Oral Surg 36:701–705, 1978.
5. Langer B: Dental implants used for periodontal patients. J Am Dent Assoc 121:505–510, 1990.
6. Langer B, Calagna L: Subepithelial connective tissue graft to correct ridge concavities. J Prosthet Dent 44:363, 1980.
7. Langer B, Calagna L: The subepithelial connective tissue graft. A new approach to the enhancement of anterior cosmetics. Int J Periodont Restor Dent 2:23, 1982.
8. Langer B, Langer L: Subepithelial connective tissue graft technique for root coverage. J Periodontol 56:715–720, 1985.
9. Nabers JM: Free gingival grafts. Periodontics 4:243, 1966.
10. Sullivan H, Atkins J: Free autogenous gingival grafts: I. Principles of successful grafting. Periodontics 6:121, 1968.
11. Tarnow DP, Scharf DR: Modified roll technique for localized alveolar ridge augmentation. Int J Periodont Restor Dent 12:415, 1992.

Study Questions

1. Describe the location of incisions for placement of implants into the anterior mandible and posterior mandible.

2. Why is a vestibuloplasty necessary for many patients whose anterior mandible has high muscle attachments? What procedure is recommended?

3. When exposing implants for abutment connection, how do you preserve and reposition keratinized gingiva?

4. Why should you avoid using the tissue punch for exposing posterior mandibular implants?

5. Given the situation of 8-mm thick tissue in the edentulous maxilla, how do you expose implants that result in 3-mm soft tissue pockets?

6. For anterior maxillary aesthetic restorations, describe two techniques for bulking the ridge resulting in a convex, aesthetic appearing ridge form.

CHAPTER 15

Placement of Implants into Extraction Sites

Michael S. Block

Treatment Planning
   Immediate Placement
   Delayed Placement
Extractions with Simultaneous Implant
     Placement
   Anterior Maxilla
References

Because of the success with osseointegrated implants, treatment consisting of extraction and replacement by endosseous implants is being planned for teeth in cases in which prognoses are guarded. Placement of endosseous implants in fresh extraction sites can result in integration as determined by histologic evidence of bone closely adapted to the implant's surface and lack of clinical mobility.[3, 5, 10, 11, 16, 17]

TREATMENT PLANNING

Immediate Placement

The advantages of placing implants immediately after tooth extraction include avoiding potential narrowing of the alveolus from labial plate resorption that naturally occurs after tooth extraction, and less time between extraction and final restoration. Successful immediate placement of an implant at the time of tooth extraction relies on excellent soft and hard tissue quality and quantity. Patients must also fulfill the selection criteria for edentulous patients previously described.[6]

Based on our clinical experiences over the last 12 years, the indications for the placement of implants immediately into extraction sites are:

1. Traumatic loss of teeth with a small amount of bone loss.
2. Teeth lost because of gross decay without the presence of purulent exudate or cellulitis.

3. Inability to complete endodontic procedures.
4. Presence of severe periodontal bone loss without purulent exudate.
5. Adequate soft tissue health and quantity to obtain a complete crestal primary wound closure.
6. Bone availability apical to the extraction site for stabilization of the implant.
7. Appropriate location of extracted tooth for planned restoration.

Contraindications for immediate placement of implants into fresh extraction sites include:

1. Presence of purulent exudate at the time of extraction.
2. Adjacent soft tissue cellulitis and granulation tissue.
3. Lack of adequate bone apical to the extraction site.
4. Adverse location of the mandibular neurovascular bundle, maxillary sinus, or nasal cavity.
5. Anatomic configuration of remaining bone or potential location of the implant preventing ideal prosthetics.
6. Any clinical condition that prevents primary soft tissue wound closure.

The presence of infection contraindicates implant placement. The infected tooth should be extracted and the site allowed to heal 6 to 8 weeks with complete resolution of the infection before grafting or implant placement. Previously infected sites may require reconstruction of ridge contour because of bone resorption to provide appropriate ridge form and aesthetics, i.e., convexity for anterior maxillary cases. Soft and hard tissue alveolar ridge preparation to provide an ideal implant site for optimal placement is required and may delay implant placement until ridge form is re-established.[2, 8, 9]

Delayed Placement

If any of the six aforementioned contraindications is present, delayed placement of the implant is indicated. The teeth are extracted, the socket is cleaned of soft tissue debris, and the site is allowed to heal for at least 6 weeks before placement of dental implants.[5, 16, 17] By delaying the implant placement, the surgeon avoids potential infections and places the implant into healthier tissue.[16]

If there is a large defect in the bone or if the tooth sockets are significantly larger than the diameter of the implant, one may delay implant placement until the extraction socket has filled in with bone. The decision whether to allow the socket to heal and fill in with bone without simultaneous implant placement or to place a graft with simultaneous implant placement to reestablish adequate bone is based on the ability to stabilize the implant by engaging bone within or apical to the socket and satisfying the mechanical requirements for predictable integration.

EXTRACTIONS WITH SIMULTANEOUS IMPLANT PLACEMENT

The most common location for placing implants into fresh extraction sites is the anterior (first premolars, canines, and incisors) maxilla and the anterior (anterior to the mental foramen) mandible. These anterior regions do not have anatomic constraints such as the maxillary sinus or the inferior alveolar nerve, which complicate immediate placement after extraction.

Extraction of anterior mandibular incisors, canines, or the first premolars is common in preparation for the placement of two or more implants for either overdenture retention or a fixed prosthesis. Reflection of the labial and lingual periosteum allows for direct visualization of the bone during atraumatic extraction of the teeth. After extractions, remnants of soft tissue are removed and sharp edges of the bone are smoothed. The implant sites are prepared using the same protocol recommended by the implant manufacturer as when placing implants into edentulous bone.

When the diameter of the root site is less than the diameter of the implant, no crestal bone defect results after placing the implant (Fig. 15–1).

A small crestal bone defect, usually labial, may be present after implant placement. With small (i.e., less than 4 mm) bone defects, adequate bone is usually present along the rest of the implant's surface to allow for implant stabilization

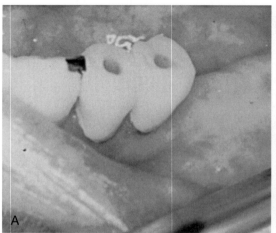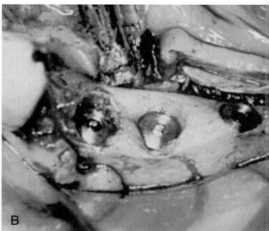

Figure 15–1. *A,* This woman was referred for extraction of the left mandibular premolars with simultaneous placement of implants. The gingiva was healthy without purulence or gingivitis. *B,* An incision was made around the necks of the teeth and a full-thickness mucoperiosteal flap raised. Then the teeth were extracted atraumatically. The extraction sites were prepared and implants placed, each countersunk 2 mm. The incisions were closed primarily. No graft or membrane was used because there was no bone defect adjacent to the implants.

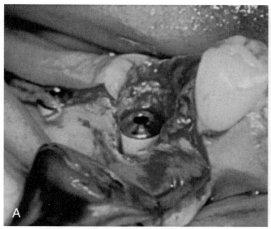
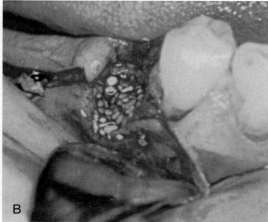

Figure 15–2. *A,* This woman had a mandibular second premolar extracted and an implant placed. A 3-mm labial dehiscence was present after the implant placement. *B,* 2040-mesh HA particles were gently compacted into the bone defect as a graft. The incisions were closed primarily.

and subsequent integration. If present after implant placement the crestal bone defect should be grafted to prevent epithelial migration down the implant's surface, which ultimately creates an infrabone pocket. These small defects can be obliterated by grafting with alloplasts (hydroxylapatite [HA]) (Fig. 15–2). Recall of patients with small defects treated with or without grafting indicates significant benefit from grafting the defects (Table 15–1).[5]

A third condition occurs when after implant placement the bone defect is large, compromising the amount of bone-implant interface available for integration. These large defects require grafting with particulate autogenous bone, allogeneic demineralized bone, or a combination of autogenous and allogeneic demineralized bone to develop bone along the implant surface and to achieve integration. Guided tissue regeneration techniques are useful to exclude epithelial invagination during the healing period and to promote bone production (Figs. 15–3 through 15–5).

Large defects require grafting before or during placement of the implants. These bone grafts restore bone bulk and form to place the implants into an ideal position. Bone loss from tooth fractures or periodontal-endodontic lesions is typically extensive, requiring reconstruction of vertical and horizontal defects. Onlay grafts or grafts using guided tissue regeneration can restore ridge anatomy for proper restoration. Often it is preferred to place the graft and allow for consolidation before placing the implants. Implants can be placed during the grafting only if mechanical stabilization of the implant is obtainable by engaging the patient's basal bone.

Anterior Maxilla

The placement of implants into the anterior maxilla must be combined with an aesthetic examination of the planned restoration. This clinical and radiographic examination should include:

1. Determination of available hard tissue.
2. Determination of available keratinized soft tissue.
3. The relationship of the hard and soft tissue to the planned restoration.
4. The relationship of the planned restoration to the lip-aesthetic zone.

Preoperative planning should include the fabrication of the planned restoration and duplication of the planned restoration in clear acrylic as a template. The clear template can then be used to determine the exact soft and hard tissue

Table 15–1. Relation of Bone Defect and Grafting to Crestal Bone Loss				
No.	Defect	Graft	Mean Bone Loss (mm)	Standard Deviation
14	None	None	1.05°	0.57
6	Yes	None	2.52°†	1.42
9	Yes	HA	1.07†	0.71

°P <0.001, Student's T-test.
†P <0.01, Student's T-test.
From Block MS, Kent JN: Placement of endosseous implants into tooth extraction sites. J Oral Maxillofac Surg 49:1269–1276, 1991.

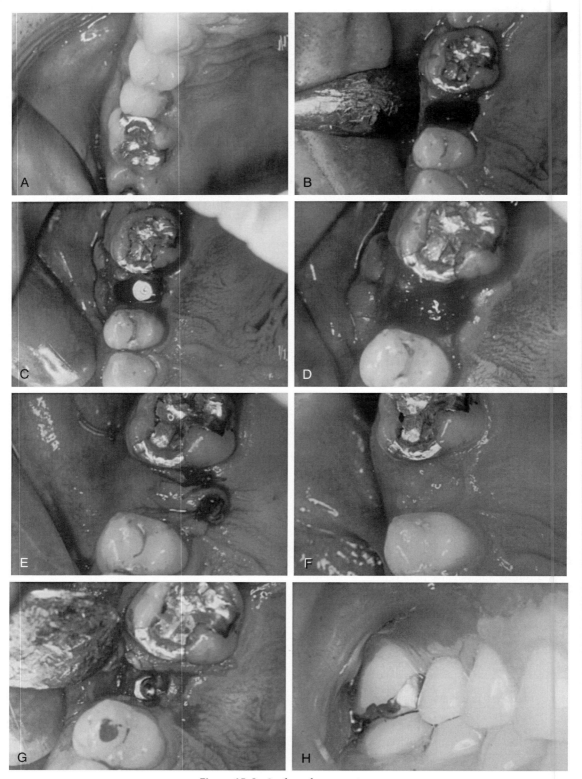

Figure 15–3. *See legend on opposite page*

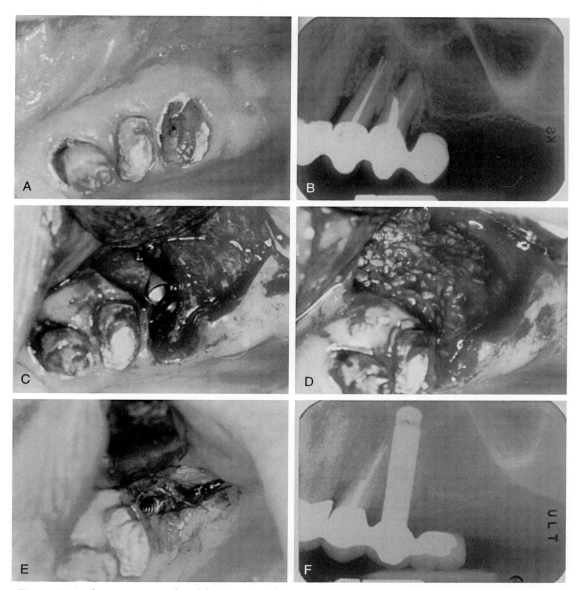

Figure 15–4. This woman was referred for extraction of the right maxillary second premolar. The adjacent first premolar and canine were restorable. Her dentist requested placement of one implant into the extraction site. *B,* This periapical radiograph indicates the reason the second premolar needed to be extracted. Note that there is bone present apical to the tooth to be extracted. *C,* An incision is made around the neck of the tooth to be extracted, with vertical release. There was a large facial and palatal bone defect after the implant had been placed. The implant engaged 4 mm of bone apical to the root. *D,* Demineralized bone was placed to graft the bone defects. The periosteum was released, and the incisions were closed primarily. *E,* Sixteen weeks later, bone was found adjacent to the implant. *F,* A 3-year follow-up radiograph showing excellent bone maintenance adjacent to the implant. (Prosthetics by Dr. Robert Charbenot.)

Figure 15–3. *A,* This 49-year-old man required extraction of his maxillary second premolar secondary to caries. *B,* Incisions were made around the neck of the tooth, and the tooth was removed with sectioning techniques, preserving the facial bone. *C,* The implant site was prepared and the implant placed. Notice the large gap, both facial and palatal, to the implant after the implant was placed. *D,* Demineralized bone powder (500-μm to 1-mm diameter) was used to graft the defect. *E,* The periosteum was released and the adjacent tissue rotated over the extraction site for primary closure. *F,* Four months later, the patient returns for exposure, with preservation of the keratinized tissue along the palatal aspect of the ridge. *G,* On reflection, bone was seen 1- to 2-mm thick along the facial aspect of the implant. *H,* A single crown was fabricated and cemented in place. (Prosthetics by Dr. Gerald Chiche.)

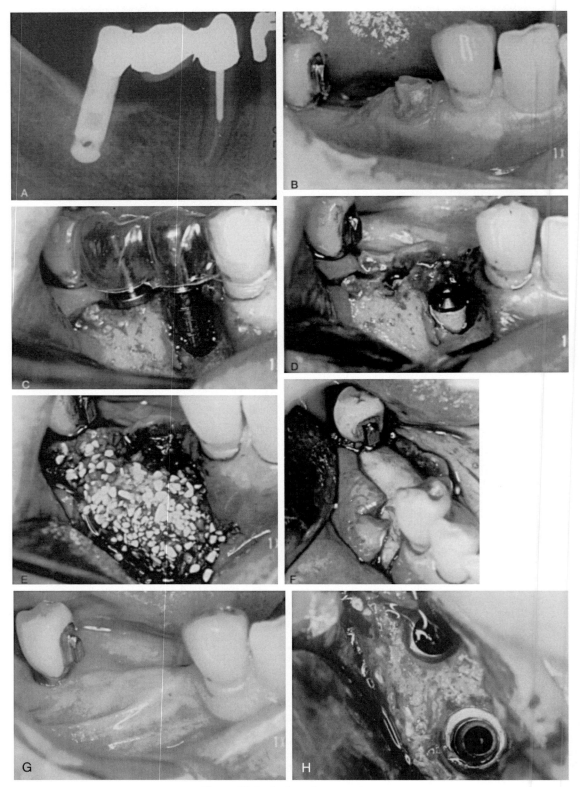

Figure 15–5. *See legend on opposite page*

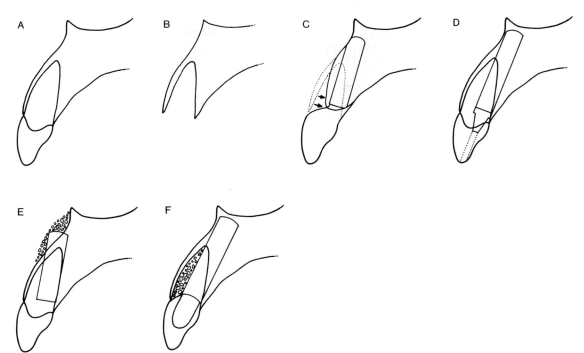

Figure 15–6. *A,* Cross section of a central incisor. *B,* The tooth has been extracted, and the clinician must now choose the location for implant placement. *C,* One option is to delay placement for 6 months. The labial bone, however, remodels toward the palate, leaving the implant, if placed in the available bone, palatal to the ideal restoration. This results in excessive facial emergence profiles or ridge lapping, which are not ideal aesthetically or hygienically. *D,* The implant can be placed totally within the alveolus, but this may position the retaining screw through the incisive edge of the crown. *E,* If the implant is placed more upright with the retaining screw emerging through the cingulum, a portion of the implant extends through the labial cortex. A graft is indicated to cover the implant's surface. *F,* In most situations, the implant can be placed completely within the alveolar bone. This requires labial augmentation with a graft material (HA or bone) to create the appropriate convex ridge form. A cemented restoration is indicated in these patients.

augmentation requirements. The template can be coated with barium sulfate–impregnated varnish, made with 30% barium sulfate by weight combined with clear acrylic, or made with gutta percha–filled hollow shell crowns. These radiopaque, nonmetallic templates are used with reformated computed tomography (CT), before surgery, to determine the exact location and dimensions of the alveolar bone with regard to the necessary implant size, length, and location related to the final restoration. A preoperative conference with the surgeon and the restorative

dentist is useful to plan the final restoration properly.

Implant site development relies on the hard tissue foundation and the soft tissue drape (Fig. 15–6). Hard tissue grafts may restore ridge width and height, but often after the hard tissue grafts consolidate, refinement of the soft tissue is still required for ideal results.

For the ridge that has sufficient hard tissue for implant placement but is deficient in form, i.e., it is concave or flat rather than convex, soft tissue augmentation is indicated. Soft tissue grafts may

Figure 15–5. *A,* This patient had one implant placed with the prosthesis nonrigidly connected to an adjacent tooth. To prevent intrusion of the natural tooth over time, the nonrigid attachment was placed on the implant crown, upside-down. After 2 years, the natural tooth fractured, necessitating extraction. *B,* The fractured tooth in relation to the implant crown and attachment. The tooth was extracted using sectioning techniques to preserve all of the facial bone. *C,* Using a surgical template, the implant sites are prepared, and confirmed by using parallel pins and implant body analogs to ensure proper positioning. *D,* The implants are placed, one in the edentulous region and one in the extraction site. This defect requires grafting both vertical and horizontal deficits. *E,* A mixture of HA and demineralized bone is used for this patient. *F,* Lyophilized dura was used as a resorbable membrane. It was placed over the defect, the incisions released, and periosteum scored, then closed primarily. *G,* After 16 weeks the soft tissue was healed without dehiscence of the lyophilized dura. *H,* After 16 weeks for graft consolidation, the implants were exposed. Note the dense, hard bone material around the implant placed into the extraction site.

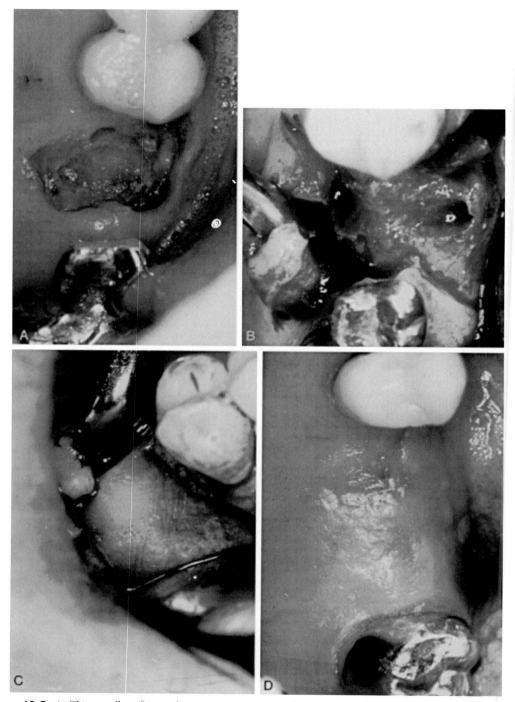

Figure 15–7. A, This maxillary first molar requires extraction. The treatment plan was to extract the tooth, place a membrane for optimal bone fill of the extraction site, and after 3 months place two implants for a two-unit fixed partial denture. B, The extraction site showing the sockets. C, A collagen membrane (Biomend, Calcitek, Inc, Carlsbad, CA) was used as a resorbable membrane. D, After 3 months, the edentulous site is ready to receive implants.

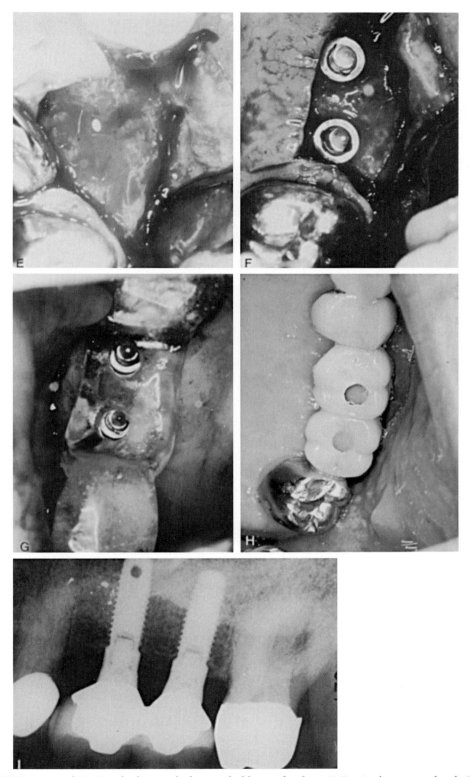

Figure 15–7 *Continued. E,* Bone healing resulted in an ideal bone ridge form. *F,* Two implants were placed. *G,* Here the implants can be seen through the occlusal holes of the template, used to position the implants properly. *H,* This is the final prosthesis showing the ideal location of the retaining screws. (Prosthetics by Dr. Troy Patterson.) *I,* One-year follow-up radiograph.

be harvested from the palate or rotated into the labial aspect of the ridge from the palate. Two methods have been used and are described in Chapter 14.

If adequate bone height is present, one may decide to place an implant into a freshly extracted maxillary molar site. Typically the most bone is found around the palatal root because the facial bone is thin over the buccal root sockets. When an implant is placed into the palatal root socket, the occlusal retaining screw emerges over the working, palatal cusps of the molar crown. In addition, the palatal location of the implant requires special considerations to avoid ridge lapping to allow the patient excellent access to the implant for oral hygiene. Proper angulation prevents prosthetic problems and allows proper emergence profiles of the crowns. The crown should emerge from the gingiva with a smooth transition without the need for ridge lap or overcontouring. To maintain ridge form and prevent facial bone loss from the buccal root site, particulate HA is placed into the empty buccal root socket.

Often the bone remaining after molar extraction is not ideal for simultaneous placement of an implant. The socket is allowed to heal; however, labial bone resorption may occur along with epithelial invagination, decreasing final bone height. A suggested treatment is the placement of a resorbable, collagen membrane using the principles of guided tissue regeneration. The membrane excludes epithelial invagination and allows for optimal bone fill. After 3 months the implant is placed in a position ideal for the planned restoration (Fig. 15–7).

References

1. Anneroth G, Hedstrom KG, Kjellman O, Kondell P-A, Nordenram A: Endosseous titanium implants in extraction sites. Int J Oral Surg 14:50–54, 1985.
2. Ashman A: An immediate tooth root replacement: An implant cylinder and synthetic bone combination. J Oral Implantol 16:28–38, 1990.
3. Barzilay I, Graser G, Iranpour B, Natiella J, Proskin H: Histologic and clinical assessment of implants placed in extraction sockets (abstract 1452). J Dent Res 69 (spec iss): 290, 1990.
4. Becker W, Becker BE: Guided tissue regeneration for implants placed into extraction sockets and for implant dehiscences: Surgical techniques and case reports. Int J Periodont Restor Dent 10:377–391, 1990.
5. Block MS, Kent JN: Placement of endosseous implants into tooth extraction sites. J Oral Maxillofac Surg 49:1269–1276, 1991.
6. Kent JN, Block MS, Finger IN, et al: Biointegrated hydroxylapatite coated dental implants—five year clinical observations. J Am Dent Assoc 121:138–144, 1990.
7. Lazzara RJ: Immediate implant placement into extraction sites: Surgical and restorative advantages. Int J Periodont Restor Dent 9:333–343, 1989.
8. Mentag PJ, Kosinski T: Hydroxyapatite-augmented sites as receptors for replacement implants. J Oral Implantol 15:114–123, 1989.
9. Mentag PJ, Kosinski TF, Sowinski LL: Dental implant reconstruction after endodontic failure: Report of case. J Am Dent Assoc 121:241–244, 1990.
10. Nail GA, Stein S, Kohri M, Waite DE: Evaluation of endosseous implants placed in fresh extraction sites in dogs (abstract 1906). J Dent Res 69 (spec iss):347, 1990.
11. Niznick GA: The Core-Vent implant system. J Oral Implantol 10:379–418, 1982.
12. Quayle AA, Cawood JI, Smith GA, Howell RA: The immediate or delayed replacement of teeth by permucosal intra-osseous implants: The Tubingen implant system. Part 2: Surgical and restorative techniques. Br Dent J 166:403–410, 1989.
13. Ross SE, Strauss T, Crossetti HW, Gargiulo AW: The immediate placement of an endosseous implant into an extraction wound: A clinical case report using the RosTR system. Int J Periodont Restor Dent 9:35–41, 1989.
14. Scott RF, Razzoog ME, Yaman P: Consequences of inadequate bone healing before implant surgery. J Prosthet Dent 61:399–401, 1989.
15. Sevor J, Meffort R, Block C: The immediate placement of dental implants into fresh maxillary extraction sites. Pract Periodont Aesthet Dent 3:55–59, 1991.
16. Yukna RA: Clinical comparison of hydroxyapatite-coated titanium dental implants placed in fresh extraction sockets and healed sites. J Periodontol 62:468–472, 1991.
17. Yukna RA: Placement of hydroxylapatite-coated implants into fresh or recent extraction sites. Dent Clin North Am 36:97–116, 1992.

Study Questions

1. For carious and periodontally involved teeth, what are your strategies for timing extraction and implant placement into those sites?

2. When placing an implant into a recent extraction site, how would you treat, at the time of implant placement, small bone defects?

3. When placing an implant into a recent extraction site and encountering a large bone defect, what do you do, and why?

CHAPTER 16

Implants and Orthodontics

David R. Hoffman
Revised by Michael S. Block

Compliance
Implants in Orthodontics—Animal Studies
Implants in Human Orthodontic Treatment

Osseous Handles
Onplant
References

It is significant that implants offer to solve one of the orthodontist's greatest dilemmas: anchorage control. Since the earliest days of the specialty, orthodontists have sought to avoid the reciprocal nature of forces. This quest has fostered many schemes that purport to defy the physical realities of Newton's law. The innate stability of an osseointegrated implant device can provide this advantage to the orthodontist. The reliance on patient cooperation would be minimized because the use of headgear and elastics would be eliminated or greatly decreased. Treatment could proceed more rapidly with highly predictable results. Tooth extractions solely for treatment side effects could be avoided. Dental arches could be lengthened by bodily distalization of the posterior teeth. The danger and inconvenience of extraoral headgear devices could be avoided.

COMPLIANCE

Achieving adequate patient compliance is the most difficult part of orthodontic treatment.[9, 29] Of a large group of postorthodontically treated patients, a mere 4% faithfully followed their orthodontist's instructions.[7] An additional 22% complied "most of the time." This left 74% of the patients admitting to having worn their headgear or elastics less than one-half the time requested.[5]

IMPLANTS IN ORTHODONTICS— ANIMAL STUDIES

There are several major differences between a prosthetic implant and an implant used for orthodontic anchorage. The prosthetic implant is stressed with intense interrupted forces directed generally along its long axis. The implant used for orthodontic treatment needs to resist less intense but continual forces that may be perpendicular to its long axis. The key to the implant's stability is the lack of a complete fibrous capsule. Adell et al[2] found that an osseointegrated implant did not move regardless of the force vector or magnitude when subjected to orthodontic forces. Vitreous carbon implants can resist movement if allowed to heal before being loaded with forces up to 200 g for as long as 7 months.[16, 21] Studies by Roberts et al[22–27] demonstrated that a longer healing period would result in a higher degree of success.

Roberts et al[26] inserted commercially pure titanium screw-shaped implants into the femurs of rabbits. After healing for 6 to 12 weeks, the paired implants were loaded with 100 g of force for 1 to 12 weeks. Histologic assessment revealed an increase in the bone mass in the area of the loaded implant. This is consistent with Wolff's law, which simply states that ". . . bone mass will increase in response to stress."[27] Helm et al[10] corroborated this finding when they noted a doubling of the remodeling rate of loaded bone. Gray et al[8] also found a lack of fibrous encapsulation of loaded bioglass implants. All surfaces of the coated implants were immediately adjacent to compact bone. This occurred on both the pressure and the tension sides of the device. There was no evidence of osteoclastic reaction to the applied forces.

IMPLANTS IN HUMAN ORTHODONTIC TREATMENT

The greatest obstacle of widespread use of implants in current orthodontic protocols is the size and shape of the current implant designs. Conventional prosthetic endosseous implant designs have limited applications in the adolescent patient.

Dolder[6] states that 3.4% of the population is missing a permanent tooth other than a third molar. In some cases, orthodontists close the edentulous spaces to avoid a fixed prosthesis on an adolescent patient. The success rate of prosthetic implants has given the orthodontist an acceptable alternative to fixed bridgework.[15] An implant in an edentulous space can also be used as an anchor unit for tooth movement. Because

orthodontic closure of the space would have protracted the treatment time, the case can be concluded more quickly. Once orthodontic treatment is completed, the implant avoids the need to prepare the adjacent, often virgin, teeth for fixed bridgework. The bulk of the implant and the occlusal load it transmits to the alveolar bone preclude the unsightly ridge atrophy that usually occurs in the pontic area.

Implants placed into a growing individual do not move with the vertically lengthening alveolus (Fig. 16–1). Vertical elongation of the alveolar

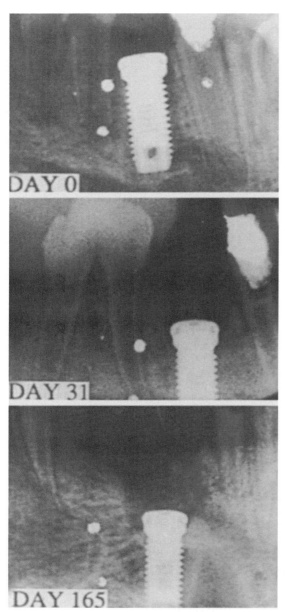

Figure 16–1. The dentoalveolar development between days 0 and 165 for this fixture. Through alveolar process growth, the implants remained static in position, as referenced to the intrabony bone maskers. (From Ödman J, et al: The effect of osseointegrated implants on the dento-alveolar development—a clinical and radiographic study in growing pigs. Eur J Orthod 13:279–286, 1991. By permission of Oxford University Press.)

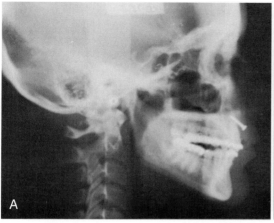

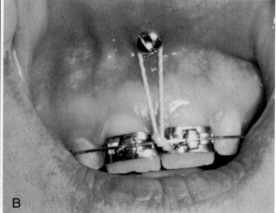

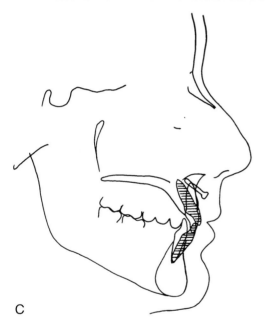

Figure 16–2. *A,* This cephalometric radiograph shows a surgical Vitallium screw placed into the anterior nasal spine region for skeletal anchorage for incisor intrusion. *B,* Light elastic thread tied from head of screw to archwire. *C,* Superimposition before and after 1 year of treatment, showing the amount of elevation and torque of upper incisors achieved. (From Creekmore TD, Eklund MK: The possibility of skeletal anchorage. J Clin Orthod 17:266–269, 1983.)

ridge as a result of a normal growth process can be a complication if implants are used during the developmental period. The implant becomes *submerged* similar to an ankylosed tooth.[19]

Virtually all conventional implant types have been successfully used as orthodontic anchors[14, 20] (Figs. 16–2, 16–3). If an implant used for orthodontic purposes is later used as a prosthetic abutment, there would be no additional cost to the patient. If, however, the implant is to be used only to anchor orthodontic tooth movement, the cost of the implant may be a factor. Because the fate of a "slept" implant is unknown, retrieving the orthodontic implant should be considered. It is anticipated that once the use of implants in orthodontic treatment becomes routine, the cost will be offset by the rapidity of treatment.

OSSEOUS HANDLES

The most dramatic use of the orthodontic implant may be to guide orthopedic development.[3] Often the skeleton is the basis for severe malocclusion. Contemporary force delivery systems designed to guide the vector and velocity of skeletal jaw growth are usually applied to the teeth.[1, 11, 12, 13, 17, 18, 22] These forces are retransmitted to the bones. The intention is to alter the pattern of jaw development.

In a classic study, Smalley et al[28] dramatically demonstrated the potential of implants for orthopedic movement (Fig. 16–4). They placed Brånemark implants into the maxilla, zygomas, and orbital and occipital bones of four monkeys. By means of an external protraction device attached

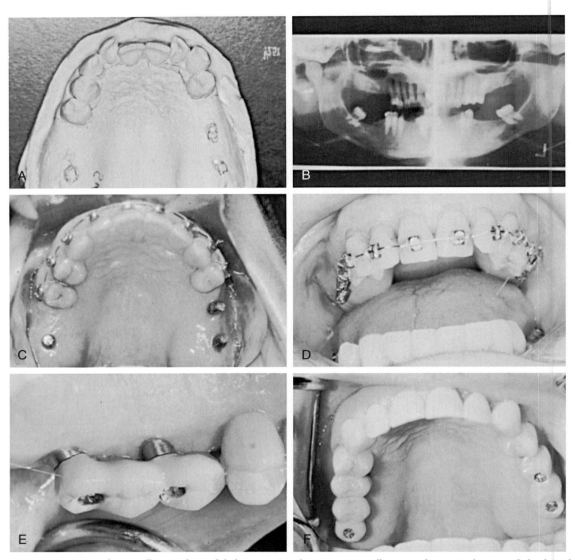

Figure 16–3. *A,* This maxillary study model demonstrates the anterior maxillary crowding. Distalization of the lateral incisors, canines, and premolars required implant placement in the posterior regions. *B,* Preoperative panoramic radiograph showing multiple missing teeth and significant peridontal disease. *C,* Orthodontic treatment progressed rapidly using implant abutments as anchorage sources. *D,* Orthodontic retraction of the teeth is occurring without flaring of central incisors. *E,* Final posterior restoration after completion of prosthesis. *F,* Final appearance after completion of prosthetics. (Surgery by Dr. A. Aceredo, prosthetics by Dr. Israel Finger.)

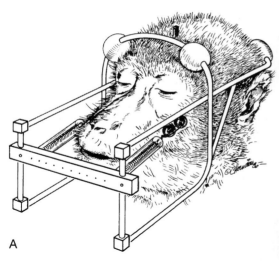

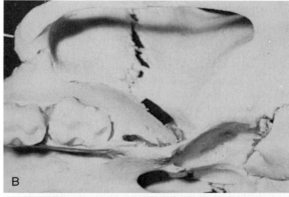

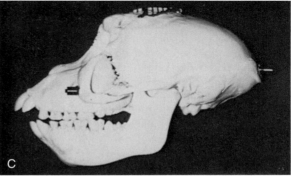

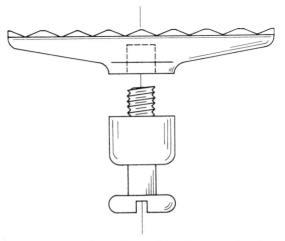

Figure 16–4. *A,* An extraoral traction appliance. The framework was rigidly attached with self-curing acrylic resin to the four cranial titanium implants. A precision coil spring with a protective tube was fastened bilaterally from the adjustable anterior horizontal bar of the framework to the facial titanium implants. *B,* Dry skull preparation showing the effect when the protraction force was applied to titanium implants in the maxilla and the zygomatic bones. Traction delivered to the maxillary implant resulted primarily in significant separation of the zygomaticomaxillary suture. In contrast, as seen here, traction applied to the zygomatic implant changed the morphology of the zygomatic bone substantially and nearly disarticulated the sphenozygomatic and zygomaticotemporal sutures. *C,* Dry skull preparation showing the left side from one of the experimental animals. It shows considerable skeletal remodeling, sutural expansion, and an excessively class II occlusion. (From Smalley WM, et al: Osseointegrated titanium implants for maxillofacial protraction in monkeys. Am J Orthod 94:285–295, 1988.)

to the orbital and occipital implants, a constant force of 600 g per side was applied to the maxillary or zygomatic bones for 12 to 18 weeks (Fig. 16–4A). They demonstrated a 12-mm widening of the zygomaticomaxillary suture, a 16-mm widening of the zygomaticotemporal suture (Fig. 16–4B), a change from a class I to a class II dental relationship, and an increase of overjet of 5 to 7 mm (Fig. 16–4C).

ONPLANT

Although materials and surgical techniques have been perfected, endosseous implant design, size, and alveolar ridge deficiency remain as deterrents to widespread use in orthodontic treatment. Block and Hoffman[4] have designed, developed, and tested a thin, surface-adherent titanium disc as a subperiosteal orthodontic anchor (Fig. 16–5). It is referred to as an *onplant* because it is not embedded into bone but becomes biointegrated onto the surface of bone. The onplant's surface adjacent to the bone is textured and coated with hydroxylapatite (HA).

The opposing titanium surface facing soft tissue is smooth and has an internally threaded hole in the center that can accept a variety of abutments to accept wires, bars, or other attachments.

The surgical placement of the onplant is

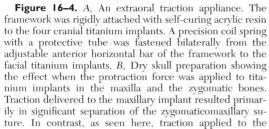

Figure 16–5. The onplant and the abutment. This abutment shown is designed to receive a 0.051-inch wire.

through a well-defined subperiosteal tunnel. A healing time of 3 to 4 months is sufficient for biointegration to occur. A small trephine is used to remove a circular patch of tissue over the healing screw. An abutment head that protrudes through the tissue into the oral cavity is screwed into place.

A monkey study was designed to mimic a situation commonly encountered in orthodontics. Five adult monkeys had all four upper premolars extracted and a single onplant device inserted subperiosteally onto the palate medial to the permanent first molars. After 12 weeks the onplants were exposed, and abutments were inserted in four of the animals. Cast transpalatal bars were soldered to a first molar on one side and to a second molar on the other side. The cast transpalatal bars were screwed to the abutment (Fig. 16–6). Springs were ligated bilaterally between the first molars and canine. The springs were maintained at approximately 250 g of force. The monkeys were sacrificed after 6 months.

The anchored molars moved mesially an average of 1.2 mm. The nonanchored molars moved mesially an average of 4.1 mm. The canines on both sides moved distally an average of 1.9 mm. The effective anchorage was significant. From a

practical point of view, the cast bar forces the orthodontist to detour from standard practices. It is not common for orthodontists to use cast devices. In addition, the use of a screw to secure the cast bar creates a bulky profile, which could be uncomfortable for the patient.

Four women participated in a pilot trial (Fig. 16–7). They were already wearing orthodontic appliances, were reluctantly wearing a headgear, had critical anchorage requirements, and welcomed an alternative form of treatment. A single onplant was surgically inserted subperiosteally in the midpalatal region. After 4 months, the onplant was exposed, and a grooved abutment was inserted. Stainless steel bands were fitted to the maxillary first molar and a polyvinylsiloxane impression technique was used to transfer the bands and abutment location to a working cast. A 0.051-inch stainless steel wire that rested against the posterior surface of the abutment was soldered to the bands. The appliance was cemented into the mouth. The upper second molars were bonded, and a full-arch continuous archwire was inserted.

En masse bodily retraction of the anterior segment was initiated without the aid of elastics or headgear. The onplant was the sole source of

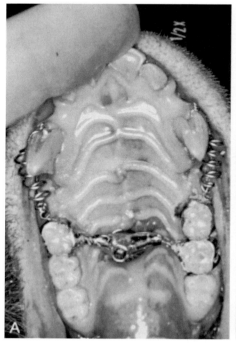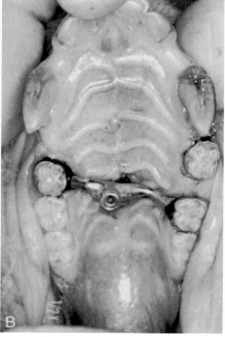

Figure 16–6. *A,* A cast bar has been fabricated in the laboratory and secured to the onplant with a screw, with the bands cemented to the molar teeth. The first molar on one side is anchored by the onplant, and the first molar on the opposite side is not anchored. *B,* Six months later, it can be seen that the anchored tooth has not moved. The nonanchored first molar has moved to the canine.

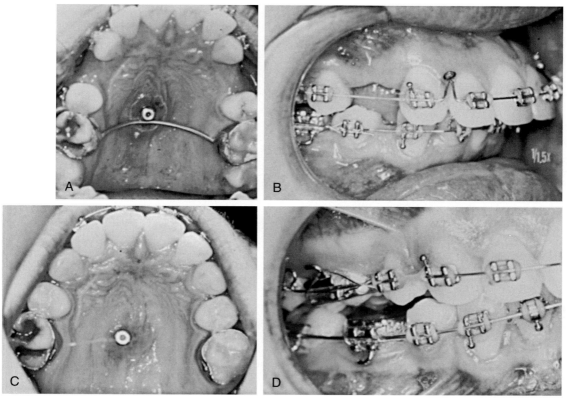

Figure 16–7. *A,* Immediately after placement of the transpalatal 0.051-inch wire. Note the 8-mm space, which must be entirely used by the canine retraction. *B,* Lateral view. Note the class I molar relationship before receiving the onplant and initiating anterior en masse retraction. *C,* The occlusal view 12 months later. The anterior teeth have been retracted 8 mm without mesial migration of the molars. *D,* Lateral view. Note maintenance of the class I molar relationship.

stabilization. Without anchorage reinforcement, at least 50% of the extraction site is usually lost from mesial movement of the posterior buccal segments. The patient demonstrated incisor retraction using the onplant as the sole source of anchorage control. It took 11 months to close the extraction site. There was no forward movement of the posterior segments. There was total utilization of the extraction site from unilateral distal movement of the anterior segment.

References

1. Adams CD, Meikle MC, Norwwick KW, Turpin DL: Dentofacial remodelling produced by intermaxillary forces in Macaca mulatta. Arch Oral Biol 17:1519–1535, 1972.
2. Adell R, Lekholm U, Rockler B, Branemark P: A 15-year study of osseointegrated implants in the treatment of the edentulous jaw. Int J Oral Surg 10:387–416, 1981.
3. Arbuckle GR, Nelson CL, Roberts WE: Osseointegrated implants and orthodontics. Oral Maxillofac Clin North Am 3:903–919, 1991.
4. Block MS, Hoffman DR: A new device for absolute anchorage for orthodontics. Am J Orthod Dentofacial Orthop 107:251–258, 1995.
5. Clemmer EJ, Hayes EW: Patient cooperation in wearing orthodontic headgear. Am J Orthodont 75:517–524, 1979.
6. Dolder E: Deficient dentition. Dent Rec 57:142, 1937.
7. Egolf RJ, BeGole EA, Upshaw HS: Factors associated with orthodontic patient compliance with intraoral elastic and headgear wear. Am J Orthodont 97:336–348, 1990.
8. Gray JB, Steen ME, King GJ, Clark AE: Studies on the efficacy of implants as orthodontic anchorage. Am J Orthodont 83:311–317, 1983.
9. Grewe JM, Hemanson PC: Influence of severity of malocclusion on the duration or orthodontic treatment. Am J Orthodont 63:533–536, 1973.
10. Helm FR, Poon LC, Marshall KJ, Gongloff RJ, Roberts WE: Bone remodeling response to loading of rigid endosseous implants. J Dent Res 66:186, 1987.
11. Hickham JH: Maxillary protraction therapy: Diagnosis and treatment. J Clin Orthodont 25:102–113, 1991.
12. Irie M, Nakamura S: Orthopedic approach to severe skeletal class III malocclusion. Am J Orthodont 67:377–392, 1975.
13. Ishii H, Morita S, Takeuchi Y, Nukamura S: Treatment effect of combined maxillary protraction and chincap appliance in severe skeletal class III cases. Am J Orthodont 92:304–312, 1987.
14. Kraut RA, Hammer HS, Wheeler JJ: Use of endosteal implants as orthodontic anchorage. Comp Contin Educ Dent 9:796–801, 1988.

15. Lanzi GL, Seran CC, Cohen SR: Prosthetic replacement of congenitally missing teeth using single-tooth osseointegrated implants: A case report. Comp Contin Educ Dent 11:548–554, 1990.
16. Mendez-Villamil C, Oliver S, Evans C, Schnitman P: Periodontometric evaluation of mobility changes in stressed vitreous carbon implants. J Dent Res 59A:280, 1980.
17. Mermigos J, Full CA, Andreasen G: Protraction of the maxillofacial complex. Am J Orthodont 98:47–55, 1990.
18. Mitani H, Fukazawa H: Effects of chincap force on the timing and amount of mandibular growth associated with anterior reversed occlusion (class III malocclusion) during puberty. Am J Orthodont 90:454–463, 1986.
19. Ödman J, Gröndahl K, Lekholm U, Thilander B: The effect of osseointegrated implants on the dento-alveolar development. A clinical and radiographic study in growing pigs. Eur J Orthodont 13:279–286, 1991.
20. Ödman J, Lekholm U, Jemt T, Brånemark P, Thilander B: Osseointegrated titanium implants—a new approach in orthodontic treatment. Eur J Orthodont 10:98–105, 1988.
21. Oliver S, Mendez-Villamil C, Evans C, Schnitman P, Shulman L: Change in position of vitreous carbon implants subjected to orthodontic forces. J Dent Res 59A:280, 1980.
22. Ritucci R, Nanda R: The effect of chin cup therapy on the growth and development of the cranial base and midface. Am J Orthodont 90:475–483, 1986.
23. Roberts WE: Bone tissue interface. J Dent Educ 52:804–809, 1988.
24. Roberts WE, Helm FR, Marshall KJ, Gongloff RK: Rigid endosseous implants for orthodontic and orthopedic anchorage. Angle Orthodont 59:247–256, 1989.
25. Roberts WE, Marshall KJ, Mozsary PG: Rigid endosseous implant utilized as anchorage to protract molars and close atrophic extraction site. Angle Orthodont 60:135–152, 1990.
26. Roberts WE, Smith RK, Zilberman Y, Mozsary P, Smith R: Osseous adaptation to continuous loading of rigid endosseous implants. Am J Orthodont 86:95–111, 1984.
27. Roberts WE, Turley PK, Brezniak N, Fielder P: Bone physiology and metabolism. Calif Dent Assoc J 15:54–61, 1987.
28. Smalley WM, Shapiro PA, Hohl TH, Kokich VG, Brånemark PI: Osseointegrated titanium implants for maxillofacial protraction in monkeys. Am J Orthodont 94:285–295, 1988.
29. White LW: The editor's corner–"Don't force it." J Clin Orthodont 25:9–10, 1991.

Study Questions

1. Why can implants be used for anchoring tooth movements?

2. If you have a patient with malposed teeth and edentulous spaces that have sufficient bone for implant placement, how would you, step-by-step, plan for the treatment of this patient?

CHAPTER 17

Inferior Alveolar Nerve Repositioning Procedures for Placement of Dental Implants

James D. Ruskin
Revised by John N. Kent

Indications for Repositioning
Surgical Procedures
Evaluation and Treatment of Nerve Injuries
    following Placement of Dental Implants
    Radiographic Evaluation
Treatment Algorithms
    Recognized Injuries during
        Instrumentation and Placement of
        Implants

Nerve Injuries Identified after Placement
    of Implants
    Injuries following Nerve Lateralization
References
Suggested Reading

In many posterior edentulous areas of the mandible a saddle deformity is generally observed following extractions and alveolar bone resorption, leading to diminished ridge height and width over several years. This may preclude placement of even the smallest endosseous implant without potentially damaging the inferior alveolar nerve. In an effort to increase the utilization of implants in these cases, the technique of nerve repositioning has been advocated. The purpose of this section is to review the rationale and describe the techniques of nerve repositioning as an adjunct for implant placement.

INDICATIONS FOR REPOSITIONING

1. Severe resorption of the residual alveolar ridge in which the neurovascular bundle rests on the crest of the ridge and is characterized by complaints of pain over the mental nerve distribution when the denture is compressed, as during mastication. In this case, the nerve bundle is "scooped off" the ridge and placed lateral to the mandible during endosseous implant placement.
2. Inadequate alveolar bone is present between the crest of the ridge and the inferior alveolar canal for placement of necessary implant length. This condition is seen with free-end saddle removable partial denture. Accurate determination of the alveolar bone height and width is necessary since magnification of techniques is up to 25% for panoramic radiographs.
3. There is inadequate anterior space between the two mental foramina for placement of the planned number of implants and a fixed bridge or spark erosion prosthesis is planned. Distalization of the mental foramen may be necessary to provide adequate space, and the presence of an anterior loop of the inferior alveolar nerve up to 5 mm must be considered.

1. The inferior alveolar neurovascular bundle is protected from damage during implant placement.
2. Nerve repositioning allows the full height of the mandible to be used for longer implant placement. Otherwise, primary implant length and stability would be compromised without engaging the inferior cortex of the mandible.
3. Implants can be placed with the proper angulation adding to stability and longevity, rather than using angled implants attempting to avoid hitting the neurovascular bundle or using offset prosthetic designs.
4. Nerve repositioning provides an alternative to augmentation bone grafting to increase the height above the mandibular canal. Bone graft procedures often require a second surgical site for harvesting bone, with the procedure performed in an operating room under general anesthesia, and are susceptible to resorption.
5. Nerve repositioning can be performed at the same time as implant placement, in the office under intravenous sedation, with less cost and potential morbidity to the patient.

SURGICAL PROCEDURES

Patient cooperation is essential to minimize risk to the contents of the mandibular canal, and intravenous sedation is routinely used. Two

Disadvantages of Inferior Alveolar Nerve Repositioning

1. Nerve repositioning may produce short-term or even protracted paresthesia (abnormal sensation without being unpleasant or painful) or dysesthesia (unpleasant or painful sensation). Although the intent of nerve repositioning is to remove the contents of the mandibular canal without injury to any of the structures, surgery may produce changes in the microarchitecture of the nerve resulting in these neurosensory disturbances. Short-term neurosensory changes following surgery are common.
2. Nerve repositioning increases the length of the procedure, requiring the use of intravenous sedation.

different surgical techniques are described. The first, or anterior approach, is used for placement of implants close to the region of the mental foramen and anterior loop of the inferior alveolar nerve. The second, or posterior approach, is primarily used for implants placed into the posterior molar region.

With the anterior approach, careful flap design incision and tissue dissection are essential to avoid injury to the branches of the mental nerve (Fig. 17–1). A mucoperiosteal flap is developed inferiorly down to the level of the mental foramen to identify the nerve. A suture followed by an elastic vessel loop may be placed around the nerve to aid in retraction and protection, while further dissection is completed to expose the entire foramen and branches of the nerve. The mental foramen is now probed with a blunt periodontal probe to determine the course of the canal and identify an anterior loop or prominent incisive branch of the inferior alveolar nerve.

A surgical hand piece with a round bur is used to remove bone over the top of the canal. A probe and other wider instruments are used to mark the location of the canal as well as to protect the contents from injury as bone is removed in a posterior direction past the last planned implant site. With the nerve gently retracted out of the way, the implant site is prepared and the implant placed (Fig. 17–2). The nerve is allowed to return to that portion of the canal not occupied by the implant as long as the nerve is not in direct contact with the implant, since this may promote neurosensory disturbances. Autogenous particulate bone, allogeneic bone, and resorbable hemostatic agents are used to isolate the nerve from the implant.

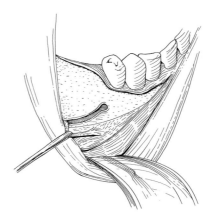

Figure 17–1. After sufficient removal of bone proximal to the last planned fixture site, the nerve is gently teased from the canal. The incisive branch may need to be sacrificed in some cases to allow for sufficient retraction of the nerve to allow fixture placement.

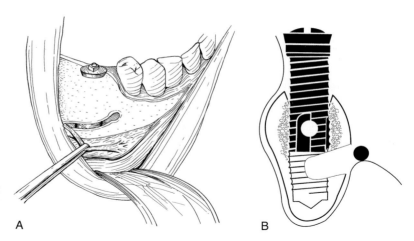

Figure 17–2. *A* and *B*, Implant placement of the fixture is completed with the nerve retracted.

A   B

A careful posterior flap design is similar to the anterior approach if the posterior arch is edentulous. If posterior dentition remains, the flap is modified to allow for primary closure over the implant fixture (Fig. 17–3). The mental nerve and foramen are identified as before and a probe placed to determine the location of the mandibular canal. With a surgical hand piece and a fissure bur, a cortical window with horizontal superior and inferior cuts is outlined encompassing the area of the nerve to be repositioned. A fine chisel is to remove the cortical plate (Fig. 17–3). Small curets are then used to remove any residual cortical or cancellous bone to allow for complete visualization and mobilization of the nerve. The vessel loop is placed, and the neurovascular bundle is gently retracted for implant site preparation and the implant placement (Fig. 17–4). The cortical plate may be ground into small particles and placed over the implant to isolate it from the nerve (Fig. 17–5). Additional material should be placed over the top of the nerve to prevent adhesions from developing between the neurovascular bundle and the periosteum.

The postoperative course, including use of chlorhexidine rinses and antibiotics, is monitored as a means of following return of sensation, or lack of it, should a deficit be noted after the procedure. At the first postoperative visit, it should be determined if a neurosensory deficit is present. The patient usually states if a deficit is present. More quantitative testing, directional sense, light touch, and algometry can be carried out to determine the degree of dysfunction. Paresthesia lasting longer than 4 months or the presence of dysesthesia should prompt referral of the patient to a specialist skilled in the diagnosis and treatment of nerve injuries. Good oral hygiene optimizes wound healing and decreases the risk of wound infection.

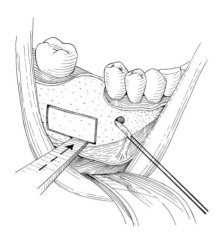

Figure 17–3. A fine chisel is placed into the inferior and superior cuts only to remove the cortical plate.

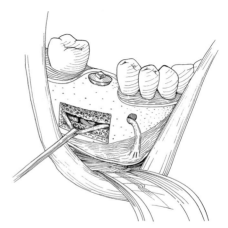

Figure 17–4. Placement of the fixture is completed with the nerve retracted.

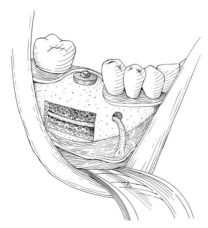

Figure 17–5. After fixture placement, the nerve is replaced as much as possible back into the inferior alveolar canal. The remainder of the nerve is allowed to rest gently against the fixture or suitable filler material that has been placed between the implant and the nerve.

EVALUATION AND TREATMENT OF NERVE INJURIES FOLLOWING PLACEMENT OF DENTAL IMPLANTS

Injuries to the inferior alveolar and lingual nerves have been associated with the removal of third molars, mandibular fractures, osteotomies, and neoplastic disease. Of late, nerve injuries have been seen with increasing frequency in conjunction with the placement of osseointegrated implants. The student is urged to review basic anatomy and structural arrangement of peripheral nerves (Fig. 17–6).

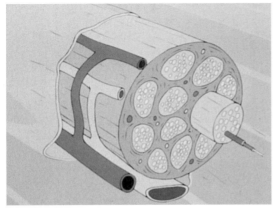

Figure 17–6. Anatomic arrangement of neural and connective tissue components of a peripheral nerve. Longitudinal view.

Nerve injuries are classified as follows[1, 2]:
1. First-degree injury: Those injuries in which there is a temporary interruption of conduction without loss of axonal structural continuity. A localized conduction block occurs as a result of decreased axoplasmic flow or localized demyelination. This usually results following indirect pressure as in retraction during surgery or from edema or hematoma postoperatively. Injuries of this type usually resolve within 3 to 6 weeks with complete recovery of neurosensory function.
2. Second-degree injury: Those injuries in which complete obstruction of axoplasmic flow occurs with degeneration of the distal nerve segment. No disruption of the endoneurium, perineurium, or epineurium occurs, however. This injury usually occurs as a result of vigorous retraction or compression during surgery. Complete recovery is expected, because the endoneurium and the surrounding supporting structures are intact.
3. Third-degree through fifth-degree injury: Those injuries in which the contents of the nerve trunk are severed to various degrees and the endoneurium has been disrupted. A fourth-degree injury is one in which the endoneurium and perineurium have been disrupted. Complete severance of the entire nerve is classified as a fifth-degree injury. Recovery from these injuries is variable and depends on the degree of regeneration (Fig. 17–7).

The physiology of degeneration and regeneration is necessarily understood by the surgeon performing nerve repairs.[3]

Nerve repair may be classified as primary, delayed primary, or secondary. Primary nerve repair affects anastomosis of the divided nerve at or soon after the original time of injury. A surgical field with an undistorted view of anatomic structures is available at this time, as opposed to the distorted view of anatomic structures following healing. Most nerve injuries in which clean severance has been noted, without concomitant crush or avulsion of tissue, are amenable to primary repair.

Nerve injuries in which an unknown amount of nerve damage is present are best treated by secondary repair. This usually occurs within 3 to 4 months following the original injury, depending on the nerve injured and type of injury suspected. Nerve repair should not be delayed more than 4 to 6 months to attain the best possible chance for successful reinnervation. This tech-

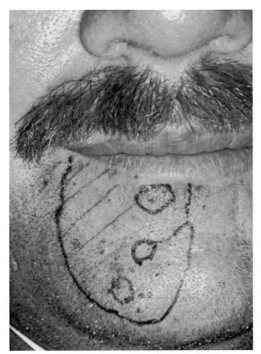

Figure 17–7. Marking on patient with mixed neurosensory dysfunction. Areas that are anesthetic, paresthetic, and dysesthetic are marked differently and photographed for future comparison.

nique is usually reserved for those injuries in which there is known damage to the nerve that could not be repaired at the time of the injury. If any doubt exists whether nerve damage has occurred, secondary repair at a later time is indicated.

Radiographic Evaluation

Although some implant manufacturers recommend that no postoperative radiographs be taken until the time of abutment placement, radiographic evaluation should be undertaken in patients who complain of neurosensory disturbances following implant placement. This is done to ascertain the relative position of the inferior alveolar nerve to the implant. The term *relative position* is used because the radiograph is only a two-dimensional representation of a three-dimensional object. From a periapical or panoramic radiograph, it is possible to determine the depth of the implant but not the buccal lingual relationship of implant to nerve (Fig. 17–8). If precise information is required as to the exact location of the implant, computed tomography

(CT) may be employed. This study has the ability to be reformatted to provide not only axial images but also cross sections through the implant site itself.

TREATMENT ALGORITHMS

Injuries to the inferior alveolar nerve secondary to implant placement may be divided into two major groups—those occurring during instrumentation and placement of implants that are recognized and those that manifest after completion of the procedure.

Recognized Injuries during Instrumentation and Placement of Implants

During instrumentation for placement of a dental implant, a nerve injury should be suspected if copious hemorrhage is encountered from the preparation site. At this point the procedure should be terminated and the hemorrhage controlled with pressure over the site. No attempt should be made to place an instrument into the site nor should an implant be placed into the site in an attempt to control hemorrhage, because this may cause further damage to the neurovascular bundle. Gentle packing of the site with hemostatic material such as methylcellulose or fibrillar collagen may be carried out after initial control of the bleeding has been obtained, but should not extend to the depth of the preparation to avoid compressing the nerve. Once the hemorrhage has been controlled an attempt may be made to visualize the nerve. If an injury is identified and the operator is skilled in microsurgery, immediate repair of the nerve is indicated. If the nerve is not able to be visualized, the

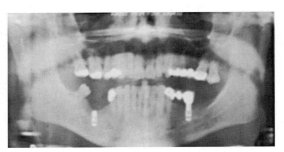

Figure 17–8. Panoramic radiograph identifying two endosseous implants. The implant on the left is noted to be above the inferior alveolar canal, whereas the implant on the right appears to be below the inferior alveolar canal.

implant procedure should be terminated and the patient informed of the possibility of a nerve injury.

The patient should be seen in 1 week and evaluated as previously outlined. If neurosensory dysfunction is detected, the patient should be followed on a weekly basis for the first month. A neurosensory evaluation should be carried out at each visit and the results documented in the patient's chart. Simply relying on the patient's perception of whether he or she is getting better or not should be avoided because the patient may perceive that the condition is unchanged, yet objective evidence may show improvement. If at the end of the month the patient is not showing definite signs of improvement, he or she should be referred to a specialist trained to diagnose and treat nerve injuries of this type for more definitive evaluation and treatment as necessary. If the patient is noted to be improving, he or she should be followed and re-evaluated on a monthly basis until the injury has resolved. If improvement reaches a plateau with no further improvement over two consecutive visits, or within 3 months, the patient should be referred for more definitive evaluation and treatment. An immediate referral is indicated if the patient develops nerve pain (dysesthesia) at any time during the recovery process (Fig. 17–9).

Nerve Injuries Identified after Placement of Implants

Some nerve injuries are not recognized until after the procedure has been completed. At the first indication of the presence of an injury, the situation should be evaluated both clinically and radiographically. The clinical evaluation has been described previously. Radiographs of the implant site in question should be obtained and evaluated for proximity of the implant to the nerve. For injuries that are recognized before significant os-

seointegration, if the implant is found to be at or below the level of the neurovascular canal, it should be removed and replaced with a shorter implant that does not encroach on the canal. Replacement of the implant is indicated only if a shorter implant does not compromise the planned prosthetic restoration. In no case should additional site preparation be performed, because this may cause further damage to the neurovascular structures. The patient is then observed for the first month on a weekly basis and signs of improvement in the neurosensory status evaluated. As for recognized injuries, if no definite signs of improvement are noted at the end of the first month, the patient should be referred to the specialist for further evaluation and treatment. If signs of improvement are noted, the patient is followed as noted previously for recognized injuries.

Occasionally patients do not complain about nerve dysfunction for weeks to months following implant placement. In these cases the implant may be well on its way toward osseointegration or it actually may be osseointegrated. Situations such as this pose a dilemma for the practitioner. Should one take out an integrated implant that is in proximity to the neurovascular canal in a patient with complaints of sensory dysfunction? In this situation, CT of the area, reformatted to provide cross-sectional views, may be beneficial to determine the exact position of the implant. If the canal has been entered and the implant is integrated, the implant should be left alone and the patient referred to a specialist skilled in nerve grafting. The nerve can usually be isolated both proximal and distal to the implant and repaired without sacrificing the implant itself. Attempts to remove an integrated implant in the vicinity of the neurovascular canal may result in additional damage to the nerve (Fig. 17–10).

Injuries following Nerve Lateralization

Although the intent of nerve repositioning is to remove the contents of the neurovascular canal without injury, changes to the microarchitecture or in some cases macroarchitecture of the nerve occur that may result in neurosensory dysfunction. With minor alterations to the microarchitecture, most sensory deficits have been reported to resolve with return to normal sensation within 6 months to a year. More major changes or gross alteration to the nerve may produce a wide array of sensory disturbances, some of which may re-

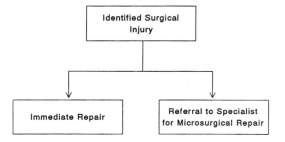

Figure 17–9. Treatment algorithm for injuries identified during instrumentation and implant placement.

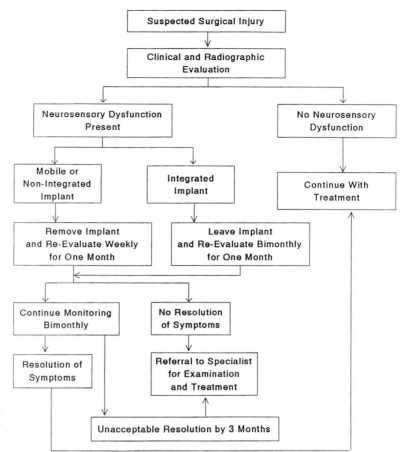

Figure 17–10. Treatment algorithm for injuries identified after implant placement.

quire operative intervention. When nerve lateralization procedures are being performed, it is important to note any alterations to the neurovascular bundle that occur during the procedure. In cases in which gross disruption of the nerve occurs, immediate repair by a practitioner skilled in nerve repair is indicated. If this is not possible, the patient should be referred as soon as possible for nerve repair.

Injuries that were not obvious at the time of the procedure are handled in much the same manner as occult injuries. Again, most of these sensory disturbances resolve spontaneously; however, close postoperative follow-up and appropriate referral are necessary (Fig. 17–10).

In summary, nerve injuries as a result of placement of dental implants are increasing rapidly. The biologic basis for nerve injury and repair has been reviewed, and a rational approach to the management of patients with neurosensory disturbances has been presented. Treatment algorithms have been proposed for various types of injuries and are based on the personal experience

of the author as well as that of others skilled in the area of nerve repair. With continuing research in this area, it is anticipated that revisions to these algorithms will occur. As with other areas of therapy, meticulous attention to detail and careful treatment planning are the best methods to prevent injuries from occurring.

References

1. Seddon HJ: Three types of nerve injury. Brain 66:237–288, 1943.
2. Sunderland S: Nerves and Nerve Injuries, ed 2. Edinburgh, Churchill Livingstone, 1978.
3. Upton LG, Rajvanakarn M, Hayward JR: Evaluation of the regenerative capacity of the inferior alveolar nerve following surgical trauma. J Oral Maxillofac Surg 45:212–216, 1987.

Suggested Reading

Friberg B, Ivanoff CJ, Lekholm U: Inferior alveolar nerve transposition in combination with Brånemark implant placement. Int J Periodont Restor Dent 12:441, 1992.

Gregg JM: Abnormal responses to trigeminal nerve injury: Clinical syndromes, surgical pathology and neural mechanisms. Oral Maxillofac Clin North Am 4:339, 1992.

Jensen O, Nock D: Inferior alveolar nerve repositioning in conjunction with placement of osseointegrated implants: A case report. Oral Surg Oral Med Oral Pathol 63:263, 1987.

Rosenquist B: Fixture placement posterior to the mental foramen with transpositioning of the inferior alveolar nerve. Int J Oral Maxillofac Impl 7:45, 1992.

Stella JP, Tharanon W: A precise radiographic method to determine the location of the inferior alveolar canal in the posterior edentulous mandible: Implications for dental implants: I. Technique. Int J Oral Maxillofac Impl 5:15, 1990.

Study Questions

1. Describe the method for respositioning the inferior alveolar nerve and implant placement.

2. You place an implant into the posterior mandible. The patient calls you the next day complaining of intense pain on the lip and chin. What do you think may be happening, and what is your plan?

3. The same situation as question 2, but the patient complains that there is absolutely no sensation in the lip and chin. What do you do?

CHAPTER *18*

Guided Bone Regeneration and Implants: History and Case Reports

PART *1*

Guided Bone Regeneration in Conjunction with Dental Endosseous Implants

Richard F. Caudill
Revised by Michael S. Block

Part 1. Guided Bone Regeneration in Conjunction with Dental Endosseous Implants
  Background: Evolution of the Concept of Guided Tissue Regeneration around Natural Teeth
  Evolution of the Concept of Guided Bone Regeneration in Skeletal Bones
  Evolution of the Concept of Guided Tissue Regeneration around Endosseous Implants
  Gore-Tex Augmentation Material: Description and Clinical Guidelines
  Summary of Prerequisites for Successful Guided Bone Regeneration Using a Barrier
  References
Part 2. The Use of Membrane Technique to Regenerate Bone with Endosseous Dental Implants
  Indications for Guided Tissue Regeneration

Considerations in the Use of Expanded Polytetrafluoroethylene Membranes in Osteopromotion
Postoperative Considerations and Follow-up Care in Guided Bone Regeneration
Premature Exposure of the Expanded Polytetrafluoroethylene Membrane
Removal Procedure for Expanded Polytetrafluoroethylene Membrane
Case Reports: Guided Bone Regeneration
  Case History 1. Cortical Dehiscence Defect
  Case History 2. Intraosseous Defect
  Case History 3. Cortical Dehiscence Defect (Mandible)
  Case History 4. Fenestration Defect (Multiple Congenitally Missing Teeth)
References

BACKGROUND: EVOLUTION OF THE CONCEPT OF GUIDED TISSUE REGENERATION AROUND NATURAL TEETH

The concept of *guided bone regeneration* around dental implants originally evolved from animal investigations that found enhanced osteogenesis in surgically created defects involving skeletal bones. When various barriers were used to create selective wound healing compartments, tissues other than bone were excluded from the arena of regeneration, resulting in unusually copious amounts of new bone growth.[30, 33, 34]

Guided tissue regeneration (GTR) principles are used in regeneration of periodontal supporting structures around natural teeth that have been lost as a result of periodontitis. The exclu-

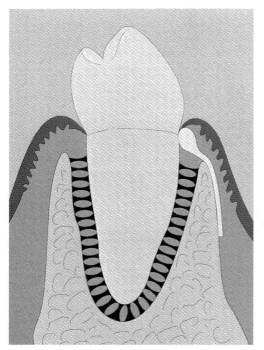

Figure 18–1. Result of periodontal regeneration when using a barrier in human periodontitis defects.

sion of both epithelium and gingival connective tissue was the objective of both animal and human experiments that used barriers of various materials for that purpose (Fig. 18–1). These included Millipore filters (Millipore, Bedford, MA)[3, 21, 31, 32, 35, 38, 40] polylactic acid membranes,[31] polyglactin sheets,[25, 31, 47] collagen membranes,[7, 8, 12, 18, 39, 41, 42] Biobrane,[2, 17] dura mater,[19, 51] human periosteum,[29] and expanded polytetrafluoroethylene* (Fig. 18–2). By allowing selective repopulation of cells from remaining bone and periodontal ligament around natural teeth, the surgically placed barrier permitted the formation of a greater amount of new bone, cementum, and inserting fibers than would have been the case without the barrier. A diagrammatic portrayal of the expected result of using a barrier in humans is depicted in Figure 18–1.

Following extensive animal and human clinical research, a Teflon material of expanded polytetrafluoroethylene (e-PTFE) was introduced as a periodontal barrier for guided tissue regeneration.

A number of human studies have documented clinical and histologic new attachment using Gora-Tex Periodontal Material (GTPM) in in-

*References 1, 4, 5, 6, 9–11, 13, 20, 22, 23, 27, 28, 36, 43–46, 48–51.

frabony periodontal defects as well as in furcations and recession defects.* Gottlow et al[22] presented several cases of GTPM application in random sites of advanced periodontitis around 12 teeth from 10 patients. After removal of the membranes 3 months following their initial placement, teeth were observed for an additional 3 months, at which time clinical photographs and measurements were recorded. In addition, five other teeth were removed en bloc for histologic analysis, one of which received no e-PTFE barrier. Clinically the membrane-treated teeth showed phenomenal regrowth of new attachment, although there was considerable variation in the amount of new attachment formed. Histologically, new cementum was seen in areas previously devoid of attachment from periodontitis; however, new bone growth was seldom noted except in areas with pre-existing infrabony defects. Becker et al[6] also presented histologic evidence of new attachment following Gore-Tex therapy with GTPM. The newly regenerated tissue probed on removal of the membrane was not characteristic of bone but was firmly attached to the tooth and resisted penetration by a periodontal probe. In a subsequent study, Becker et al[4] reported on GTR-treated class II and class III furcations and vertical osseous defects. They found gains in probing attachment levels of 4.5 mm for vertical osseous lesions, 2.3 mm for class II furcations, and 1.3 mm for class II furcations. The predictability of filling class II furcations was evident as corroborated by other investigators,[1, 11, 27, 28, 46] with a considerably less predictable outcome when class III furcations were treated. The same general findings were reported by Pontoriero et al.[43–45] They showed that of 21 class II furcations treated with GTPM, 14 had been

*References 1, 4, 6, 13, 22, 23, 27, 28, 36, 43–46, 48–50.

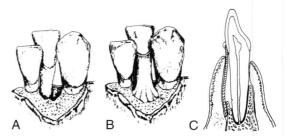

Figure 18–2. First reported use of the Millipore filter for human periodontal GTR. *A*, Intraosseous defect distal to mandibular incisor. *B*, Millipore filter luted in place. *C*, Side view of wound healing compartment created by the barrier. (From Nyman S, et al: New attachment following surgical treatment of human periodontal disease. J Clin Periodontol 9:290–296, 1982.)

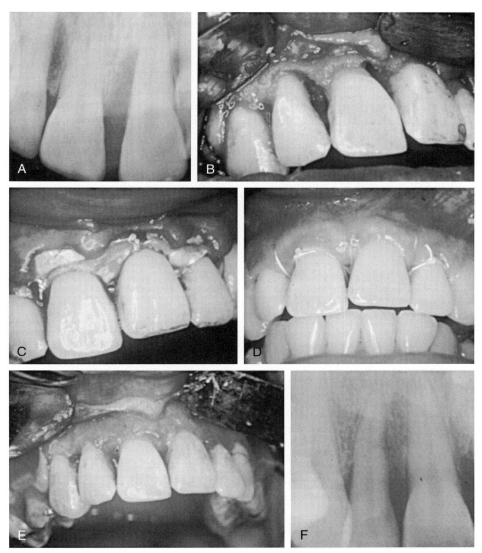

Figure 18–3. *A,* Radiographic representation of bony defects in a localized juvenile periodontitis patient. *B,* Clinical view of bony defects depicted radiographically in *A. C,* Gore-Tex Periodontal Material adapted over osseous defects that had been filled with demineralized freeze-dried bone. *D,* Gingival flaps sutured with e-PTFE sutures. *E,* Appearance of regenerated tissue after Gore-Tex removed at 4 weeks. *F,* Radiographic evidence of bone fill in localized juvenile periodontitis defects 6 months postoperatively. (Courtesy of Dr. Mark Zablotsky, Sacramento, Calif.)

completely resolved as compared with 2 of 21 control furcations without a barrier.[43] The same authors demonstrated a phenomenal 8 of 21 class III furcations completely filled after GTPM treatment, whereas none of the 21 control furcations was closed with debridement alone[44] (Fig. 18–3).

A wide variety of resorbable barrier materials have been used for GTR around periodontitis-affected teeth.[2, 7, 8, 12, 17, 19, 25, 31, 39, 41, 42, 47, 51] Magnusson et al[31] used polylactic acid membranes in dogs and reported newly formed cementum with

inserting collagen fibers covering 46% of the surgically created buccal bone defects and newly formed bone covering 39%. Control roots without barriers manifested only minor new attachment (12%). Pitaru et al[41, 42] described the effectiveness of collagen membranes in preventing apical growth of junctional epithelium in dogs. Closure of the periodontal defect was accomplished by partial regeneration of the periodontium and formation of a long junctional epithelium in the coronal 25% of the defect with a connective tissue adhesion in the remaining portion. Blumenthal[7] placed collagen membranes in dogs and reported 0.24 to 0.28 mm of spontaneous regeneration in untreated defects, 0.46 to 0.49 mm of regeneration in debrided-only defects, and 1.84 to 1.89 mm of regeneration when collagen membranes were employed. Pfeifer et al[39] histologically documented the merits of collagen barriers to treat chronic periodontal defects in dogs. Chung et al[12] clinically compared the use of a biodegradable type I bovine collagen membrane for GTR in human osseous defects versus using no barrier and found a gain in clinical attachment levels when the membrane was employed but a loss of attachment without it. Similarly, collagen membrane barriers manifested a distinct advantage in human infrabony defects.[8] Disappointing results have been reported,[8] when intraosseous periodontal defects were treated with collagenous membranes along with citric acid root conditioning and osseous grafting. The degree of collagen cross-linkage determines its resorption time and is variable according to the chemical used by the manufacturer for cross-linkage. Assuming the collagen barrier stays in place, it can be expected to block the downgrowth of epithelium and produce more new periodontium than flap procedures without barriers.

Obviously the main advantage of using absorbable materials for GTR is not having to remove them during a second-stage surgical procedure only for that purpose. Designing an absorbable barrier with predictable absorption time has presented a challenge for membrane manufacturers.

EVOLUTION OF THE CONCEPT OF GUIDED BONE REGENERATION IN SKELETAL BONES

The early use of guided tissue regeneration for nonunion fractures of long bone involved separating the regenerating bone from the influence of adjacent nonmineralized connective tissues. Linghorne[30] created 15-mm gaps in dog fibulae and placed a polyethylene tube in one fibula to bridge the gap but no tube in the other side. A bone union was seen radiographically at 42 days only on the tube side, indicating that an osteogenic rather than a fibrous repair had taken place. This was corroborated histologically. Murray et al[34] removed a portion of the cortex from the femur or ilium in dogs over which they placed a fenestrated cage made of plastic material. They observed that "there seemed to be

almost no limit to the level at which bone would form under such a cage. The limiting factor in such cases was determined by the size of the cage which could be accommodated beneath the muscle and fascia tissue so that it would not cause too much pressure and ulcerate through to the skin." Melcher and Dreyer[33] likewise created cortical defects in rat femurs that were covered with a cellulose-acetate shield on one side and left "unprotected" on the other side. At varying periods up to 18 postoperative months, they observed the proliferation of new bone into the concavity of the shields in most of the animals, which protruded beyond the contour of the femur. The authors concluded that "the function of the shield in the formation of the bony protuberance is thought to be twofold, in that it protects the hematoma from invasion by nonosteogenic extraskeletal connective tissue, and that it governs the size of the hematoma and prevents its distortion by the pressure of the overlying soft tissue." More recently, investigators isolated skeletal muscle flaps from the surrounding tissues using silicone rubber molds into which demineralized bone matrix and osteogenin had been added. The result was a transformation into vascularized bone grafts.[24]

EVOLUTION OF THE CONCEPT OF GUIDED TISSUE REGENERATION AROUND ENDOSSEOUS IMPLANTS

The principle of GTR has been successfully applied to the regeneration of bone in conjunction with the placement of endosseous dental implants where insufficient bone support exists before or after placement of implants. By inhibiting ordinarily more dynamic and epithelial cells into the defect around the implant, slower osteoblasts are permitted to repopulate the defect area and form bone to approximate the implant surface.

e-PTFE membranes could regenerate bone in surgically created jaw defects[14, 15] (Fig. 18–4). Dahlin then began to investigate their use for regenerating bone around titanium implants.[16] Implants were placed using rabbit tibiae, so that three or four of the coronal threads were left exposed. Test sites were covered by a membrane, whereas control sites were covered only by the overlying flap. On re-entry after 6 weeks of healing, all threads were covered with bone on the test sites, whereas several exposed threads were

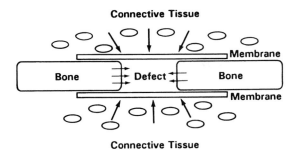

Connective Tissue

Bone   Defect   Bone

Membrane

Membrane

Connective Tissue

Figure 18–4. Design of rat model to test e-PTFE barriers in through-and-through mandibular defects. (From Dahlin C, et al: Healing of bone defects by guided tissue regeneration. Plast Reconstr Surg 81:672–676, 1988.)

still seen on the sides without barrier placement. Increased bone formation, using the membrane technique, was also evident histologically at the 6-week re-entry time frame. Photometric measurements of the newly formed bone showed 95.6% to 100% coverage in test sites compared with 38.9% to 92.4% coverage in control sites. The potential for using e-PTFE material for repairing dehiscence defects thus became evident and confirmed in other studies.[5]

Lazzara[26] was the first author to publish reports of human cases using a Gore-Tex membrane to regenerate bone around titanium implants placed into maxillary anterior extraction sockets. Soon to follow were two case reports presented in a single publication.[37]

GORE-TEX AUGMENTATION MATERIAL: DESCRIPTION AND CLINICAL GUIDELINES

As a result of animal studies and clinical cases, Gore-Tex Augmentation Material (W. L. Gore and Associates Inc., Flagstaff, AZ) (GTAM) (Fig. 18–5) was developed specifically for use in regenerating bone in osseous defects. GTAM is made from medical grade e-PTFE, which is inert and biocompatible. Expansion of the material creates a mazelike structure with a series of interconnected nodes. It is engineered with two different microstructures to meet the specific demands for its application, an inner portion and an outer portion. The inner portion has a minimal internodal distance of less than 8 μm, rendering it occlusive. This prevents connective tissue cells from the overlying flap from entering the wound site. It is somewhat stiff to maintain a space under which osteoblastic cells can migrate. If clinical exposure occurs, the more occlusive

structure may restrict the ingress of contaminants and reduce plaque accumulation. The outer, more peripheral portion of GTAM is more flexible, allowing it to drape easily over the defect margins for facilitated flap closure. Although it does not allow cells to move through the material, its open microstructure of approximately 25 μm internodal distance allows tissue integration for enhanced wound stabilization and prevents lateral ingrowth of connective tissue between the material and bone surface during the healing phase (Figs. 18–6 to 18–10).

Primary coverage of the mucosa overlying the membrane is recommended for the period the GTAM is to remain in place. Once the membrane is exposed clinically, it can be left in place (1) if the area is kept free of acute infection and (2) if connective tissue integration of the open microstructure portion seals off the epithelialized pocket such that its base does not approach the periphery of the membrane. Primary coverage of the membrane can always be attained by flap manipulation that includes periosteal release and supraperiosteal dissection, allowing for tension-free closure. Should the membrane become exposed clinically, a mouth rinse such as 0.12% chlorhexidine gluconate can be used twice a day by the patient, and the antibiotic regimen can be continued as needed. Patients with exposed membranes should be observed at weekly intervals to ensure the cleanliness of the site to ensure that an abscess does not form in the space between the membrane and flap.

If the membrane is removed at an earlier time such as 4 weeks after placement, a granulation tissue appearance is normal with marked erythema and friable texture. This is especially the case when the tissue underneath the membrane becomes contaminated, leading to clinical exposure before its removal. The mineralization potential of this granulation tissue is not as great as the tissue under a nonexposed membrane, since exposed sites collapse to a small buccolingual dimension with insufficient size for subsequent implant placement. When left completely submerged for 6 to 10 months, hard tissue bone is found.

SUMMARY OF PREREQUISITES FOR SUCCESSFUL GUIDED BONE REGENERATION USING A BARRIER

Important intraoperative considerations for the enhancement of regeneration include:

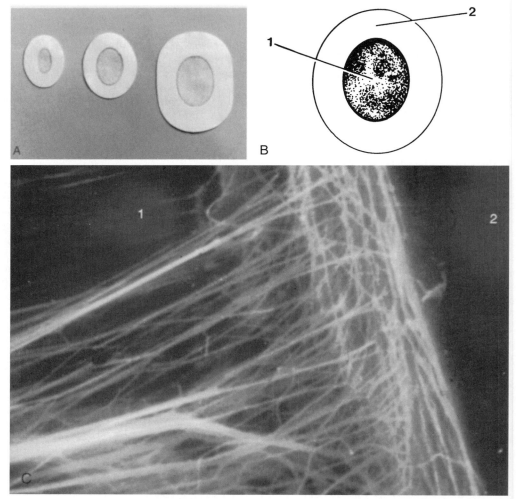

Figure 18–5. *A,* Gore-Tex Augmentation Material (available in three different sizes). *B,* Gore-Tex Augmentation Material showing inner occlusive (1) and outer open (2) microstructure portions. *C,* Scanning electron micrograph of the junction between open (1) and occlusive (2) microstructure of an e-PTFE membrane (Magnification × 3500.)

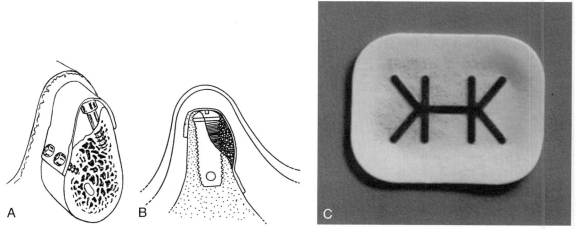

Figure 18–6. *A, B,* Representation of using bone grafting materials to create space for regeneration under a barrier using screw *(A),* grafting material *(B),* and titanium-reinforced membranes *(C).* (Courtesy of WL Gore and Associates Inc., Flagstaff, AZ.)

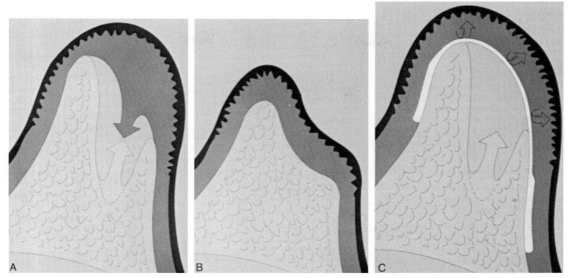

Figure 8–7. *A,* Depiction of competition between progenitor cells with potential for a residual osseous defect following tooth extraction. *B,* Alveolar ridges less suitable for implant placement following crestal resorption. *C,* Depiction of potential bone regeneration after placement of e-PTFE barrier that favors bone progenitor cells for repopulation of the space under the barrier.

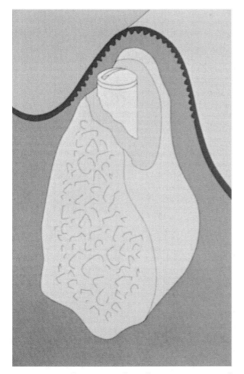

Figure 18–8. Placement of implant in a narrow alveolar ridge causing a dehiscence defect.

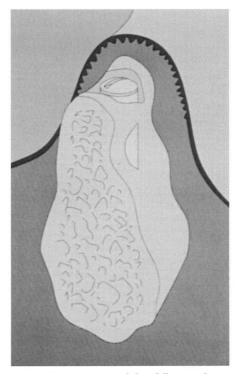

Figure 18–9. Fenestration defect following placement of fixture into alveolar ridge undercut area.

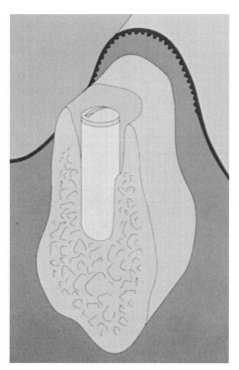

Figure 18–10. Depicting placement of endosseous implant into extraction socket.

1. Creation of adequate space for new bone to form.
2. Stabilization of the blood clot.
3. Debridement of all soft tissues from bone surfaces on which osteogenesis is to occur.
4. Provision for influx of bone progenitor cells by decortication of nonbleeding bone surfaces.
5. Prevention of contamination of the barrier.
6. Adequate coverage of the site to be regenerated underneath the barrier.
7. Primary intention closure of the mucosa overlying the membrane.

The barrier material itself should be dimensionally stable, biocompatible, capable of remaining in situ long enough for regeneration to occur, adaptable to the site as well as space-making, and if exposed, capable of excluding pathogens and epithelium, while resistant to microbial accumulation.

References

1. Anderegg CR, Martin SJ, Gray JL, Mellonig JT, Gher ME: Clinical evaluation of the use of decalcified freeze-dried bone allograft with guided tissue regeneration in the treatment of molar furcation invasions. J Periodontol 62:264–268, 1991.
2. Aukhil I, Pettersson E, Suggs C: Guided tissue regeneration—an experimental procedure in beagle dogs. J Periodontol 57:727–734, 1986.
3. Aukhil I, Simpson DM, Schaberg TV: An experimental study of new attachment procedure in beagle dogs. J Periodont Res 18:643–654, 1983.
4. Becker W, Becker BE, Berg L, Prichard J, Caffesse R, Rosenberg E: New attachment after treatment with root isolation procedures: Report for treated class III and class II furcations and vertical osseous defects. Int J Periodont Restor Dent 8:8–23, 1988.
5. Becker W, Becker B, Handlesman M, et al: Bone formation at dehisced dental implant sites treated with implant augmentation material: A pilot study in dogs. Int J Periodont Restor Dent 10:92–101, 1990.
6. Becker W, Becker BE, Prichard JF, Caffesse R, Rosenberg E, Gian-Grasso J: Root isolation for new attachment procedures: A surgical and suturing method: Three case reports. J Periodontol 58:819–826, 1987.
7. Blumenthal NM: The use of collagen membranes to guide regeneration of new connective tissue attachment in dogs. J Periodontol 59:830–836, 1988.
8. Blumenthal N, Steinberg J: The use of collagen membrane barriers in conjunction with combined demineralized bone-collagen gel implants in human infrabony defects. J Periodontol 61:319–327, 1990.
9. Caffesse RG, Nasjileti CE, Anderson GB, Lopatin DE, Smith BA, Morrison EC: Periodontal healing following guided tissue regeneration with citric acid and fibronectin application. J Periodontol 62:21–29, 1991.
10. Caffesse RG, Smith BA, Castelli WA, Nasjleti CE: New attachment achieved by guided tissue regeneration in beagle dogs. J Periodontol 59:589–594, 1988.
11. Caffesse RG, Smith BA, Duff B, Morrison EC, Merrill D, Becker W: Class II furcations treated by guided tissue regeneration in humans: Case reports. J Periodontol 61:510–514, 1990.
12. Chung KM, Salkin LM, Stein MD, Freedman AL: Clinical evaluation of a biodegradable collagen membrane in guided tissue regeneration. J Periodontol 61:732–736, 1990.
13. Cortellini P, Pini Prato GP, DeSanctis M, Baldi C, Clauser C: Guided tissue regeneration procedure in the treatment of a bone dehiscence associated with a gingival recession: A case report. 11:461–467, 1991.
14. Dahlin C, Gottlow J, Linde A, Nyman S: Healing of maxillary and mandibular bone defects using a membrane technique. An experimental study in monkeys. Scand J Plast Reconstr Surg 24:13–19, 1990.
15. Dahlin C, Linde A, Gottlow J, Nyman S: Healing of bone defects by guided tissue regeneration. Plast Reconstr Surg 81:672–676, 1988.
16. Dahlin C, Sennerby L, Lekholm U, Linde A, Nyman S: Generation of new bone around titanium implants using a membrane technique: An experimental study in rabbits. Int J Oral Maxillofac Imp 4:19–25, 1989.
17. Flanary DB, Twohey SM, Gray JL, Mellonig JT, Gher ME: The use of a synthetic skin substitute as a physical barrier to enhance healing in human periodontal furcation defects: A follow-up report. J Periodontol 62:684–689, 1991.
18. Garrett S, Loos B, Chamberlain D, Egelberg J: Treatment of intraosseous periodontal defects with a combined adjunctive therapy of citric acid conditioning, bone grafting, and placement of collagenous membranes. J Clin Periodontol 15:383–389, 1988.

19. Garrett S, Martin M, Egelberg J: Treatment of periodontal furcation defects. Coronally positioned flaps versus dura mater in class II defects. J Clin Periodontol 17:179–185, 1990.

20. Gottlow J, Karring T, Nyman S: Guided tissue regeneration following treatment of recession-type defects in the monkey. J Periodontol 61:680–685, 1990.

21. Gottlow J, Nyman S, Karring T, Lindhe J: New attachment formation as the result of controlled tissue regeneration. J Clin Periodontol 11:494–503, 1984.

22. Gottlow J, Nyman S, Lindhe J, Karring T, Wennstrom J: New attachment formation in the human periodontium by guided tissue regeneration: Case reports. J Clin Periodontol 13:604–616, 1986.

23. Handelsman M, Davarpanah M, Celletti R: Guided tissue regeneration with and without citric acid treatment in vertical osseous defects. Int J Periodont Restor Dent 11:351–363, 1991.

24. Khouri RK, Koudsi B, Reddi H: Tissue transformation into bone in vivo. A potential practical application. JAMA 266:1953–1955, 1991.

25. Kon S, Ruben MP, Bloom AA, Mardam-Bey W, Boffa J: Regeneration of periodontal ligament using resorbable and non-resorbable membranes: Clinical, histological, and histometric study in dogs. Int J Periodont Restor Dent 11:58–71, 1991.

26. Lazzara RJ: Immediate implant placement into extraction sites: Surgical and restorative advantages. Int J Periodont Restor Dent 9:333–343, 1989.

27. Lekovic V, Kenney EB, Carranza FA Jr, Danilovic V: Treatment of class II furcation defects using porous HA in conjunction with a polytetrafluoroethylene membrane. J Periodontol 61:575–578, 1990.

28. Lekovic V, Kenney EB, Kovacevic K, Carranza FA Jr: Evaluation of guided tissue regeneration in class II furcation defects: A clinical re-entry study. J Periodontol 60:694–698, 1989.

29. Lekovic V, Kenney EB, Carranza FA, Martignoni M: The use of autogenous periosteal grafts as barriers for the treatment of class II furcation involvements in lower molars. J Periodontol 62:775–780, 1991.

30. Linghorne WJ: The sequence of events in osteogenesis as studied in polyethylene tubes. Ann NY Acad Sci 85:445–460, 1960.

31. Magnusson I, Batich C, Collins BR: New attachment formation following controlled tissue regeneration using biodegradable membranes. J Periodontol 59:1–6, 1988.

32. Magnusson I, Nyman S, Karring T, Egelberg J: Connective tissue attachment formation following exclusion of gingival connective tissue and epithelium during healing. J Periodont Res 20:201–208, 1985.

33. Melcher AH, Dreyer CJ: Protection of the blood clot in healing circumscribed bone defects. J Bone Joint Surg (Br) 44B:424–430, 1962.

34. Murray G, Holden R, Roachlau W: Experimental and clinical study of new growth of bone in a cavity. Am J Surg 93:385–387, 1957.

35. Nyman S, Gottlow J, Karring T, Lindhe J: The regenerative potential of the periodontal ligament: An experimental study in the monkey. J Clin Periodontol 9:257–265, 1982.

36. Nyman S, Gottlow J, Lindhe J, Karring T, Wennstrom J: New attachment formation by guided tissue regeneration. J Periodont Res 22:252–254, 1987.

37. Nyman S, Lang NP, Buser D, Brägger U: Bone regeneration adjacent to titanium dental implants using guided tissue regeneration: A report of two cases. Int J Oral Maxillofac Impl 5:9–14, 1990.

38. Nyman S, Lindhe J, Karring T, Rylander H: New attachment following surgical treatment of human periodontal disease. J Clin Periodontol 9:290–296, 1982.

39. Pfeifer J, Van Swol RL, Ellinger R: Epithelial exclusion and tissue regeneration using a collagen membrane barrier in chronic periodontal defects: A histologic study. Int J Periodont Restor Dent 9:262–273, 1989.

40. Pini-Prato GP, Cortellini P, Clauser C: Fibrin and fibronectin sealing system in a guided tissue regeneration procedure. A case report. J Periodontol 59:679–683, 1988.

41. Pitaru S, Tal H, Soldinger M, Azar-Avidan O, Nuff M: Collagen membranes prevent the apical migration of epithelium during periodontal wound healing. J Periodont Res 22:331–333, 1987.

42. Pitaru S, Tal H, Soldinger M, Grosskopf A, Noff M: Partial regeneration of periodontol tissues using collagen barriers. Initial observations in the canine. J Periodontol 59:380–386, 1988.

43. Pontoriero R, Lindhe J, Nyman S, Karring T, Rosenberg E, Sanavi F: Guided tissue regeneration in degree II furcation-involved mandibular molars. A clinical study. J Clin Periodontol 15:247–254, 1988.

44. Pontoriero R, Lindhe J, Nyman S, Karring T, Rosenberg E, Sanavi F: Guided tissue regeneration in the treatment of furcation defects in mandibular molars. A clinical study of degree III involvements. J Clin Periodontol 16:170–174, 1989.

45. Pontoriero R, Nyman S, Lindhe J, Rosenberg E, Sanavi F: Guided tissue regeneration in the treatment of furcation defects in man: Short communication. J Clin Periodontol 14:618–620, 1987.

46. Schallhorn RG, McClain PK: Combined osseous composite grafting, root conditioning, and guided tissue regeneration. Int J Periodont Restor Dent 8:8–31, 1988.

47. Schulz AJ, Gager AH: Guided tissue regeneration using an absorbable (polyglactin-910) and osseous grafting. Int J Periodont Restor Dent 10:8–17, 1990.

48. Stahl SS, Froum SJ: Healing of human suprabony lesions treated with guided tissue regeneration and coronally anchored flaps. J Clin Periodontol 18:69–74, 1991.

49. Stahl SS, Froum S: Histologic healing responses in human vertical lesions following the use of osseous allografts and barrier membranes. J Clin Periodontol 18:145–152, 1991.

50. Stahl SS, Froum S, Tarnow D: Human histologic responses to guided tissue regenerative techniques in intrabony lesions. Case reports on 9 sites. J Clin Periodontol 17:191–198, 1990.

51. Zaner DJ, Yukna RA, Malinin TI: Human freeze-dried dura mater allografts as a periodontal biological bandage. J Periodontol 60:617–623, 1989.

PART 2

Use of Membrane Technique to Regenerate Bone with Endosseous Dental Implants

Jay P. Malmquist
Revised by Michael S. Block

INDICATIONS FOR GUIDED TISSUE REGENERATION

Guided bone regeneration has been recommended for isolated localized bone defects or defects associated with dental implant placement. Specifically, residual osseous defects (Fig. 18–11) or extraction defects (Fig. 18–12) can be treated by means of localized guided bone regeneration. Defects associated with dental implants may be divided into several different categories: dehiscence defects (Fig. 18–13), residual intraosseous defects (Fig. 18–14), fenestration defects

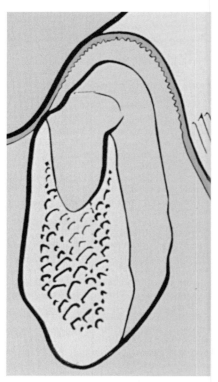

Figure 18–12. Extraction defect.

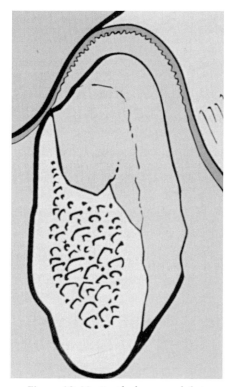

Figure 18–11. Residual osseous defect.

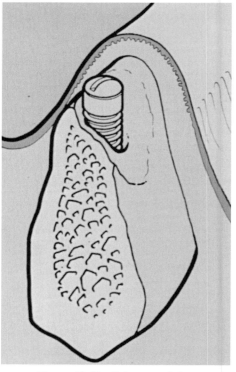

Figure 18–13. Dehiscence defect.

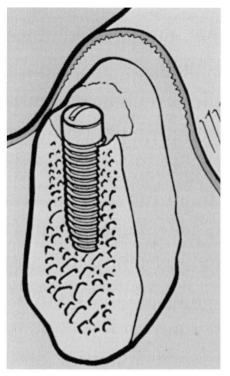

Figure 18–14. Residual osseous defect.

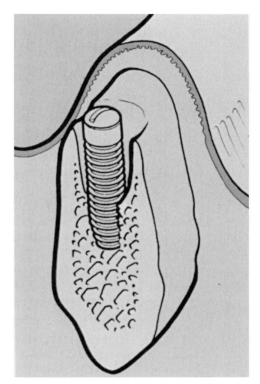

Figure 18–16. Extraction socket defect.

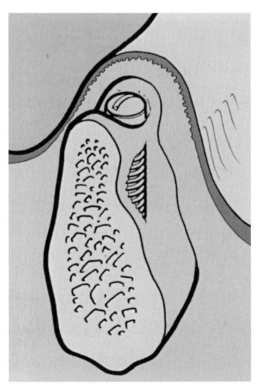

Figure 18–15. Fenestration defect.

(Fig. 18–15), and extraction socket defects (Fig. 18–16).[7] Each of these defects can adversely affect the prognosis of an implant through the lack of bone volume and quality.

The dehiscence defect (see Fig. 18–13) is the most common bone anomaly. It is often a defect of cortical bone resulting from bone loss through natural resorption, trauma, or tooth removal. The resulting bone loss creates a negative environment for implant placement and can lead to the unnecessary exposure of threads, plasma spray surface, or hydroxylapatite (HA) coating. This may lead to mucogingival problems and ultimately compromise the implant. The anterior maxilla is particularly impacted because exposed threads can lead to significant aesthetic problems with graying of the tissue through submucosal exposure of the implant surface.

The residual intraosseous defect (see Fig. 18–14) often associated with dental implants results from incomplete healing of the alveolus after us surgery or tooth removal. This may lead to exposure of implant threads or surface coating, resulting in a surgical compromise. Additional uneven contours may also lead to a compromise of the aesthetics with aberrations in the existing bone morphology.

The fenestration defect (see Fig. 18–15) often seen in the anterior maxilla results from resorption or from the normal alveolar contours of the pre-

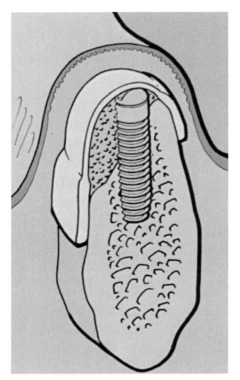

Figure 18–17. e-PTFE membrane in place with bone-grafting materials.

non-implant–isolated defect, as in an alveolar ridge defect, it is necessary for a space to be present beneath the membrane. The space allows for formation of a blood clot and the subsequent emergence of cells, which can promote new bone formation. The ultimate bone architecture of the defect is determined by the space between the membrane and the underlying bone or bone and implant. This space must be maintained throughout the initial healing period, preferably the 4 to 6 months the implant is allowed to osseointegrate. Because the membrane is flaccid and does not support the overlying soft tissue, the space may be lost beneath the membrane through collapse. Often the space must be maintained by some maintenance material, such as demineralized bone products or bone grafting materials (Fig. 18–17). There are, however, conditions when the membrane is supported by the surrounding bone architecture, and thus a space is maintained without materials. Such defects are called natural space-making defects (Fig. 18–18). Those defects that require support of the membrane are non–space-making defects (Fig. 18–19). These defects always require support through material such as bone grafts or bone grafting products. The single most important concept in guided bone regeneration

maxilla as seen in the canine fossa. Often in an attempt to place an implant ideally for aesthetic and functional reasons, the anterior portion of the implant fenestrates the bone tissues, resulting in a compromised placement. Exposure of the threads in this region leads to soft tissue color changes, tissue perforations, or a lack of implant stability.

The extraction socket defect (see Fig. 18–16) can lead to poor bone contours when the implant is placed immediately. Primary closure can be difficult owing to lack of soft tissue apposition. A staggered approach may be used in which the tooth is extracted and the soft tissue is allowed to heal. At subsequent implant placement, there is often an underlying bone defect. Again the lack of bone apposition to the implant surface and the potential invasion of soft tissue may lead to a compromise functionally and aesthetically.

CONSIDERATIONS IN THE USE OF EXPANDED POLYTETRAFLUOROETHYLENE MEMBRANES IN OSTEOPROMOTION

For osteopromotion to occur in relation to a defect associated with a dental implant or in a

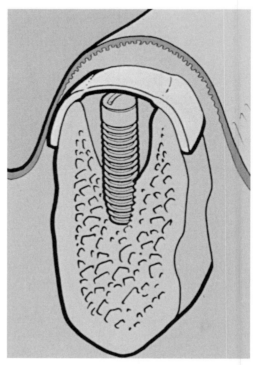

Figure 18–18. Natural space-making defect.

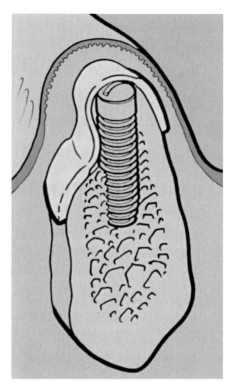

Figure 18–19. Non-space–making defect.

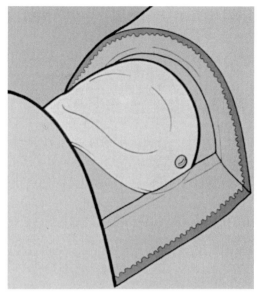

Figure 18–20. e-PTFE membrane stabilization with miniscrew.

is the maintenance of a space beneath the membrane so new bone formation may occur.[2, 4, 8]

Another concept in osteopromotion is the membrane placement and stabilization (Figs. 18–20 and 18–21). Lack of stabilization of the membrane creates micromovement at the interface of the defect and the membrane. This creates a soft tissue layer between the new bone and the membrane and reduces the potential bone fill. It is advised to keep the membrane away from the incision and tooth by approximately 1 to 2 mm (Fig. 18–22). This ensures proper long-term maintenance of the site through the healing period. Generally the healing period for the membrane is thought to be the 4 to 6 months needed to allow for osseointegration of the implant. The membrane, however, can be removed as early as 2 months or as late as 9 months.[1]

POSTOPERATIVE CONSIDERATIONS AND FOLLOW-UP CARE IN GUIDED BONE REGENERATION

The single most important factor in good follow-up is close patient observation.[3, 7] Antibiotics

are an individual decision of the surgeon. The routine use of chlorhexidine rinse is advocated until primary closure and healing of the soft tissue are complete.[3, 7, 8] Patients who wear pros-

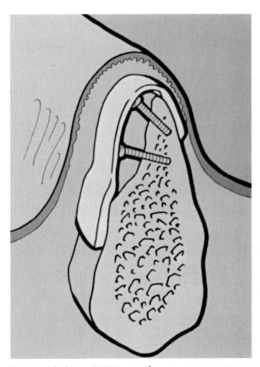

Figure 18–21. e-PTFE membrane space maintenance with miniscrew "tenting" technique.

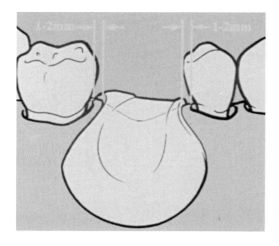

Figure 18–22. e-PTFE membrane positioning 1.2 mm away from adjacent teeth.

thetic devices should have them adjusted so as not to pressure the tissue adversely. Nonresorbable sutures should be removed only when they no longer provide support to the wound. This is usually at 2 weeks after placement of the membrane.

PREMATURE EXPOSURE OF THE EXPANDED POLYTETRAFLUOROETHYLENE MEMBRANE

Although it is recommended that the membrane be maintained for the period of 4 to 6 months to allow osseointegration of the implants, premature exposure can occur. When this occurs, several factors are important in considering the best outcome for the patient. Exposure of the

membrane does not necessarily mean that the membrane will need to be removed.[8] Often the exposure of the center allows the membrane to be maintained with good monitoring and careful maintenance of the site with chlorhexidine rinses. If, however, there is evidence of infection or significant inflammation with the exposed center portion or if an edge or corner of the membrane becomes exposed, it is imperative that the membrane be removed.[5, 6]

REMOVAL PROCEDURE FOR EXPANDED POLYTETRAFLUOROETHYLENE MEMBRANE

Generally the e-PTFE membrane is removed at the time of the second-stage implant surgery.

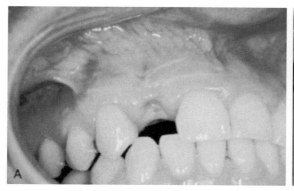
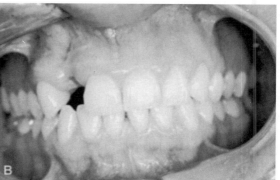

Figure 18–23. Postextraction defect with loss of labial contours of bone resulting in compromise for implant placement. *A,* Closeup of defect. *B,* Relationship of defect to remaining dentition.

This may range from 4 to 6 months depending on the placement of the implant and course of desired healing. The advantage of leaving the membrane in position until the second-stage surgery is that it reduces the need for a third surgical procedure, and the osseous tissue is more mature at the time of removal. Removal requires a surgical procedure and should be planned for at the second-stage abutment surgery. The newly regenerated tissues should not be disturbed because many times the tissue is not fully mature and breaks down if traumatized, especially when the membrane is removed before the second-stage surgery.

CASE REPORTS: GUIDED BONE REGENERATION

Case History 1
CORTICAL DEHISCENCE DEFECT

The preoperative photograph of the area of missing tooth no. 7 illustrates the loss of labial contours, resulting in a compromised area for the placement of an implant (Fig. 18–23). There is a loss of bone and soft tissue as a result of the multiple surgical procedures performed to try to maintain tooth no. 7 in the dental arch. Ideal placement of the implant leaves multiple threads of the implant visible, thus creating a compromised implant (Fig. 18–24). Augmentation of the implant site with inorganic bovine bone (Bio-Oss) and placement of the ePTFE membrane create an ideal tissue contour (Fig. 18–25). At 6 months, the soft tissue has healed nicely, and the implant is ready for uncovering. The uncovering procedure is coupled with removal of the membrane, showing excellent bone consolidation and good tissue contour (Fig. 18–26). Subsequent restoration of the implant with an aesthetic abutment gives the patient excellent function and aesthetics. A 1-year follow-up photograph and radiograph show excellent stability to the result (Figs. 18–27A,B).

Case History 2
INTRAOSSEOUS DEFECT

The patient had tooth no. 11 removed 6 months before the placement of an endosseous implant. A residual defect was present. Ideal placement of the implant resulted in excessive thread exposure on the facial aspect of the implant (Fig. 18–28). The area of the thread exposure was augmented with inorganic bovine bone (Bio-Oss), and a contoured membrane was placed over the graft material (Figs. 18–29 and 18–30). Note the placement of the membrane and the relationship to the adjacent teeth and to the incision site (Fig. 18–30). Primary closure was accomplished, and the tissue was allowed to heal for 6 months. At re-entry, there was excellent bone consolidation and marked improved contours of the hard tissue relative to the implant (Fig. 18–31). The implant was then restored with an aesthetic crown, giving the patient an excellent result (Fig. 18–32).

Case History 3
CORTICAL DEHISCENCE DEFECT (MANDIBLE)

This case represents the loss of buccal mandibular bone and a subsequent defect created with placement of two osseointegrated implants to restore partially the left mandibular dentition. The patient had previously worn a partial denture, resulting in normal remodeling of the ridge with associated bone loss (Fig. 18–33). Ideal placement of the two implants resulted in buccal dehiscence of the threads and potential mucogingival problems associated with pocketing and lack of hard tissue coverage (Fig. 18–34). The buccal aspects of the implants were augmented with inorganic bovine bone (Bio-Oss) (Fig. 18–35), and a membrane was carefully placed over the grafted site (Fig. 18–36). Primary closure was accomplished, and the area was allowed to heal for 4 months during the first phase of osseointegration. On re-entry, there was marked bone formation and improved tissue contours (Fig. 18–37). The patient was then treated with aesthetic restorations (Fig. 18–38).

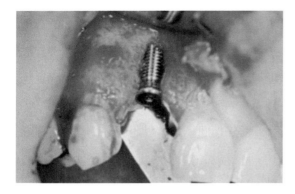

Figure 18–24. Exposed implant threads with ideal placement.

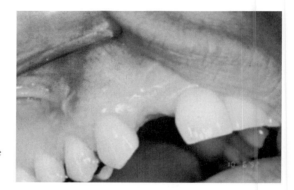

Figure 18–25. e-PTFE membrane placement with inorganic bovine bone for space maintenance.

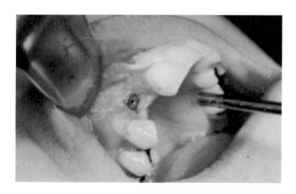

Figure 18–26. Bone contour at the time of membrane removal.

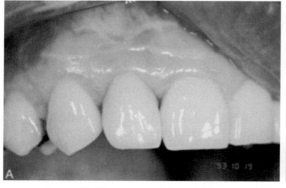

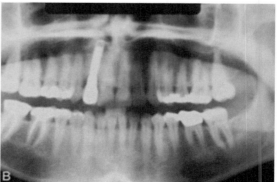

Figure 18–27. One-year follow-up photograph (A) and radiograph (B) showing excellent stability of result.

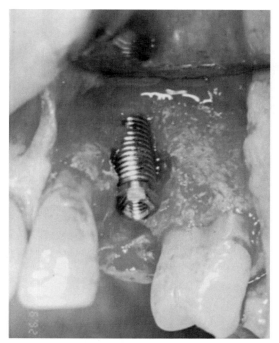

Figure 18–28. A residual defect from poor bone healing resulted in excessive thread exposure at placement of implant.

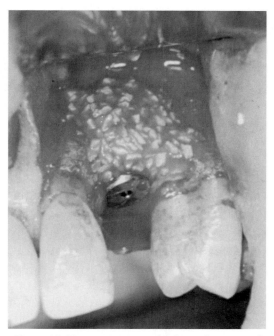

Figure 18–29. Augmentation of defect with inorganic bovine bone.

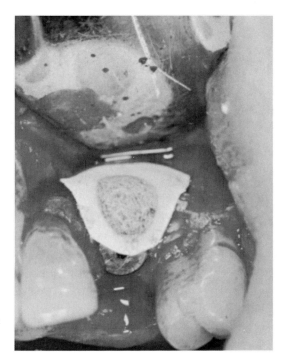

Figure 18–30. e-PTFE membrane coverage of defect with graft material in place.

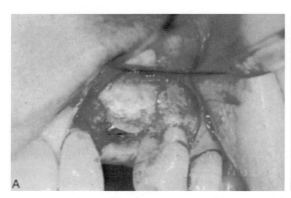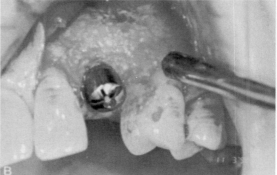

Figure 18–31. Excellent bone contours and bone consolidation at re-entry. *A,* Membrane in place. *B,* Membrane remover; temporary gingival abutment placed.

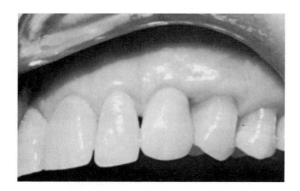

Figure 18–32. Aesthetic result with implant fully restored.

Figure 18–33. Radiograph of thin ridge contours in post-mandibular partial denture after 20 years.

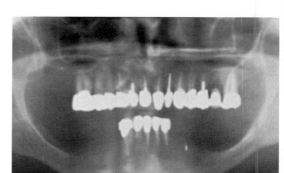

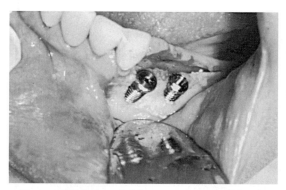

Figure 18–34. Buccal dehiscence of the threads of two implants ideally placed.

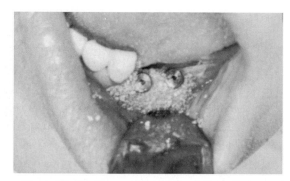

Figure 18–35. Augmentation of the defect with inorganic bovine bone.

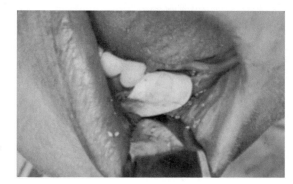

Figure 18–36. e-PTFE membrane placement over the grafted site.

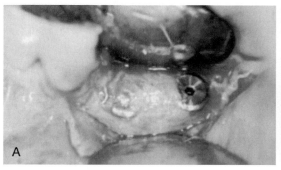

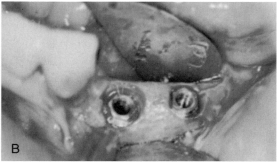

Figure 18–37. At re-entry, there was increased bone (A) and improved bone contours (B).

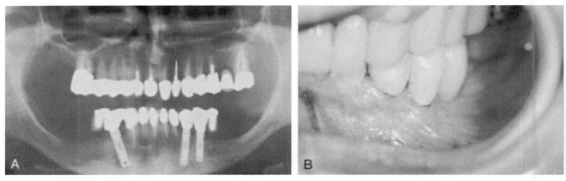

Figure 18–38. Restoration of the implants with aesthetic restorations. *A*, Postoperative radiograph. *B*, Clinical photograph.

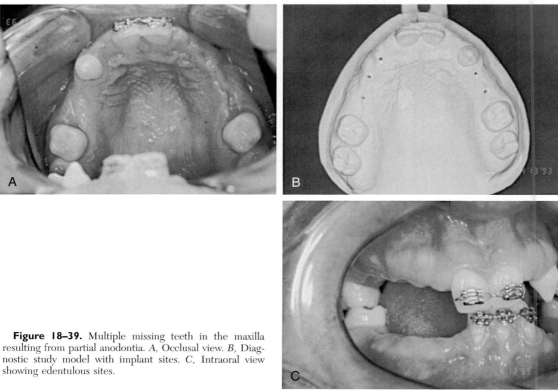

Figure 18–39. Multiple missing teeth in the maxilla resulting from partial anodontia. *A*, Occlusal view. *B*, Diagnostic study model with implant sites. *C*, Intraoral view showing edentulous sites.

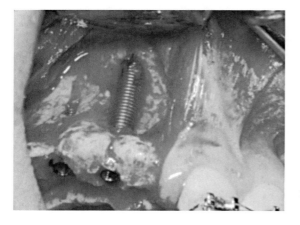

Figure 18–40. Ideal fixture placement results in significant fenestration of cortical plate.

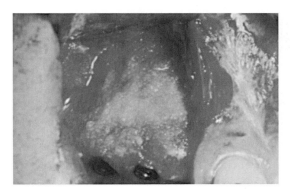

Figure 18–41. Grafted defect with demineralized freeze-dried bone and e-PTFE membrane.

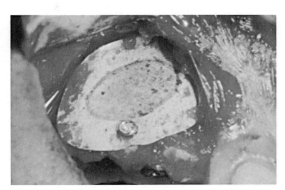

Figure 18–42. Membrane is stabilized with small mini-screw.

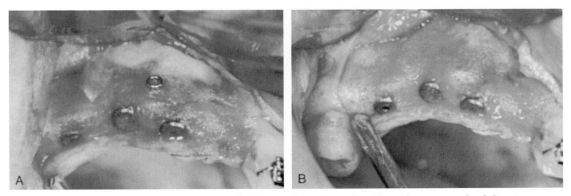

Figure 18–43. *A*, Membrane exposure and (*B*) removal reveal significant bone formation at the defect site.

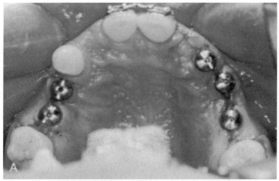

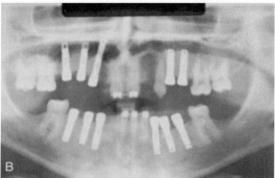

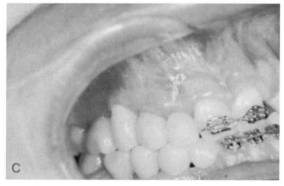

Figure 18–44. *A*, Hard tissue contours are now compatible with proper soft tissue architecture and aesthetics. *B*, Postexposure panoramic radiograph. *C*, Final restoration.

in the maxilla (Fig. 18–39) can be replaced with osseointegrated fixtures. Proper placement of the fixtures creates a sizable fenestration of the cortical plate (Fig. 18–40). The defect is grafted with demineralized freeze-dried bone and an e-PTFE membrane (Fig. 18–41). Note that the membrane is stabilized with a small miniscrew (Fig. 18–42) to ensure that the membrane does not move during the 6-month healing period. The soft tissue at 6 months is well healed, and there was no sign of membrane exposure. Exposure of the implant and removal of the membrane reveal significant bone formation at the prior fenestration defect (Fig. 18–43). The hard tissue contours are now compatible with proper soft tissue architecture for a good aesthetic result (Fig. 18–44).

In summary, the use of membrane techniques has been well documented as a viable adjunct therapy for endosseous implant reconstruction. A procedure is now available that allows patients to be predictably treated in compromised situations. Guided bone regeneration allows the clinician the opportunity to develop treatment plans that provide predictable tissue contours and increased bone volume. The envelope of implant reconstruction and bone grafting has been enhanced by the use of these compartmentalization techniques. Future considerations will stress further advancements in these areas with exploration of resorbable membranes and reinforced shapable membranes. Implant surgery, however, has truly been advanced by osteopromotion and regenerative membranes.

References

1. Buser D, Dula K, Belser U, Hirt H-P, Berthold H: Localized ridge augmentation using guided bone regeneration: I. Surgical procedure in the maxilla. Int J Periodont Restor Dent 13:29–45, 1993.
2. Buser D, Hirt H-P, Dula K, Berthold H: GBR-technique/implant dentistry. Schweiz Monatsschr Zahnmed 102:1491–1501, 1992.
3. Dahlin C: Creation of new bone at dental implant by an osteopromotive membrane technique. Rivista Italiana di Osteointegrazione 1:14–27, 1991.
4. Dahlin C, Alberius P, Linde A. Osteopromotion for cranioplasty. An experimental study in rats using a membrane technique. J Neurosurg 74:487–491, 1991.
5. Jovanovic SA, Spiekermann H, Richter E-J, Koseoglu M: Guided tissue regeneration around titanium dental implants. *In* Laney WR, Tolman DE (eds): Tissue Integration in Oral, Orthopedic and Maxillofacial Reconstruction (Proceedings of the Second International Congress on

Case History 4
FENESTRATION DEFECT (MULTIPLE CONGENITALLY MISSING TEETH)

Congenitally missing teeth are a common finding and create a real treatment planning problem with regard to aesthetics and function. Often, missing teeth correspond to an underdeveloped alveolar ridge. This creates a problem in implant placement, leading to structural abnormalities in the proper placement of the implant. Multiple missing teeth

Tissue Integration in Oral, Orthopedic, and Maxillofacial Reconstruction. Mayo Medical Center, Rochester, Minn, 1990). Carol Stream, Ill, Quintessence, 1992, pp 208–215.

6. Mellonig JT, Triplett RG: Guided tissue regeneration and endosseous dental implants. Int J Periodont Restor Dent 13:108–119, 1993.

7. Procedural Guidelines. *In* GOR-TEX. Augmentation Material Technical Manual. Flagstaff, Ariz, WL Gore & Associates, 1991. Gore Item No. 10044 Rev. 5/91.

8. Shanaman RH: The use of guided tissue regeneration to facilitate ideal prosthetic placement of implants. Int J Periodont Restor Dent 12:257–266, 1992.

Study Questions

1. Why does guided tissue regeneration result in bone and not soft tissue under the membranes?

2. You place an implant and 10 threads are exposed through the labial plate of bone. Describe how you would use GTR to increase your long-term success with this patient's implant restoration.

3. Discuss the rationale for maintaining space under a membrane and the rationale for using different materials to enhance bone formation under the membrane.

CHAPTER 19

Maxillary Sinus Bone Grafting

Michael S. Block
John N. Kent

Treatment Planning
Choice and Behavior of Graft Materials
Surgical Procedure

Clinical Results
Complications
References

Bone availability is the key for successful placement of endosseous implants in the posterior maxilla. When the thickness of bone between the sinus and alveolar crest is less than 10 mm, increasing the thickness of the sinus floor or alveolar crest is advantageous to necessarily allow placement of implants greater than 8 mm long for prosthetic restoration.

Creating maxillary bone for the placement of implants relies on onlay grafts, interpositional (Lefort I) grafts, or inlay grafts for nasal floor and sinus grafting. Only small amounts of bone may form in the sinus floor by intruding teeth, stress stimulation on the alveolar ridge, or elevation of the sinus membrane.

Tatum first performed sinus graft augmentations for implant retention.[19] Boyne and James were the first to report their 4-year experiences with autogenous bone placed into the sinus and allowed to heal for 6 months, which was followed by the placement of blade implants.[3] Tatum, in 1986, reported his techniques for raising the sinus membrane from a lateral approach as well as raising the membrane from an inferior approach through the implant preparation site.[19] Misch reported in 1987 a 98% success rate of 170 sinuses grafted with tricalcium phosphate combined with demineralized bone and blood.[14] Smiler and Holmes, in 1987, reported early results using porous hydroxylapatite (HA) particles as the sinus graft material.[17] Case reports by Wood and Moore demonstrated the potential for using ramus or coronoid bone as the graft source.[23] Kent and Block, in 1989, reported 4-year follow-up using autogenous hip bone as the graft source.[10] To date, bone grafts have originated from the hip

(anterior and posterior crests), ramus, coronoid process, tuberosity, chin, calcarium, and rib. Unfortunately not all authors report long-term follow-up data (Table 19–1).

TREATMENT PLANNING

Patients referred for implant placement with concomitant sinus grafting must have preoperative planning similar to placement of dental implants in other locations such as:
1. Avoidance of smoking.
2. Palpation of the ridge to determine both ridge contour and width.
3. Panoramic radiographs to determine available bone height. In some cases the use of reformatted computed tomography (CT) can aid in absolute determination of available bone height and width.
4. A surgical guide with radiopaque markers used during the CT to help provide information on the location of bone and implant to satisfy prosthetic requirements.
5. Intranasal observation to determine the size of the inferior turbinates and the position of the nasal septum, which, if abnormal, may contraindicate sinus grafting surgery.
6. Once the physical determination of bone availability has been completed, a thorough dental examination to exclude other dental pathology.

For proper diagnosis, the intended prosthesis should be carried through the tooth setup stage. This allows direct visualization of the location of the prosthetic teeth to the underlying bone as

Table 19–1. Review of Sinus Graft Implant Literature

Authors	Follow-up Period	No. of Patients	No of Sinus Grafts	Material	Success Rates/ Grafts	Success Rates/ Implants
Boyne & James, 1980[3]	?–4 years	11	?	Autogenous hip	?	?
Tatum, 1986[19]	?	?	?	Autogenous ?	?	?
Misch, 1987[14]	?–4 years	?	170	TCP ± DMB + blood	98%	?
Smiler & Holmes, 1987[17]	4–6 months	4	5	Porous HA particles	100%	100%
Wood & Moore, 1988[23]	6 months	2	2	Autogenous ramus coronoid	100%	100%
Kent & Block, 1989[10]	1–4 years	11	18	Autogenous hip marrow	100%	100%
Whittaker et al, 1989[22]	6 months	1	1	Osteogen + DMB	100%	100%
Jensen et al, 1990[6]	10–29 months	5	10	Autogenous post hip marrow	?100%	75%
Hall & McKenna, 1991[4]	1–26 months	15	30	Autogenous hip	100%	90%
Hirsch & Ericsson, 1991[5]	?	?	?	Autogenous chin blocks	?	?
Wagner, 1991[21]	?–3.5 years	?	63	Osteogen + blood	90/95	?
Jensen & Sindet-Pedersen, 1991[7]	6–32 months	22	31	Chin	93.5%	?
Smiler et al, 1992[18]	?–6 years	36	66	Porous HA	?	?
Smiler et al, 1992[18]	?–2.5 years	?	21	Bio-Oss + DMB 3:1	?	95%
Smiler et al, 1992[18]	?–4.5 years	?	106	Osteogen + blood + collagen	?	?
Smiler et al, 1992[18]	?	72	81	Osteogen + DMB	?	?
Tidwell et al, 1992[20]	12–32 months	26	48	Autogenous marrow + nonresorptive HA	?	93.6%
Loukota et al, 1992[11]	?5 months	7	?	Autogenous hip blocks	?	?
Jenson et al, 1992[8]	18 months	1	1	Mineralized allogeneic bone	100%	80%
Block & Kent, 1993[2]	1–10 years	32	51	Autogenous Hip alone Hip/DMB Chin/DMB Tuberosity + DMB DMB alone	94.4% 100% 100% 100% 75%	100% 100% 100% 100% 75%

? = unknown; TCP = tricalcium phosphate; DMB = demineralized bone.

well as the skeletal relationship of the atrophic maxilla to the planned restoration (Table 19–2).

For those maxillae with narrow alveoli from facial bone resorption, a decision must be made concerning the location of implants faciopalatally. At least 2 mm of facial bone should remain after

Table 19–2. Assessment of Maxillary Bone Parel Classification

Class I	Alveolar bone height normal—patient missing only teeth; alveolus is intact
Class II	Moderate alveolar bone resorption—patient needs restoration of alveolus either with denture flange or bone graft
Class III	Severe alveolar bone resorption—all alveolar bone resorbed; patient requires restoration with denture material or bone graft

implant placement to preserve crestal bone that will be mechanically tested by opposing occlusion. For most overdentures, implants can be positioned along the palatal aspect of the posterior maxillary ridge engaging the cortical palatal bone. For fixed restorations requiring placement of implants within the fossae of the planned crowns, the narrow, palatally oriented ridge should be grafted facially to place the implants in the ideal location.

For those patients with anterior maxillary deficiencies resulting in a class III skeletal relationship between the maxilla and mandible, treatment plans include (1) maxillary repositioning with bone grafts, (2) mandibular setback, or (3) onlay grafting to reconstruct the deficient alveolar bone.

For those patients who have lost alveolar height with resultant excessive interridge height, either an onlay graft or a sinus graft, or both, can be used, depending on the type of prosthesis desired. Large interridge space results in a thicker, heavier prosthesis requiring more retentive aids. Onlay grafts and inferior maxillary repositioning can both reconstruct the missing interridge space that resulted from alveolar bone resorption; however, both have advantages and disadvantages.

Onlay grafts involve harvesting a large cortical-cancellous piece of iliac bone, meticulous attention to rigid fixation of the graft to the maxilla, and closure of the incision site without tension.[1, 9] The most common problem with onlay grafts is incisional dehiscence resulting in chronic infection and loss of part or all of the graft. Onlay grafts by themselves or osteotomies designed to widen the anterior maxillary crest[16] can restore small anteroposterior deficits. Large anteroposterior discrepancies must be corrected by maxillary advancement surgery combined with bone grafts.

The following sections and accompanying figures describe sinus grafting surgical procedures that can be used for both totally and partially edentulous patients. (Figs. 19–1 to 19–4)

CHOICE AND BEHAVIOR OF GRAFT MATERIALS

The grafting material chosen must provide bone to stabilize the implant and encourage osseointegration. Materials available for sinus grafting include autogenous bone, allogeneic bone, and alloplastic materials. Criteria for the graft include:
1. The ability to produce bone in the sinus by cellular proliferation from viable transplanted osteoblasts or by osteoconduction of cells along the graft's surface.
2. The ability to produce bone in the sinus by osteoinduction of recruited mesenchymal cells.
3. Remodeling of the initially formed bone into mature lamellar bone.
4. Maintenance of the mature bone over time without loss through function.
5. The ability to stabilize implants when placed simultaneously with the graft.
6. Low infection liability.
7. Ease of availability.
8. Low antigenicity.
9. High level of reliability.

Autogenous bone harvested from the patient is ideal and serves as the standard with which all other graft materials are compared. Autogenous bone grafts that are primarily cancellous revascu-

larize quickly; provide phase 1 (immediate) bone production; can be harvested in multiple forms (particles, strips, blocks); are available from the iliac crest, tuberosity, symphysis, or ramus of the jaws; have no adverse antigenicity because they originate from the patient; and are extremely reliable[12, 13] (Figs. 19–5 and 19–6).

Cortical-cancellous block grafts have an advantage because they are strong and can be shaped to match the host site. Large grafts must be harvested from the anterior or posterior ilium (Figs. 19–7 and 19–8), and smaller grafts can be harvested from the symphysis. Traditionally, cortical-cancellous block grafts are known to maintain more of their bulk compared with cancellous grafts when used as onlays.[1] It is unknown whether a cancellous or cortical-cancellous graft maintains bone better when placed into the sinus and then has implant forces transmitted into the graft.

Autogenous cancellous bone can be harvested from any bone with a marrow space, including the chin, retromolar region, and maxillary tuberosity. The bone from the symphysis has been advocated for both sinus grafts and onlay grafting because it is membranous bone and presumably less prone to resorption compared with iliac crest bone.[5]

Allogeneic grafts are those taken from the same species but transferred to a different individual, have the advantage of ease of access, and have no donor-site morbidity. Allogeneic bone graft materials are available in solid or particle forms and are available from several bone banks. The material is packaged in a lyophilized state and therefore must be reconstituted before use. In general, one allows 30 minutes of sterile saline reconstitution.

Freeze-dried (lyophilized) bone may be mineralized or demineralized. Mineralized freeze-dried bone is not osteoinductive, but does retain certain osteoconductive qualities. When used as a graft material it is slowly resorbed; its mineralized skeleton acts as the support for new bone formation. Vascularization must occur before the production of new bone. Mineralized allogeneic bone is not indicated for sinus grafts because it revascularizes slowly by *creeping substitution*. This is a lengthy process sometimes associated with an increased chance of infection when this graft material is placed in regions of low vascularity, such as the sinus.

Demineralized bone is bone that has had its mineral removed through an acid treatment, then washed and lyophilized until reconstituted for use. When donor bone is demineralized, the remaining organic substrate contains bone mor-

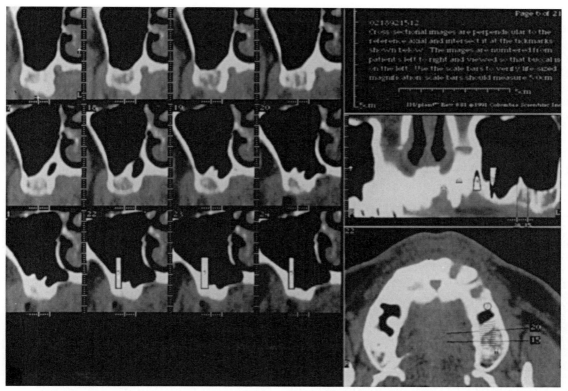

Figure 19–1. Reformatted CT scan indicates the amount of bone in the maxillary tuberosity region *(top row)*, compared with lack of bone in the first molar location *(bottom row)*. An implant is simulated in its desired location, allowing the surgeon, the restorative dentist, and the patient an opportunity to appreciate the need for a bone graft.

phogenetic protein. Neighboring mesenchymal cells receive a signal from this protein complex, which tells these cells to differentiate into bone-producing cells. The process of bone production from osteoinduction, however, depends on oxygen tension, which in turn depends on the vascular status of the wound and the amount of BMP in the allograft.

Because the amount of available autogenous bone from the jaws may be limited, demineralized bone is combined with autogenous bone to expand the graft's volume.

Alloplastic materials, specifically calcium phosphate ceramics, have been used alone, in combination with autogenous bone, or in combination with allogeneic bone for sinus grafting.[21,22] HA either as dense or porous particles is believed to provide the matrix for bone development because of the osteoconductive nature of these materials. *Resorbable HAs,* such as Bio-Oss (Walter Lorenz Corp, Jacksonville, FL) and Osteograf/N (CeraMed Corp, Denver, CO) are calcium-deficient carbonate apatites originating from bovine bone. These materials are resorbed by osteoclasts and presumably replaced by new bone. One hypothesis for bone replacement of these

materials is that these crystals act as a mineral reservoir and contribute to bone production by their osteoconductive properties and as such are advocated for sinus grafting under the assumption that bone follows their resorption. These low crystalline and amorphous phases of HA are resorbable, in contrast to highly crystalline, sintered HA.

Sintered HA particles in porous form have been placed as a graft into the sinus. Approximately 20% to 30% of the graft volume became filled with bone. The amount of bone that formed within the porous HA augmentation of the sinus is believed to depend on the ability of the host's cells to migrate into or between the particles and then form bone. Most investigators agree that more bone is found close to the patient's intact sinus floor and less as the distance from the sinus floor increases, as has been shown with porous HA grafts in the sinus.

Biopsy cores of patients grafted with HA alone (6 months after graft), HA combined with autogenous chin bone (6 to 10 months after graft), or HA combined with demineralized bone (8 months after graft) were evaluated using histo-

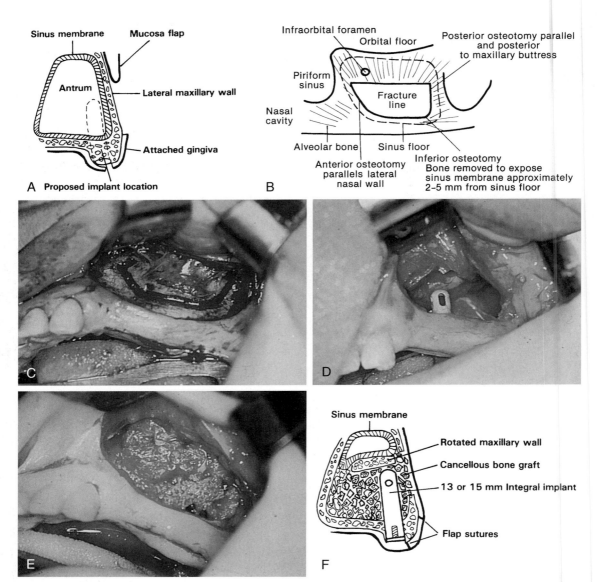

Figure 19–2. Incision design—wide band of attached gingiva. *A,* Location of the incision and osteotomies when there is a wide band of attached gingiva in the posterior edentulous maxilla. *B,* Lateral diagram shows the desired locations for the osteotomy cuts. *C,* Location of the incision at the junction of the attached and unattached gingiva with the osteotomy performed, just before reflecting the sinus membrane. *D,* After the sinus membrane and lateral wall have been rotated medially into the sinus, the implant site is prepared and the medial part of the sinus grafted. The implant is then placed. *E,* After the implant has been placed, the remaining lateral part of the sinus defect is grafted with bone. *F,* Bone graft placed medial to the implant and then over the facial aspect of the implant.

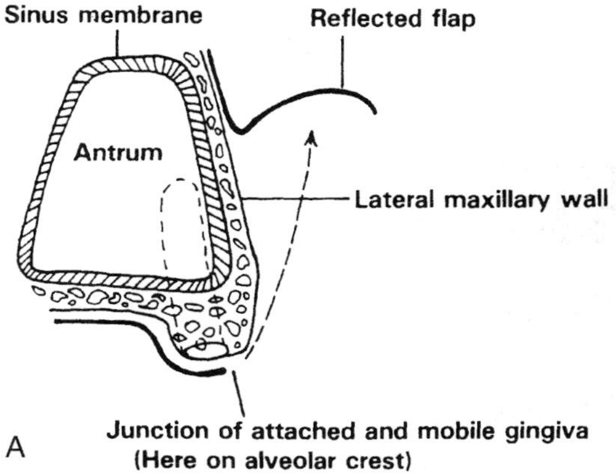

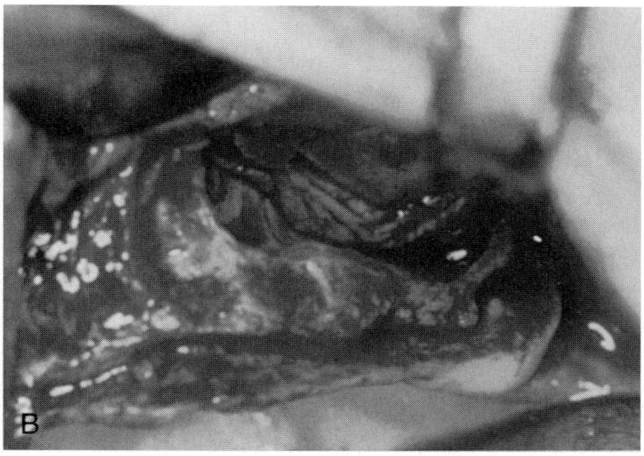

Figure 19–3. Incision design–thin band of attached gingiva. *A*, A crestal incision is made, and with vertical extensions, the lateral aspect of the maxilla is exposed. Then the osteotomy is completed. Location of the incision and reflection of the palatal gingiva for placement of the implant. *B*, Crestal incision approach. Note how the sinus membrane can fold on itself when reflected medially.

morphometric analysis. The HA graft alone had 20.3% bone, the HA/chin graft had 44.4% bone, and the HA/demineralized bone graft had 4.6% bone.[15] These results indicate that the use of autogenous bone increased the amount of bone formed within the sinus.

SURGICAL PROCEDURE

A consent form is signed indicating the chances for failure, infection, oral antral fistula, sinusitis requiring drainage, and potential loss of bone and teeth.

Bilateral sinus grafts requiring a large amount of autogenous bone are performed in the hospital under general anesthesia by oral and maxillofacial surgeons. Unilateral sinus grafts with autogenous bone harvested from the oral cavity (maxillary tuberosity or mandibular symphysis) can be performed in the clinic under local anesthesia with or without intravenous conscious sedation or in the hospital under general anesthesia.

The sinus surgery is performed first. After the membrane is elevated and the lateral maxillary wall rotated medially, the thickness of the alveolus is assessed, and the proper bone graft can be harvested.

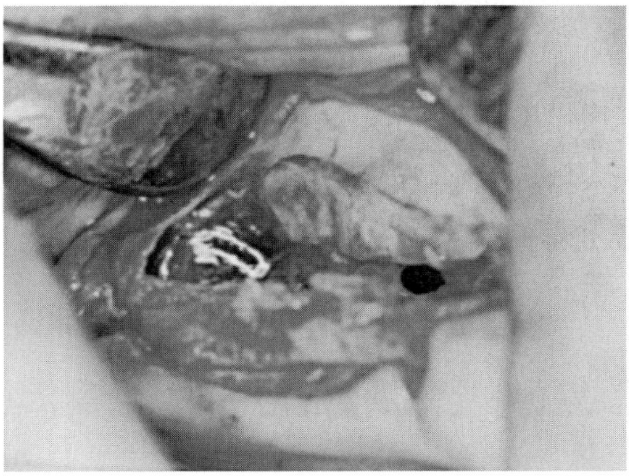

Figure 19–4. Perforations of the sinus membrane can occur. Small ones as shown here are easily obturated by foldings of the membrane itself or pieces of graft material. Larger sinus membrane perforations are obturated by resorbable materials, such as Gelfilm or collagen membranes.

CLINICAL RESULTS

Table 19–1 summarizes the literature concerning sinus grafting. In the earliest reports by Boyne and Tatum, both used autogenous bone harvested from the patient's hip as the source. Implant placement was delayed after the graft had consolidated. Because some patients did not desire to use the hip as a donor site, clinical use of alloplastic materials began to be reported. Unfortunately there are few if any well-documented, long-term reports. Currently, autogenous bone transplanted from the patient's hip or jaws is the graft source preferred until long-term well-documented reports demonstrate adequate results with alloplasts or allografts used alone.

We have used sinus grafts for treatment of totally edentulous and partially edentulous patients in our institution for the past 13 years. The use of intraoral bone as the graft material began in 1987. A total of 173 implants have been placed into 51 grafted sinuses in 32 patients who have

Text continued on page 220

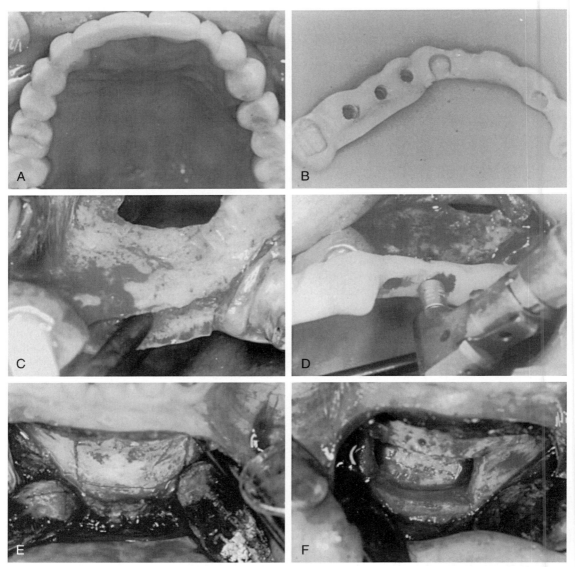

Figure 19–5. *A,* The use of sinus grafts in a partially edentulous patient. The patient had a fixed bridge removed and treatment planning performed to determine the teeth to be extracted and the condition of the remaining teeth. *B,* The duplicated temporary bridge has had the planned implant sites prepared with the intermediate-sized drill to guide the surgeon in precise location and angulation of the implants at placement. *C,* A crestal incision has been made and the sinus membrane and lateral wall have been rotated medially within the sinus. Note the thin ridge. *D,* The template is in place over the tooth preparations with the intermediate drill used to create the proper implant sites. *E,* The chin was chosen as the bone graft donor site. Shown here is the anterior aspect of the symphysis with the corticotomy scored before removing the cortical plate to gain access to the cancellous bone. *F,* After the cortex is removed, the cancellous bone is removed with the aid of curets and osteotomes.

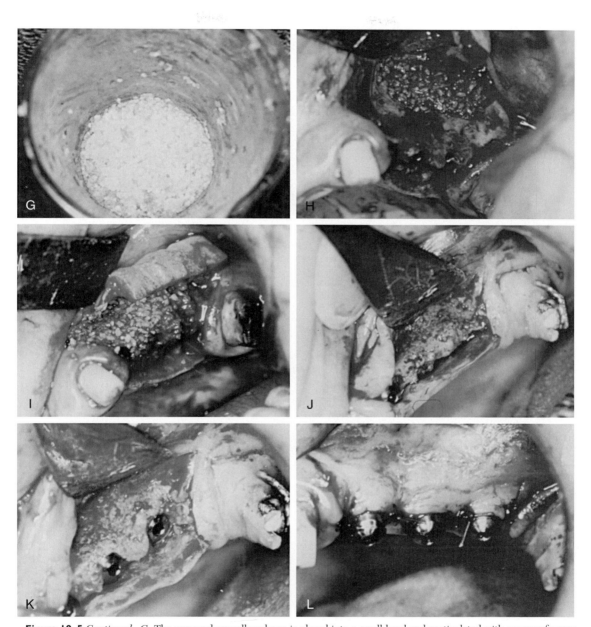

Figure 19–5 *Continued.* *G,* The removed cancellous bone is placed into a small bowl and particulated with rongeur forceps, and an equal volume of demineralized bone is added to expand the graft's volume. *H,* The medial aspect of the sinus is grafted, and the implants are placed. Then the space between the implants and the lateral aspect of the sinus is grafted. *I,* Because of the thin ridge present in this patient, the lateral aspect of the ridge is also grafted. Then the flaps are relieved and closed primarily. *J,* Six months later on exposure of the ridge, excellent bone formation is noted with two of the implants covered with bone. *K,* The healing screws are exposed. *L,* Abutments are placed and the attached tissue is transposed labially.

Illustration continued on following page

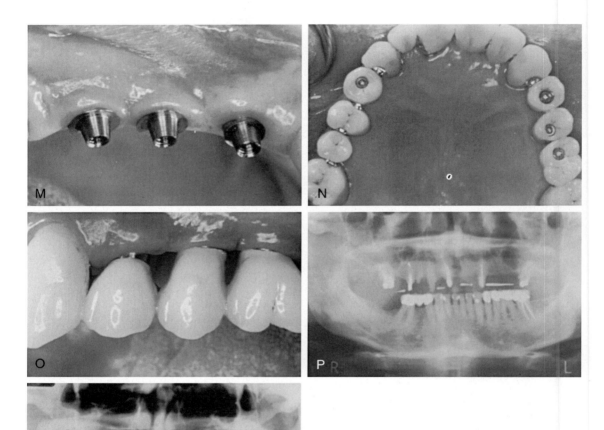

Figure 19–5 *Continued.* M, After several weeks, abutments are chosen and placed. Note the excellent gingival healing and preservation of the keratinized gingiva. N, Occlusal view of final restoration. O, The lateral view demonstrates the increased embrasure form recommended in the posterior maxilla to provide easy access for the patient's oral hygiene. P, Preoperative radiographs. Q, Final radiograph. (Prosthetics by Dr. Gerald Chiche.)

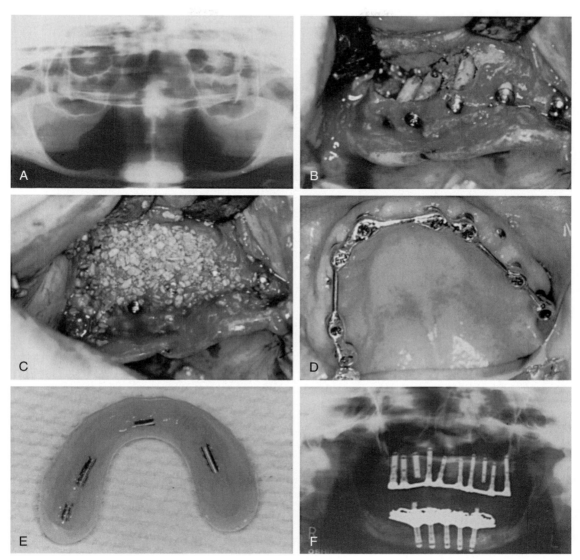

Figure 19–6. *A,* This 56-year-old woman requested implants placed to provide her with a fixed mandibular denture. The preoperative panoramic radiograph indicated extreme mandibular and maxillary atrophy. Implants were placed with a bone graft to the mandible and a fixed prosthesis fabricated. After a year of function, the patient requested a similar procedure performed in the maxilla. Because of severe maxillary atrophy and skeletal ridge relationships, an overdenture was planned. *B,* Autogenous bone was harvested from the iliac crest combined with an equal volume of demineralized bone. The sinus membrane and lateral wall have been medially rotated into the sinus, the bone graft placed, and the implants carefully positioned. Small pieces of bone were placed between the implants to aid in maintenance of parallelism. *C,* The bone graft was then placed over the implants and thin alveolar ridge. *D,* After 6 months for bone graft consolidation and implant integration, the implants are exposed and restored. The bar is designed to accept clips within the denture. An occlusal view demonstrates cross-arch stabilization of implants to the bar. Two implants were left unrestored to allow for sufficient length of clips. *E,* Clips are placed with the maxillary overdenture for retention. *F,* The 5-year postoperative radiograph shows excellent maintenance of bone around these implants. (Prosthetics by Dr. Israel Finger.)

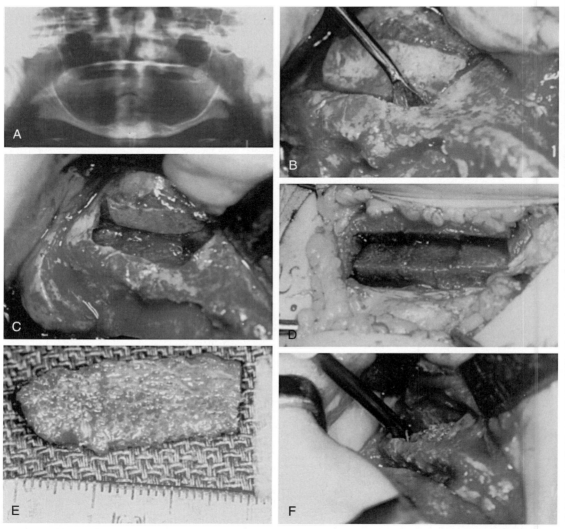

Figure 19–7. *A,* This 57-year-old woman desired a fixed prosthesis in the maxilla. Preoperative planning indicated that skeletal ridge relationships were adequate for a fixed prothesis. As seen in this preoperative panoramic radiograph, however, the maxillary bone was extremely thin. The treatment plan included bone grafting the maxillary sinuses with placement of maxillary and mandibular implants. *B,* After a crestal incision was made, a full-thickness mucoperiosteal flap was raised, exposing the lateral aspect of the maxilla. The osteotomy was completed and an elevator gently placed between the sinus membrane and the maxillary bone, allowing atraumatic membrane elevation. *C,* The lateral wall of the maxilla is rotated medially. Note the thin alveolus. *D,* The iliac crest is approached through a standard dissection and the cortical plates of the iliac crest out-fractured, exposing the cancellous bone. *E,* Osteotomes are used to remove a block of cancellous bone approximately 8 × 10 × 22 mm in dimension. Two such blocks are harvested, one for each side of the maxilla. *F,* The bone graft is trimmed as needed and placed into the sinus. The thickness of the alveolus has been increased by the bone graft. Now the implant sites are prepared.

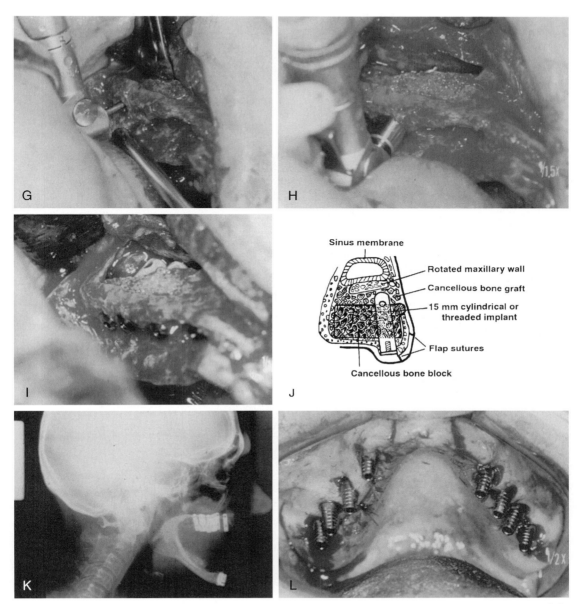

Figure 19–7. *Continued. G,* The pilot drill is used after marking the sites through the template. An elevator is needed to hold the bone graft in place during drilling. *H,* The final drill is used to complete the preparation site for the first implant. *I,* An implant body try-in is placed to help stabilize the graft. Additional sites are sequentially prepared. As each implant site is completed, an implant is placed. Once two implants are placed, the graft is quite stable in position. The final implant is then placed. Note how additional bone graft material is required to graft the apical region of the implants. *J,* Placement of the solid block of bone in relation to the implant. *K,* The lateral cephalogram demonstrates the parallelism that can be achieved in these patients. *L,* After 6 months, the implants were exposed and abutments placed. The denture was relined. The implant bodies were transferred to a model and the fixed heads minimally prepared. Then routine crown and bridge impressions were taken.

Illustration continued on following page

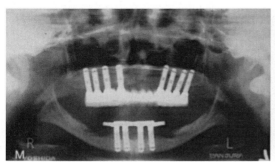

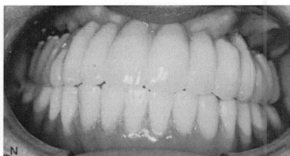

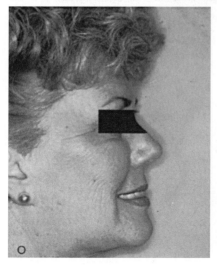

Figure 19–7 *Continued.* *M,* The patient had a one-piece porcelain-fused-to-metal restoration; 4-year panoramic radiograph. *N,* Frontal view of the final restoration. Note how by placing the implants from canine posteriorly, ridge lapping can be used anteriorly for aesthetics and phonetics. *O,* This lateral view demonstrates excellent support of the soft tissues by the prosthesis. (Prosthetics by Dr. Larry McMillen.)

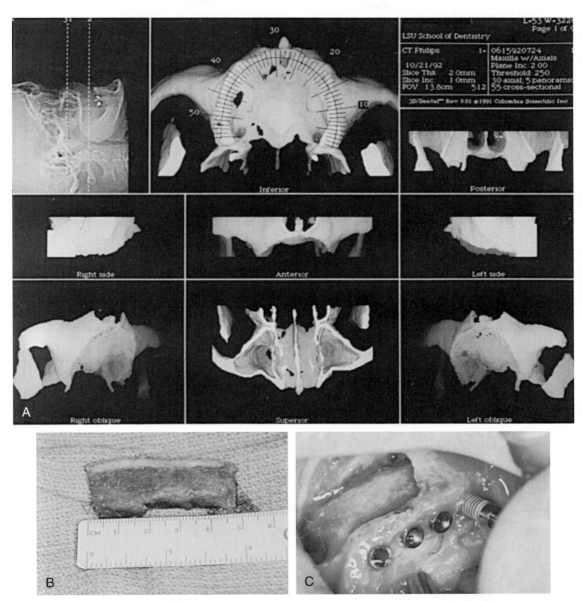

Figure 19–8. *A,* This 45-year-old man with an intact anterior mandibular dentition complained of inadequate denture retention. His combination syndrome resulted in anterior maxillary atrophy combined with posterior atrophy. These three-dimensional images (Columbia Scientific Software) show the extreme atrophy. *B,* Several blocks of iliac bone were harvested. The blocks for the sinus grafts were approximately 25 mm in length. *C,* After elevation of the sinus membrane, the iliac bone was trimmed and placed into the sinus. Four threaded HA-coated implants were then placed into the graft. The threaded implants engaged the cortex (placed superiorly in the sinus, marrow inferiorly) and rigidly fixed the grafts to the sinus floor.

Illustration continued on following page

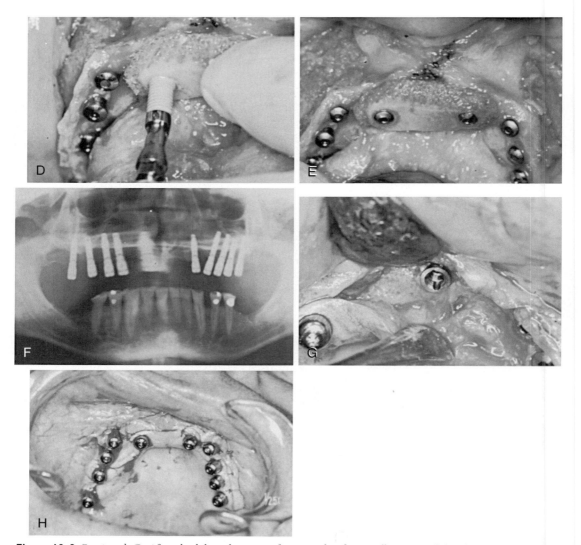

Figure 19–8 *Continued. D,* After the bilateral sinus grafts were placed, a smaller piece of iliac bone was trimmed and onlayed to the atrophic maxilla using the threaded HA-coated implants for rigid fixation. *E,* The implants were placed into the sinus grafts as well as the anterior maxillary implants. The implants all integrated, and a spark-erosion prosthesis was eventually made. *F,* Panoramic radiograph was taken immediately after exposure of the implants, 6 months after placement. *G,* Excellent healing of the onlay graft in the anterior maxilla. *H,* Using the technique of securing implants into solid pieces of bone, implants can be placed with assurance of parallelism, as demonstrated in this immediate postexposure photograph. The patient had restoration with a spark-erosion overdenture. (Prosthetics by Dr. Israel Finger.)

been followed for 5 to 13 years. Two-thirds of the grafts were iliac cancellous bone alone, 25% were iliac crest bone combined with demineralized bone, and the remainder were chin or maxillary tuberosity combined with demineralized bone. One implant was severely malposed and had to be slept; otherwise, only one implant has been lost in the grafted bone. One sinus bone graft has been lost (no implants were placed) because of a large tear in the sinus membrane and incision breakdown. One patient developed purulent sinusitis associated with the placement

of a collagen membrane to obturate a large sinus membrane tear. Aggressive incision and drainage resolved the infection. Transient sinusitis has been found in 20% of the patients and is treated with decongestants and antibiotics until resolution, typically within 10 to 14 days after the graft.

Seven patients have had only demineralized bone placed by itself as the sinus graft material. Four of these patients had only fibrous and cartilage tissue in the graft after 12 months and elected not to have another graft or implants placed. Twenty-five percent of the implants

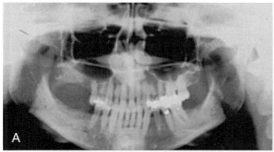

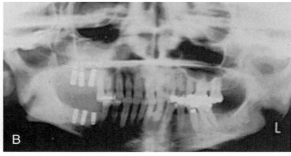

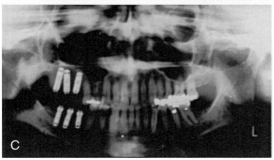

Figure 19–9. *A,* Preoperative radiograph of a 48-year-old woman before receiving a bone graft to the sinus. *B,* This 7-day postoperative radiograph demonstrates fluid within the right sinus after the graft. No obvious perforations had been seen at surgery; however, sinus congestion can occur. She was kept on an antibiotic regimen for 14 days postoperatively and given decongestants. She was instructed to avoid nose blowing and other Valsalva actions. *C,* Six months later, on exposure of the implants, a clear sinus and excellent delineation of the sinus graft can be seen.

placed into the remaining patients have subsequently been removed owing to lack of integration 4 months after their placement, which was 16 months after the graft placement.

When iliac crest bone was compared with chin/ramus/tuberosity bone as the graft material, no qualitative clinical differences have been seen with regard to implant integration or maintenance of bone.

COMPLICATIONS

In the acute phase, sinusitis is easily controlled in the first few days, and infection has not been a significant problem. Chronic sinus disease resulting from this procedure has not been found, probably because the dissection is limited to the inferior portion of the sinus and not extended to the os of the sinus adjacent to the middle meatus (Fig. 19–9).

Incision breakdown is rare but may occur, especially if the incision was placed too far palatal to the alveolar crest, owing to ischemia from a lack of blood supply coursing across the crestal tissue. Incision breakdown over the vertical shelves of the palate does not create a serious problem. Incision breakdown when the incision is placed in the maxillary vestibule, however, can result in a fistula communicating to the sinus graft, with ultimate loss of the entire graft.

Malposition of the implants is a surgical complication resulting in prosthetic compromise. Re-

sorption of facial bone after tooth extraction and atrophy of the alveolus results in thin crestal bone. Implants are then placed palatal to the thin ridge with simultaneous sinus floor augmentation. These implants are not placed in an ideal position for fixed prosthetics. Proper treatment planning predicts which patient has this potential problem, and overdentures can be planned.

Implants not properly stabilized can tilt, resulting in excessive angulation preventing restoration. Placing a block graft or staging the implant placement 6 to 9 months after the bone graft prevents this complication.

References

1. Adell R, Lekholm U, Grondahl K, Bråemark P-I, Lindstrom J, Jacobsson M: Reconstruction of severely resorbed edentulous maxillae using osseointegrated fixtures in immediate autogenous bone grafts. Int J Oral Maxillofac Impl 5:233–246, 1990.
2. Block MS, Kent JN: Maxillary sinus grafting for totally and partially edentulous patients. J Am Dent Assoc 124:139–143, 1993.
3. Boyne PJ, James RA: Grafting of the maxillary sinus floor with autogenous marrow bone. J Oral Surg 38:613–616, 1980.
4. Hall DH, McKenna SJ: Bone graft of the maxillary sinus floor for Brånemark implants. A preliminary report. Oral Maxillofac Surg Clin North Am 3:869–875, 1991.
5. Hirsch JM, Ericsson I: Maxillary sinus augmentation using mandibular bone grafts and simultaneous installation of implants. Clin Oral Impl Res 2:91–96, 1991.
6. Jensen J, Simonsen EK, Sindet-Pedersen S: Reconstruction of the severely resorbed maxilla with bone grafting

and osseointegrated implants: A preliminary report. J Oral Maxillofac Surg 48:27–32, 1990.

7. Jensen J, Sindet-Pedersen S: Autogenous mandibular bone grafts and osseointegrated implants for reconstruction of the severely atrophied maxilla: A preliminary report. J Oral Maxillofac Surg 49:1277–1287, 1991.

8. Jenson OT, Perkins S, Van De Water FW: Nasal fossa and maxillary sinus grafting of implants from a palatal approach. J Oral Maxillofac Surg 50:415–418, 1992.

9. Keller EE, Van Roekel NB, Desjardins RP, Tolman DE: Prosthetic-surgical reconstruction of the severely resorbed maxilla with iliac bone grafting and tissue integrated prostheses. Int J Oral Maxillofac Impl 2:155–164, 1987.

10. Kent JN, Block MS: Simultaneous maxillary sinus floor bone grafting and placement of hydroxylapatite coated implants. J Oral Maxillofac Surg 47:238–242, 1989.

11. Loukota RA, Isaksson SG, Linner ELJ, Blomqvist J-E: A technique for inserting endosseous implants in the atrophic maxilla in a single stage procedure. Br J Oral Maxillofac Surg 30:46–49, 1992.

12. Marx RE: The science and art of reconstructing the jaws and temporomandibular joints. In Bell WH (ed): Modern Practice in Orthognathic and Reconstructive Surgery. Philadelphia, WB Saunders, 1992, pp 1449–1452.

13. Marx RE, Saunders TR: Reconstruction and rehabilitation of cancer patients. In Fonseca RJ, Davis WH (eds): Reconstructive Preprosthetic Oral and Maxillofacial Surgery. Philadelphia, WB Saunders, 1986, pp 347–428.

14. Misch CE: Maxillary sinus augmentation for endosteal implants: Organized alternative treatment plans. Int J Oral Implantol 4:49–58, 1987.

15. Moy PK, Lundgren S, Homes RE: Maxillary sinus augmentation: Histomorphometric analysis of graft materials for maxillary sinus floor augmentation. J Oral Maxillofac Surg 51:857–862, 1993.

16. Richardson D, Cawood JJ: Anterior maxillary osteoplasty to broaden the narrow maxillary ridge. Int J Oral Maxillofac Surg 20:342–348, 1991.

17. Smiler DG, Holmes RE: Sinus lift procedure using porous hydroxyapatite: A preliminary report. J Oral Implantol 13:239–253, 1987.

18. Smiler DG, Johnson PW, Lozada JL, Misch C, Rosenlicht JL, Tatum OH Jr, Wagner JR: Sinus lift grafts and endosseous implants: Treatment of the atrophic posterior maxilla. Dent Clin North Am 36:151–188, 1992.

19. Tatum H: Maxillary and sinus implant reconstruction. Dent Clin North Am 30:207–229, 1986.

20. Tidwell JK, Blijdorp PA, Stoelinga PJW, Brouns JB, Hinderks F: Composite grafting of the maxillary sinus for placement of endosteal implants: A preliminary report of 48 patients. Int J Oral Maxillofac Surg 21:204–209, 1992.

21. Wagner J: A 3 and one half year clinical evaluation of resorbable hydroxylapatite osteogen (HA resorb) used for sinus lift augmentations in conjunction with the insertion of endosseous implants. J Oral Implantol 17:152–164, 1991.

22. Whittaker JM, James RA, Lozada J, Cordova C, GaRey DJ: Histological response and clinical evaluation of autograft and allograft materials in the elevation of the maxillary sinus for the preparation of endosteal dental implant sites. Simultaneous sinus elevation and root form implantation: An eight month autopsy report. J Oral Implantol 15:141–144, 1989.

23. Wood RM, Moore DL: Grafting of the maxillary sinus with intraorally harvested autogenous bone prior to implant placement. Int J Oral Maxillofac Impl 3:209–214, 1988.

Study Questions

1. What are the indications for a sinus graft?

2. Which patients are not candidates for sinus grafts?

3. What are the ideal requirements for a graft material for sinus floor augmentation?

4. Where can bone marrow be harvested in the human body?

5. What is the rationale for adding demineralized bone to autogenous bone grafts?

Team Management of Atrophic Edentulism with Autogenous Inlay, Veneer, and Split Grafts with Endosseous Implants

Thomas A. Collins
Gene K. Brown
Neale Johnson
William D. Nunn
Revised by Michael S. Block

Case History 1
    Chief Complaint
    Radiographic Examination
    Diagnosis
    Treatment

Case History 2
    Chief Complaint
    Physical Examination
    Diagnosis
    Treatment
    References

Autogenous corticocancellous and compressed cancellous bone grafting has become an acceptable method for anatomic replacement of lost or missing parts of the maxillofacial skeleton.[8, 9, 15, 19, 21–23] The combining of implant and grafting procedures has been a natural progression with varying but improving long-term success rates.[1–9, 14, 16–18, 20, 24] Onlay grafts include the autogenous inlay for a single tooth, the veneer graft to thicken a tall but thin ridge area, and the split graft with one onlay on each fully edentulous side as opposed to a full-arch, single-piece graft.[10–13]

Predictable success of graft/implant reconstructions crucially depends on preoperative alignment and prosthetic considerations planned by the surgeon and the restorative dentist in a *team approach*. By using a team approach that includes presurgical planning, the surgeon has an opportunity to accurately place bone grafts that allow implants to be secured in both the correct position and axis for good prosthetic restoration. With careful thought, the restorative dentist and surgeon should work together regarding the location, shape, and volume of the bone graft. The bone deficit should be discovered and analyzed in terms of the design of the graft for anatomic replacement.

Improper shape, volume, or position of bone grafts results in no benefit to the restorative dentist and the patient that the team is supposed to serve.

When autogenous grafting is required to provide necessary bone volume for implants, there are 10 distinct, equally important requirements for success.

1. *Alignment and the team approach.* Autogenous inlay, veneer, and split grafting add variables to be carefully considered for success of implant restorations. The position and axis (angulation) of proposed implants should be thoroughly discussed by the restorative dentist and the surgeon. Tracings on acetate overlays of cephalometric and panoramic radiographs, mounted study model analyses, diagnostic wax-ups when indicated, and final construction of a surgical alignment stent should be accomplished as a team. The surgical stent may be constructed of clear acrylic and should *capture the facial aspect* of the proposed final restoration. Removal of flange and cingulum area acrylic provides the surgeon with visual perspective of the facial surface of the final restoration and allows appropriate positioning and contouring of graft and implants (immediate or delayed placements) free from stent interference (Figs. 20–1 and 20–2).

2. *Anatomic replacement.* Onlay grafts should anatomically replace lost alveolar bone and sometimes associated adnexal basal bone. The surgeon needs to be cognizant of this throughout the procedure. Grafts by themselves or grafts with immediate placement of implants may be considered "successful" by the surgeon, but if implants are placed in an unusable area for the final restoration, they are considered a failure. Poorly positioned or excessively bulky grafts lead to serious restorative compromises and maintenance difficulties for the patient.

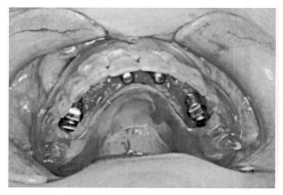

Figure 20–2. Maxillary nongraft implant stent with only the lingual area acrylic removed. Alignment stents that capture the facial surface of a future restoration should be employed both in partial and in full graft/implant reconstructions.

3. *Intimate interfacial mortising.* When onlay grafts are placed with or without immediate implant placements, the graft and host bed interfaces should be carefully adjusted to achieve complete contact between the graft and host bone. The graft should fit without rocking under finger pressure before fixation with screws or with implants. Fenestration of the native recipient site bone is unnecessary when solid interfacing is accomplished. This is especially true when there is intimate contact with cancellous graft side bone to the host bone.

4. *Rigid fixation.* The principles of rigid fixation, as popularized in trauma and orthognathic surgery, critically apply to graft/implant reconstructions. Just as *movement* between parts causes nonunions or fibrous tissue unions with fractures and orthognathic surgery, *movement* can lead to interposing fibrous tissue seams or outright failure of implants, grafts, or implant/graft combinations. Rigid fixation is essential to successful onlay grafting and is often achieved by placement of 1.5-mm diameter titanium rigid fixation screws after intimate nonrocking interfacing of graft with host bone is accomplished. On the basis of the senior author's (TAC) experience, the 1.5-mm size screws are ideal because 2-mm screws are too large. These can result in graft fracture and large residual holes when eventually removed. One-millimeter screws are too small and tend to break or loosen when used for graft fixation. The drill hole preparation for the 1.5-mm screw is accom-

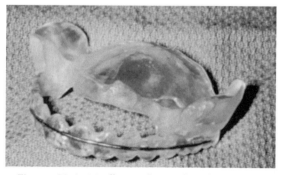

Figure 20–1. Maxillary onlay graft/implant alignment stent constructed from a clear acrylic duplicate of a patient's existing denture. Both facial flange and lingual area have been removed to allow visual perspective of missing soft and hard tissues, while retaining the ultimate tooth locations of the final planned restorations.

plished with a long-shaft 1.0-mm diameter wire passing bur without the necessity of tapping. Countersinking for flush placement of the screw head is accomplished with a medium-sized oval bur. If implants are to be placed immediately, the fixation screws should be placed first to fixate the graft rigidly. The screws and screw heads should be placed 1.5 to 2 mm away from the anticipated implant placement sites. Closer placement of the screw heads can result in a cratering defect of the surface of the graft between the screw head and the implant itself. Without rigid fixation, varying degrees of resorption or infection with failure of the graft result. Screws are removed at second-stage surgery.

5. *Solid nongraft anchorage of implant in native bone.* If implants are to be placed immediately in an onlay graft, solid anchorage of the implant in native bone is required. This often means that one-half or more of the surface of the implant must be solidly anchored in native basal bone, otherwise the implant may be lost from lack of stabilization during the resorptive phase of graft remodeling.

6. *Minimum of 1.5-mm thickness of graft bone covering implant.* When an implant is being placed in immediate or delayed fashion with an onlay graft, the implant should be covered labially and palatally by at *least* 1.5 mm of graft bone. This amount of bone was determined by experience to be the minimal amount of bone needed to prevent thread exposure as the graft matures. If such minimum coverage is not accomplished, graft resorption can occur with exposure of the implant surface (e.g., threads, coating). Graft resorption during the healing phase may be due to the somewhat compromised blood supply of the graft itself or to compromise of nutrient supply associated with the periosteal stripping associated with immediate or delayed implant placements. The fact that the surface of the graft bone is typically avascular cortical bone, compared with more vascular trabecular bone, may also contribute to such surface bone loss.

7. *Implants anchored in graft alone fail.* Implants placed at the same time as the graft, that are solely within a graft, fail. Substantial native area bone anchorage (see item no. 5) is required for success when imme-

diately placing implants into onlay bone grafts.

8. *Careful closure without tension.* The most carefully interfaced, anatomically contoured, and rigidly fixed onlay graft fails if overlying mucosa is not carefully closed without tension. The mucosal flaps should be made to drape the graft loosely with approximated margins before suturing is attempted. Periosteal release is usually necessary to achieve a passive tissue drape for tension-free closure. It is a good idea to evert wound edges slightly by combining small (5–0) mattress sutures with running sutures.

9. *Provisionals without pressure.* Pressure on grafts or transmucosal loading of implants within grafts invariably causes shrinkage of the graft and may cause loosening of the implants. This most often occurs during the first 4 months whether grafting alone, grafting with immediate implants, or implanting in a healed graft in delayed fashion. In the case of partial arch reconstructions, "flippers" or partials should not touch the reconstructed area in any way, or they should not be worn. In the case of mandibular split-onlay grafting for complete edentulism, no lower provisional should be worn at all for 4 to 6 months. Patients should understand this before surgery. For maxillary onlay grafting the patient may wear a provisional denture immediately *if the entire area of acrylic overlying the graft is cut out completely* and only the facial surfaces of teeth are retained. Such a full maxillary provisional should be virtually flange free in the graft area. The palatal and tuberosity area of acrylic should not be soft lined but should act as a "stop." Denture adhesive is necessary for retention because the cosmetic nonfunctional prosthesis has no seal. An example provisional (Fig. 20–3) is demonstrated to the patient preoperatively. The patient is informed that the provisional is not for chewing but only for show on social occasions and otherwise should not be worn. If the patient is unwilling to accept this, the full maxillary onlay graft should not be attempted.

10. *Good candidate with reasonable expectations.* Careful patient selection is necessary when choosing an implant bone graft treatment plan. Owing to the complexity of the surgery and a lower success rate

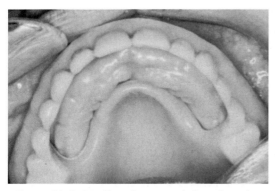

Figure 20–3. Maxillary denture with lingual acrylic removed over grafted area. The facial flange has also been reduced to prevent tissue contact. A soft liner is not employed, so the tuberosities and hard palate act as a definitive "stop." Denture is not to be worn for chewing or while sleeping.

than with implants placed into nongrafted bone, there may be significant increase in postoperative procedures, including implant removal, prosthetic revisions, and possibly even reoperation of an entire case. The patient needs to be informed that in nongraft implant cases, success percentages over 90% can be achieved, whereas in grafted cases, the percentage of successful implants may be in the low to mid 80s.[10] The patient should be informed that implants do not always "take" in grafts and that extra implants will be placed anticipating an unknown number of failures. The patient must also be informed in the case of full-arch onlay-split iliac crest graft reconstruction with implants that a screw-retained prosthesis is possible only if five implants successfully integrate in the case of the mandible and six to eight or more survive in the case of the onlay grafted maxilla. If fewer implants integrate, a removable clip-on style of prosthesis needs to be constructed. The patient also needs to know that the clip-retained overdenture may require tissue support provided by a partial or total acrylic palate. If a significant number of maxillary implants are lost, widespread tissue support by conventional full denture design becomes more necessary.

These 10 requirements for successful onlay grafting are important because failure to regard any one is likely to result in serious compromise or failure of graft or implants. The various types of onlay grafts are used singly or in combination to address bone loss and implant requirements across the spectrum of edentulism and may be combined with autogenous sinus grafts for reconstructions involving partial or total edentulism.

To illustrate the combined restorative and surgical thinking in autogenous graft/implant cases, two cases are presented; grafts involved in these cases were inlay and veneer.

Case History I

William D. Nunn
Thomas A. Collins

Chief Complaint

This 19-year-old woman involved in an automobile accident had significant oral and maxillofacial injuries. Among other injuries to the face, the patient had avulsion and partial avulsion of maxillary and mandibular anterior incisor and cuspid teeth.

At the time of trauma surgery there was substantial loss of the labial cortical bone. This would preclude placement of future dental implants unless a facial veneer grafting augmentation procedure was performed.

Radiographic Examination

Radiographs showed a large defect in the anterior maxillary region. The bone located in the anterior portion of the mandibular symphysis appeared to be of good quality and quantity for harvest of a graft.

Diagnosis

The patient was seen by the restorative dentist approximately 9 months after the original accident. The great challenge in this case was the large osseous defect of the anterior maxilla and the patient's high smile line. It was decided in consultation with the oral and maxillofacial surgeon that a facial *veneer* bone graft (Fig. 20–4) would be necessary to restore facial hard and soft tissue contours to their original anatomy to facilitate proper emergence profile of the final prosthesis. Study models were obtained, and a diagnostic wax-up was done to work out restorative details before the graft and implant surgery. The restorative dentist and the surgeon met with the

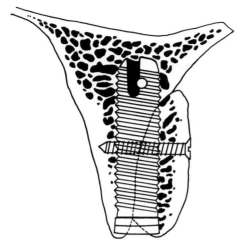

Figure 20–4. Maxillary veneer graft.

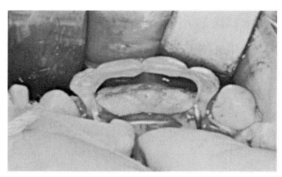

Figure 20–5. Surgical stent constructed similar to a temporary flipper partial. The stent retains the facial surface of the tooth to be restored, while allowing visual perspective for soft and hard tissue replacement. This type of stent serves as an anatomic guide during graft reconstruction as well as immediate or delayed implant placement.

laboratory technician member of the team to decide on size and contour of teeth, lip line, and lip support. When the wax-up was finalized, an impression was made, and a master cast was poured. From this model a processed surgical stent was constructed in clear orthodontic acrylic.

Treatment

The surgical stent was constructed much the same way as a temporary flipper partial. The lingual portion of the splint was cut away, leaving only the facial surfaces of the teeth to be replaced. This stent was to serve as a guide for the surgeon during surgery, bringing direct visual perspective of the planned final prosthesis for anatomic veneer grafting of the lost alveolus and for appropriate positioning and axial alignment of the endosseous implants. The stent was delivered to the surgeon a few days before surgery to make any final necessary adjustments. The stent keyed on occlusal and facial surfaces of adjacent teeth for proper stability during veneer grafting and implant placements (Fig. 20–5).

At the time of graft/implant reconstruction, the bone-deficient recipient site was first exposed through a crestal incision, examined, and carefully measured. The inferior border and anterior surface of the symphysis of the mandible were conservatively exposed through an incision low in the mandibular vestibule. The exposed thin maxillary ridge area was then carefully examined for dimensional and contour requirements for anatomic replacement of anterior bone. With use of the

dimension measured from the host site, a graft of specificdimension with the most ideal contour was then harvested from the chin utilizing no. 699 burs, thin chisels, and curets (Fig. 20–6). The graft was contoured until it was nonrocking under finger pressure at the recipient site to ensure good interface. Several 1.5-mm diameter rigid fixation screws were then used to fixate the graft rigidly. The peripheral edges of the graft were feathered down to ensure a smooth interface with adjacent bone. The surgical alignment stent was used to guide the anatomic replacement of bone as well as direct placement of three immediate implants (Nobel Biocare, Westmont, IL) (Figs. 20–7 and 20–8). Vertical incisions and periosteal release were used to allow tension-free closure. During all stages of the healing phase,

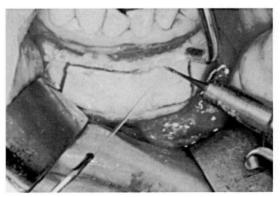

Figure 20–6. After inspection of the recipient site for contour and size requirements, an appropriate area of the anterior mandible is selected using a vestibular approach. The graft is cut to size and depth using a 699 bur.

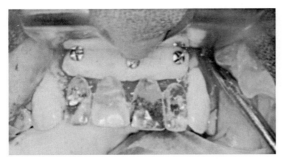

Figure 20–7. Alignment stent is constantly referred to during graft placement. The cervical margin of the maxillary left central incisor impinges on the graft. Relief must be provided in this area.

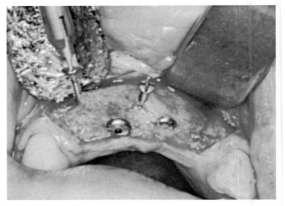

Figure 20–9. At second-stage surgery there is a well-healed graft exposed through a crestal incision that preserves the peripheral cuff of gingiva around adjacent natural teeth. Titanium screws are removed.

the patient was allowed to wear a temporary flipper partial. Stage II uncovering surgery was performed 6 months after stage I veneer grafting (Fig. 20–9).

Before construction of the final prosthesis, two different trial wax patterns were constructed to evaluate aesthetics. Changes were made before casting of the final restorations because the patient and her parents were allowed to examine critically both wax-ups in private and discuss any possible changes that they thought might improve the final restoration. After both the patient and the restorative dentist were pleased with the wax-ups, the restoration was completed in the laboratory. Shade selection was done at the laboratory with the patient in the presence of the porcelain technician. Three weeks later, the final prosthesis was delivered and secured in place by three prosthetic screws placed at 10 New-

ton-centimeters of torque. The anterior veneer graft resulted in anatomic replacement of avulsed bone and allowed natural emergence profile of the prosthetic teeth. The patient was seen 1 week postinsertion to check screw tightness and set up a regular 6-month recall and prophylactic schedule. It is now 5 years postinsertion, and the patient reports no problems with function or aesthetics (Figs. 20–10 and 20–11).

Case History 2

Neale Johnson
Thomas A. Collins
Steven P. Quinn

Chief Complaint

This patient had continued problems with retention and comfortable function of the maxillary denture.

Physical Examination

Excessive horizontal bone loss had occurred during the 10-month period following placement of the immediate denture.

Diagnosis

The continued rapid resorption of alveolar bone had created a need for some type of implant-stabilized prosthesis. Because bone bulk and form were not present to stabilize

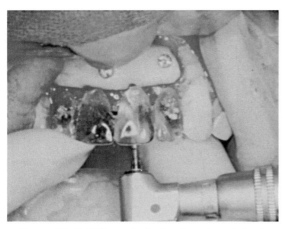

Figure 20–8. With graft sized and contoured for true anatomic replacement, implants are placed in the usual fashion. Perfection of position and axis for future prosthetic screw is achieved by reference to the guide stent during surgery.

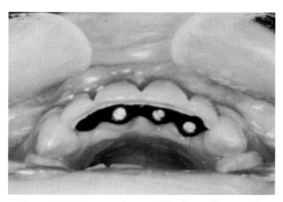

Figure 20–10. Lingual view of fixed maxillary prosthesis demonstrating lingual access and screws in satisfactory position accomplished by team approach planning for the final prosthesis.

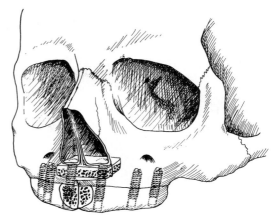

Figure 20–12. Cross-arch nasal graft—LeFort I access. The inferior portion of the nasal system is removed or dictated by height of graft.

implants in their desired positions, ridge augmentation with iliac crest veneer, cross-arch nasal floor, and sinus bone grafts would be required to establish acceptable bone volume before implant fixture placement (Figs. 20–4 and 20–12).

Treatment

A clear acrylic duplicate of the patient's existing denture was fabricated with lingual acrylic removed (Fig. 20–1) to facilitate implant or graft location. Bone was harvested from the iliac crest. Through a crestal incision, bilateral maxillary sinus–compressed cancel-

lous grafts and a cross-arch nasal floor corticocancellous block graft (Fig. 20–13) were placed. Cross-arch nasal floor grafts were rigidly fixed to prevent micromotion and graft loss. Multiple facial veneer iliac crest bone grafts were additionally placed to achieve acceptable horizontal bone volume (Fig. 20–14). The surgeon determined that implant placement was not appropriate at the time of the grafting procedure because of the lack of native area bone for implant stabilization.

The patient was initially allowed to wear the modified clear acrylic duplicate denture to maintain facial contours and vertical dimension. The duplicate had the anterior ridge

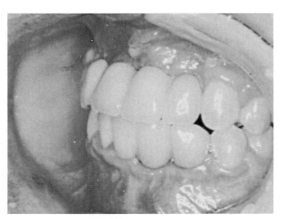

Figure 20–11. Facial view of final prosthesis; aesthetic emergence profiling.

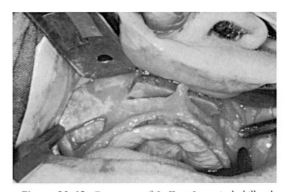

Figure 20–13. By means of LeFort I surgical skills, the floor of the nose is exposed, the inferior portion of the septum is removed, and the inferolateral corners of the pyriform aperture are squared with 699 burs. A carefully measured corticocancellous block of bone is wedged into the space created. Such bone volume receives the apical end of future implants of greater length.

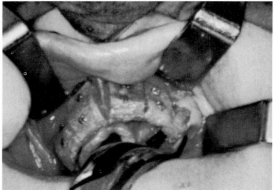

Figure 20–14. Multiple corticocancellous facial veneer segments have been fixed across the entire facial surface of the maxilla with titanium screws.

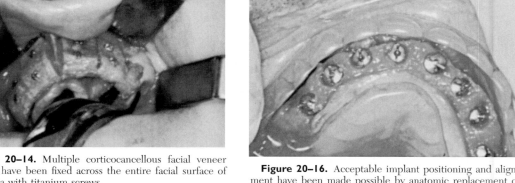

Figure 20–16. Acceptable implant positioning and alignment have been made possible by anatomic replacement of lost labial and buccal bone.

and palatal segment removed to alleviate all pressure over the graft site (Fig. 20–15). The patient's existing denture was later modified to resemble the surgical duplicate stent (similar to Fig. 20–3) to allow return to normal social activities. The patient was again advised that the denture was intended only to fill aesthetic needs and was not to be used for chewing and not to be worn during sleep. A soft lining was not provided, so the hard palatal and tuberosity area acrylic could function as a definitive stop. Denture adhesive was used because the prosthesis lacked an anterior seal. After the graft site healed for 6 months, implants were placed using the implant alignment stent for proper position and axis. Because this stent was originally used to place the grafts, there now was available bone volume in the correct anatomic position (Fig. 20–16).

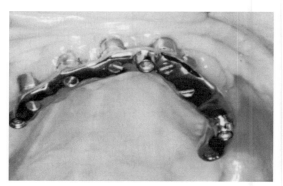

Figure 20–17. Cross-arch palladium-gold casting has been rigidly fastened to six osseointegrated implants.

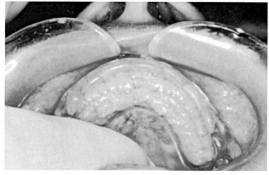

Figure 20–15. Clear acrylic implant/graft alignment stent in position at the time of suture removal. The patient's denture is relieved of all lingual acrylic in similar fashion and can be worn until final prosthetic denture is delivered (see Fig. 20–3). Graft/implant alignment stent returned to mouth at time of first-stage surgery.

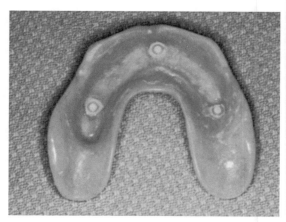

Figure 20–18. Tissue and implant–supported prosthesis retained by three extracoronal resilient attachments.

The final restoration was constructed as an overdenture. A flat 7-mm cross-arch palladium-gold casting was rigidly fastened to six osseointegrated implants (two of the original eight implants had failed to integrate) with prosthetic gold screws (Fig. 20–17). An acrylic, partially palateless tissue-borne and implant-borne prosthesis was retained by two extension extracoronal resilient attachments (ERAs) distally and one overdenture-type ERA anteriorly (Figs. 20–17 and 20–18). The patient was thereafter seen at 6-month intervals to check hygiene and tightness of components. The prosthetic framework should be removed only if there is an apparent problem. The patient has been pleased with the prosthesis. It is currently 5 years since treatment.

References

1. Adell R, Lekholm U, Grondahl K, et al: Reconstruction of severely resorbed edentulous maxillae using osseointegrated fixtures in immediate autogenous bone grafts. Int J Oral Maxillofac Impl 3:233–246, 1990.
2. Adell R, Lekholm U, Rockler B, Brånemark PI: A 15-year study of osseointegrated implants in the treatment of the edentulous jaw. Int J Oral Surg 10:387–416, 1981.
3. Albrektsson T: A multicenter report on osseointegrated oral implants. J Prosthet Dent 60:75–84, 1988.
4. Albrektsson T, Brånemark PI, Hansson HA, Lindstrom J: Osseointegrated titanium implants. Requirements for ensuring a long-lasting, direct bone anchorage in man. Acta Orthop Scand 52:155–170, 1981.
5. Albrektsson T, Dahl E, Enbom L, et al: Osseointegrated oral implants. A Swedish multicenter study of 8139 consecutively inserted Nobelpharma implants. J Periodont 59:287–296, 1988.
6. Albrektsson T, Zarb GA, Worthington P, Eriksson AR: The longterm efficacy of currently used dental implants: A review and proposed criteria of success. Int J Oral Maxillofac Impl 1:11–25, 1986.
7. Beumer J III, Lewis SG: The Brånemark Implant System—Clinical and Laboratory Procedures. St. Louis, Ishiyaku EuroAmerica, 1989.
8. Boyne PJ: Transplantation, implantation and grafts. Dent Clin North Am 15:433–453, 1971.
9. Brånemark PI: Introduction to osseointegration. In Brånemark PI, Zarb G, Albrektsson T (eds): Tissue-Integrated Prostheses. Chicago, Quintessence Publishing Company, 1985, pp 42, 47.
10. Collins TA: Brånemark—Basic and beyond. In Bell WA (ed): Modern Practice in Orthognathic Reconstructive Surgery. Philadelphia, WB Saunders, 1992, pp 1129–1139.
11. Collins TA: Onlay bone grafting in combination with Brånemark implants. Oral Maxillofac Surg Clin North Am 3:893–902, 1991.
12. Collins TA: Bone grafting with dental implants. American Association of Oral and Maxillofacial Surgeons Forum, 1992.
13. Collins TA: Implants—Onlay Bone Grafting. Oral and Maxillofacial Surgery Knowledge Update: Home Study Program. American Association of Oral and Maxillofacial Surgeons, 1994.
14. Hall DH: Particulate bone graft of the maxillary sinus and alveolar ridge for Brånemark implants. Paper presented at the Annual Meeting of the Academy of Osseointegration, Dallas, 1990.
15. Hinds EC: Bone grafts: Indications and timing. J Oral Surg Anesth Hosp Dent Serv 20:298–315, 1962.
16. Jemt T, Lekholm U, Adell R: Osseointegrated implants in the treatment of partially edentulous patients: A preliminary study on 876 consecutively placed fixtures. Int J Oral Maxillofac Impl 4:211–217, 1989.
17. Kahnberg KE, Nystrom E, Bartholdsson L: Combined use of bone grafts and Brånemark fixtures in the treatment of severely resorbed maxillae. Int J Oral Maxillofac Impl 4:297–304, 1989.
18. Keller EE, Sather H: Quadrangle Le Fort I osteotomy: Surgical technique and review of 54 patients. J Oral Maxillofac Surg 48:2–11, 1990.
19. Keller EE, Triplett WW: Iliac bone grafting: Review of 160 consecutive cases. J Oral Maxillofac Surg 45:11, 1987.
20. Keller EE, VanRoekel NB, Desjardins RP, Tolman DE: Prosthetic surgical reconstruction of severely resorbed maxilla with iliac bone grafting and tissue-integrated prostheses. Int J Maxillofac Impl 2:155–165, 1987.
21. Marx RE, Kline SN: Principles and methods of osseous reconstruction. Int Adv Surg Oncol 6:167–228, 1983.
22. Marx RE, Wong ME: A technique for the compression and carriage of autogenous bone during bone grafting procedures. J Oral Maxillofac Surg 45:988–989, 1987.
23. Tessier P: Autogenous bone graft taken from the calvarium for facial and cranial applications. Clin Plast Surg 4:531–538, 1982.
24. Waite WE: Overview and historical perspective of oral reconstructive surgery. Oral Surg Oral Med Oral Pathol 68:497, 1989.

Study Questions

1. A patient completely edentulous in the maxilla requests a fixed restoration. What should the restorative dentist provide the surgeon to ensure correct positioning of bone grafts and implants?

2. Describe three critically important landmarks that the surgical template provides the surgeon.

CHAPTER 21

Composite Graft Reconstruction of Advanced Maxillary Resorption: Autogenous Iliac Bone, Titanium Endosseous Implants

Eugene E. Keller
Revised by John N. Kent

Preoperative, Anatomic, Structural, and
    Cosmetic Considerations
Cosmetic Considerations
Bone Graft Considerations

Surgical Techniques
    Full-Arch Onlay Composite Grafts
    Sinus Inlay Composite Graft
    Interpositional Composite Graft with
        LeFort I Osteotomy
References

Reconstruction of the severely resorbed edentulous maxilla has historically presented a difficult treatment challenge because of a combination of compromised anatomy, limiting biologic factors, unfavorable biomechanics, and compromised healing.

PREOPERATIVE, ANATOMIC, STRUCTURAL, AND COSMETIC CONSIDERATIONS

Several factors consistently lead to a high incidence of advanced maxillary resorption or limit the success of maxillary surgical-prosthetic reconstructive efforts. Once the maxillary natural dentition is lost, varying degrees of bone resorption (disuse) occur regardless of the type of prosthetic reconstruction. When a mucosal-supported removable prosthesis is placed, resorptive processes may be greatly accelerated because abnormal forces can be greatly concentrated over a relatively small maxillary ridge surface area.

Maxillary bone is frequently lacking in both quantity and quality. Basal cortical bone in the maxilla is normally minimal and is confined to the hard palate–floor of nose and piriform aperture. The bone cortex of the alveolus, except on the lingual surface, is usually thin and cannot be relied on for implant stability, especially in the posterior maxilla or in patients with advanced bone resorption. Cancellous bone in the maxilla normally has low density secondary to thin, sparse trabeculae and the presence of a high percentage of marrow and fat. This poor cancellous bone quality along with thin cortices creates problems with initial implant stability.

Pneumatized bilateral antrum, midline nasal cavity, nasopalatine canal and foramen may severely limit the anatomic space to place endosseous implants.

Cosmetic Considerations

Cosmetic problems ensue with advanced maxillary bone resorption when significant loss of anterior alveolar or basal bone displaces muscle attachments of the upper lip and nose. These alter the position and form of the lip and nose (alar widening, nasal tip depression, and lip vermilion narrowing).

Cosmetic compromise is also present in patients with advanced maxillary bone resorption who are wearing a large removable prosthesis. If instability is present, compensatory, unaesthetic functional facial muscle distortions are created as the patient is required to function (speak, masticate, or swallow) and at the same time control a large, unstable prosthesis.

Bone Graft Considerations

Nonvascularized free autogenous corticocancellous block grafts are most commonly used with or before implant placement. If basal bone is completely lacking from trauma or tumor resection, vascularized composite (soft and hard tissue) grafts may be considered.

The blocks of corticocancellous bone are easier to stabilize, and are frequently stabilized with endosseous implants, allowing for a one-stage rather than a two-stage procedure (Fig. 21–1). Particulate cortical or cancellous free autogenous grafts are problematic because of lack of graft stabilization (an unstable bone graft resorbs) and adequate anatomic confinement of the graft (onlay ridge or inlay sinus) is difficult to accomplish (frequently requires cumbersome, uncomfortable splints for ridge onlay grafts).

From a theoretic standpoint, fresh autogenous bone graft, in addition to being nonantigenic, heals by bone induction, bone conduction, and survival of osteoblasts. Allogeneic bone grafts heal much more slowly and rely on bone induction and slow bone conduction. Alloplastic grafts (e.g., hydroxylapatite [HA]) may, if placed below surrounding bone contours, promote new bone formation through osteoconduction; this is not suitable, however, for onlay composite grafts.

Large corticocancellous block grafts used for maxillary composite graft reconstruction are usually harvested from the superior-medial anterior iliac crest. Anatomic sites such as calvarium, mandible, tibia, radius, clavicle, and scapula have been tried. All of these sites (except the tibia), however, would provide primarily cortical block or cortical particulate graft material. Corticocancellous grafts from these sites (e.g., mandible, tibia, and calvarium) could be used for reconstruction of small isolated maxillary defects.

SURGICAL TECHNIQUES

Full-arch onlay, sinus inlay, and interpositional composite grafts have been used in providing a

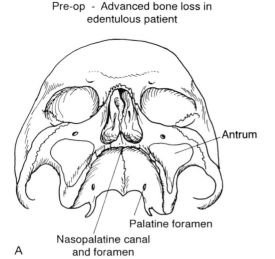
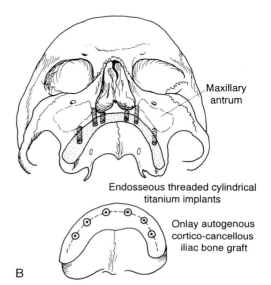

Figure 21–1. The edentulous maxilla (*A*) and the onlay composite graft for advanced maxillary alveolar-basal bone resorption (*B*). The horseshoe-shaped corticocancellous iliac bone graft is secured to the residual recipient site bone with threaded endosseous implants. These endosseous implants eventually function as bone anchorage for a fixed or fixed/removable dental prosthesis.

stable endosseous implant-supported prosthesis for patients with advanced maxillary bone resorption.

Full-Arch Onlay Composite Grafts. Breine and Brånemark[3] were the first to report reconstruction of advanced maxillary resorption via onlay composite bone grafts using autogenous tibial bone and titanium with two techniques: (1) Autogenous tibial cancellous bone chips were packed around endosseous implants into the residual bone, but high implant failure rates and significant bone graft resorption were encountered. (2) Preformed two-stage (preformation technique) onlay composite graft employed autogenous tibial bone and titanium endosseous implants in which implants were placed into the tibia 4 to 6 months before the composite bone graft transfer. Additional endosseous implants were placed at the transfer operation (second stage) to secure the composite graft to the residual maxilla. Because the implant failure rate was higher in the initially placed implants (versus those placed at the second stage), this technique was abandoned in favor of a one-stage procedure, later described by Brånemark et al in 1985,[2] that used the lateral anterior iliac bone and titanium endosseous implants.

Keller et al[9] in 1987 described a one-stage technique similar to Brånemark's by using the medial versus the lateral anterior iliac crest approach. They and others reported improved multicenter statistical analyses of implant success (80–90%). Long-term implant stability and marginal bone graft resorption rates (beyond a 5-year interval) have not been reported and theoretically would depend on proper prosthetic loading (e.g., correct occlusal force vectors, precise casting fit of osseoprosthesis) and soft tissue health (Figs. 21–1 and 21–2).

Candidates for the maxillary onlay composite grafting procedure typically are totally edentulous and have experienced extensive loss of alveolar and basal bone with anatomic deficiencies described above. Lip length and interarch space must be adequate to accommodate the onlay graft and eventual dental osseoprosthesis. If vertical dimensions are short or marginal, a nasal-antral-inlay composite graft should be considered.

Sagittal and coronal computed tomography (CT) is helpful in identifying available cortical basal bone; however, a detailed clinical examination, mounted diagnostic casts, routine radiographic imaging, and adequate surgical exposure of the residual maxilla are usually adequate. Collaborative evaluation by the prosthodontist, surgeon, and, if necessary, proper medical and psy-

chological evaluation are mandatory for the patient to have realistic expectations and understanding of the surgical-prosthetic procedures and projected treatment result.

Adequate soft tissue volume and elasticity must be available for proper flap mobilization and wound closure over the composite graft. Wound breakdown with graft and implant loss can also be caused by trauma from retained mandibular teeth, previous radiotherapy, poor flap design, and even a poor fitting interim maxillary prosthesis throughout the healing period. Various preprosthetic surgical procedures, such as scar tissue revision or excision, hyperplastic tissue removal, or mucosal or skin grafting, may be necessary before grafting in selected patients. Proper medical-surgical management must be provided to those patients with a positive history and radiographic documentation of antral disease before performance of the composite graft procedure.[1]

Sinus Inlay Composite Graft. The history, techniques, and results of grafting into the antral floor are described in Chapter 19.

Completely edentulous patients with advanced bone resorption may be candidates for this procedure for several reasons.

1. Inadequate lip length or interarch space to accommodate the full-arch onlay composite graft (described previously).
2. Lack of soft tissue volume or elasticity (secondary to postsurgical or post-traumatic scarring) to cover adequately the full-arch onlay composite graft.
3. Desire of the patient for a fixed rather than a fixed/removable dental prosthesis.
4. Inadequate alveolar bone height where placement of short implants without grafting would lead to biomechanical failure.

Harvesting of corticocancellous blocks of autogenous iliac bone for antral grafting is accomplished by exposing the anterior-superior medial iliac crest. The antral inlay graft is substantially smaller than the full-arch onlay graft, so iliac crest exposure is generally more conservative and is associated with less surgical morbidity (Figs. 21–3 to 21–5).

Interpositional Composite Graft with LeFort I Osteotomy. Obwegeser,[10] in 1969, described a LeFort I osteotomy procedure in which interpositional corticocancellous block bone grafts stabilize the maxilla following vertical or anteroposterior advancement corrections in or-

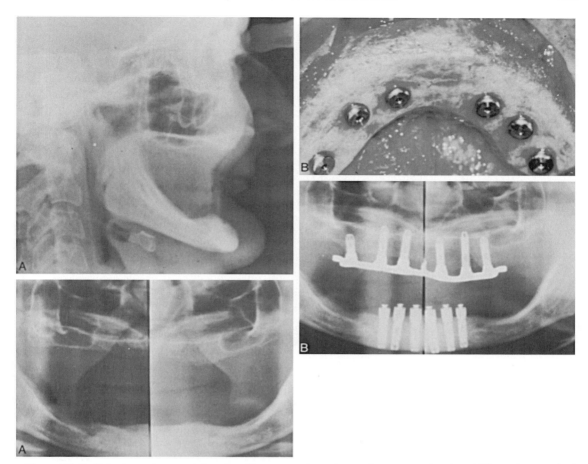

Figure 21–2. Patient no. 1 presentation (maxillary composite onlay graft reconstruction in middle-aged woman). *A,* Pretreatment lateral cephalogram *(above)* and panoramic radiograph *(below).* Note adequate interarch space for onlay graft and osseoprosthesis. Anterior maxillary residual bone was marginal in height and inadequate in width for implant placement. *B,* Surgical photograph of onlay graft *(stage-one surgery)* secured with titanium endosseous implants *(above)* and posttreatment panoramic radiograph *(below)* showing implants and incorporated bone graft following 1 year of prosthesis function.

Figure 21–3. Placement of a block cortico-cancellous iliac bone graft in floor of maxillary antrum secured with titanium endosseous threaded implants.

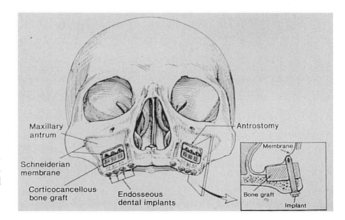

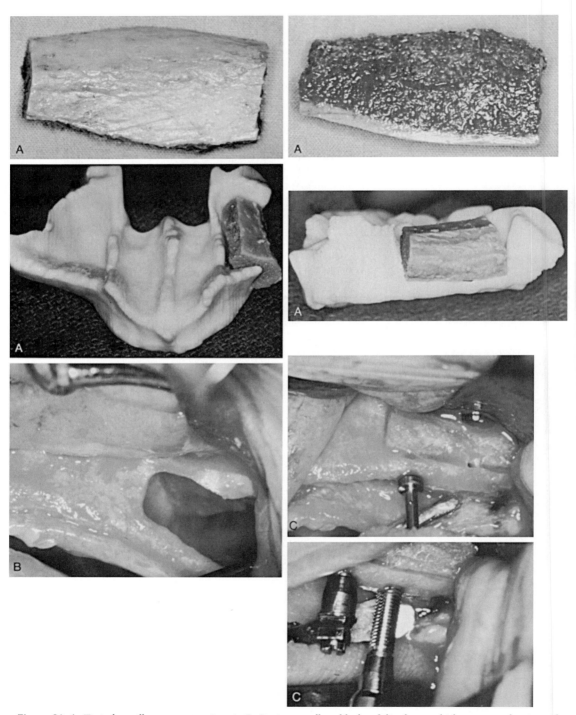

Figure 21–4. Typical maxillary reconstruction. *A, B,* Corticocancellous blocks of iliac bone, which are properly trimmed to fit into the floor of the antrum as illustrated in a computer-generated model *(below left and right). C,* Maxillary antrum following removal or inward fracture of the lateral wall and squaring and flattening of the inferior and anterior boundaries with a pear-shaped bur. Meticulous removal of antral membrane on recipient site is mandatory. Maintaining the antral membrane intact during reflection is ideal but not critical with this type of grafting procedure. Fitting of the block bone graft in the antral floor (cortex facing antrum and cancellous bone facing antral floor) and placement of stabilizing endosseous titanium implants.

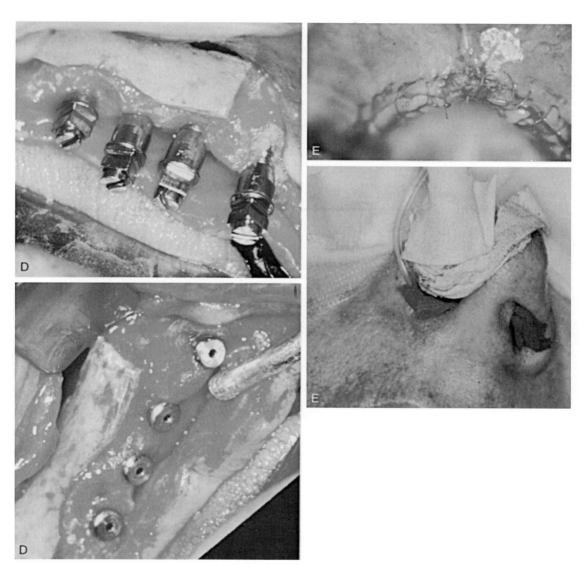

Figure 21–4 *Continued. D,* After placement of three endosseous implants through the residual ridge and into the block bone graft. One implant was placed into the residual piriform rim *(above)*. The same patient *(below)* following removal of the fixture mount and placement of healing caps. Further recontouring of the graft at this time is avoided because overcontouring to the buccal is desirable. *E,* Closure of the crestal incision following bilateral antral graft placement. Water-tight closure accomplished with absorbable horizontal mattress suture. A previously worn prosthesis can be placed immediately in most patients because the ridge shape and form have not been altered with this technique (in contrast to the full-arch onlay graft).

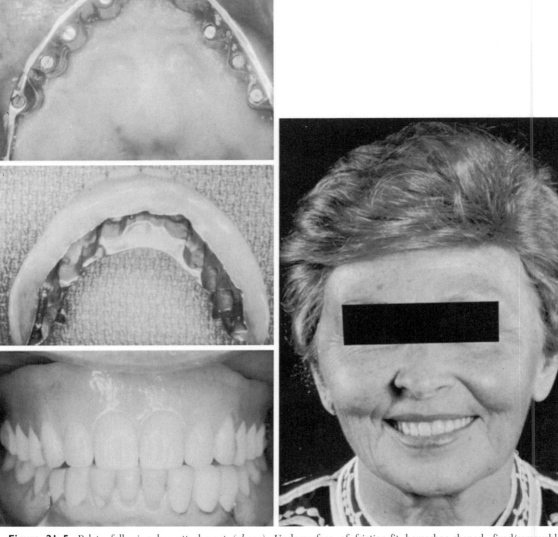

Figure 21–5. Palate following bar attachment *(above)*. Undersurface of friction-fit horseshoe-shaped, fixed/removable osseoprosthesis *(middle)*. The fixed/removable osseoprosthesis in occlusion with lower natural dentition *(below left)*. A thick labial flange was required to satisfy aesthetics and lip support requirements as illustrated in anterior facial profile. (Prosthodontics provided by Dr. W. R. Laney, Section of Prosthodontics, Mayo Clinic, Rochester, MN.)

thognathic surgery cases. However, LeFort I osteotomy procedures in edentulous patients are infrequently reported. Farrell et al[4] were the first to describe a one-stage interpositional bone grafting of the atrophic maxilla. Keller described a two-stage procedure in which titanium endosseous implants were placed through the residual maxilla and into the previously placed iliac bone graft through a LeFort I osteotomy.[8] Sailer[11] described preliminary data on five patients in whom LeFort I osteotomy with autogenous iliac interpositional block bone graft was performed and

endosseous titanium implants were simultaneously placed. Each of those bone blocks was stabilized by endosseous cylindrical threaded implants. This technique offers the advantage of a one-stage procedure but adds to the difficulty of proper implant placement and preservation of adequate blood supply for bone (osteotomy) and implant healing.

Graft materials other than autogenous bone have been used for the interpositional graft (HA, xenogenic, or allogeneic bone preparations) following LeFort I osteotomy with limited success

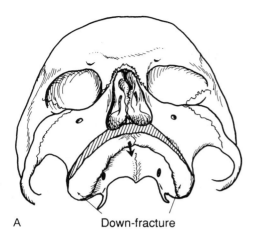

A   Down-fracture

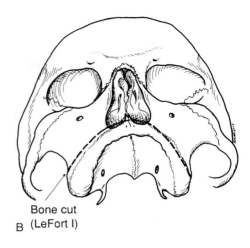

B   Bone cut
(LeFort I)

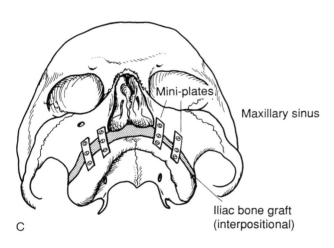

C

Mini-plates

Maxillary sinus

Iliac bone graft
(interpositional)

Figure 21–6. Stage one. LeFort I osteotomy downfracture with interpositional corticocancellous autogenous iliac bone graft. Osteotomy is at low level (*A*), and downfracture hinges on pterygoid plate (*B*) and accommodates a one-piece block bone graft (*C*) stabilized by miniplates or transosseous wire osteosynthesis. Intermaxillary fixation is used temporarily intraoperatively in edentulous patients and up to 6 weeks (light elastics) in the partially edentulous patient. The mobilized maxilla contains the palate (horizontal process of maxilla and palatine bone); e.g., the palatal depth and ridge contour do not change with this technique.

because osseointegration is required for long-term stability with physiologic functional loading of the endosseous implants and these graft material preclude their use. Adding fresh autogenous marrow or cellular-rich cancellous bone to allogeneic or alloplastic materials, however, is helpful.

The interpositional composite bone graft is indicated for edentulous patients with anterior-posterior or vertical maxillary deficiency (relative mandibular prognathism) who exhibit inadequate bone for endosseous placement. Patients who are candidates for the interpositional composite graft (rather than the onlay or inlay composite graft) generally are younger and place added emphasis on attainment of maximum cosmetic benefit and placement of a fixed rather than a fixed/removable dental prosthesis. A majority of patients in

this group are partially edentulous with posttraumatic or congenital-developmental dentofacial deformities.

Large corticocancellous blocks of autogenous iliac bone are harvested from the medial-anterior ilium and placed after advanced vertically as well as horizontally (Figs. 21–6 to 21–8).

Internal miniplate skeletal fixation is the preferred stabilization method, as it provides early rigidity to the mobilized maxilla and interpositional bone graft and eliminates need for intermaxillary fixation. An interim removable prosthesis can be constructed in the edentulous areas 2 or 3 weeks after the osteotomy procedure and used for aesthetics and pureed diet function during the initial 6 to 8 weeks.

Routine LeFort I osteotomy incisions, subperi-

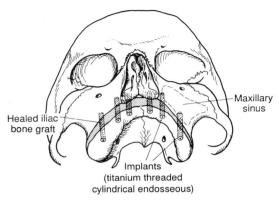

Figure 21–7. Stage two. Six months following the osteotomy procedure, threaded endosseous implants are placed through the repositioned maxilla and into the previously placed (and healed) interpositional bone graft. Previously placed transosseous wires or miniplates are removed at this time.

osteal dissection, wound closure, and preoperative, intraoperative, and postoperative medical-anesthesia-surgical protocol are followed to manage the patient and the donor/recipient wound sites.[5–8] Presurgical diagnosis management of the maxillary antrum is crucial for uncomplicated healing of the interpositional bone graft and mobilized maxilla (see previous section on antral-

inlay bone graft). Documented antral disease must be eliminated so a well-ventilated and aseptic antrum is present presurgically.[1] If residual hyperplastic antral mucosa or sepsis is encountered intraoperatively, the diseased lining is removed, and nasal antral windows are created below the inferior turbinate before interpositional graft placement and maxillary segment stabilization.

Simultaneous endosseous implant placement at the time of LeFort I osteotomy–interpositional bone graft procedure is desirable but not recommended by Keller because additional ridge and palatal mucoperiosteal reflection may unduly compromise the mobilized maxilla blood supply to compromise the predictability of bone graft healing and attainment of implant osseointegration, and this approach may compromise the ideal implant placement (angulation) for the eventual dental prosthetic reconstruction.

Endosseous threaded implants are placed (second stage) 4 to 6 months following the osteotomy–bone grafting procedure. The implant surgical-prosthetic protocol at this time is generally as in routine maxillary endosseous implant reconstructions because adequate bone volume and jaw position should be normal if the stage-one procedure was successful. Implant uncovering and abutment connection are carried out 6 months after implant placement and are generally routine except for a higher incidence of soft tissue revisions needed for scar excision or hyperplastic ridge tissue reduction.

References

1. Bell RD, Stone HE: Conservative surgical procedures in inflammatory disease of the maxillary antrum. Otolaryngol Clin North Am 9:175–186, 1976.
2. Brånemark P-I, Zarb GA, Albrektsson T (eds): Tissue-Integrated Prostheses. Osseointegration in Clinical Dentistry. Chicago, Quintessence Publishing, 1985.
3. Breine U, Brånemark P-I: Reconstruction of the alveolar jaw bone. An experimental and clinical study of immediate and preformed autologous bone grafts in combination with osseointegrated implants. Scand J Plast Reconstr Surg 14:23–48, 1980.
4. Farrell CD, Kent JN, Guerra LR: One-stage interpositional bone grafting and vestibuloplasty of the atrophic maxilla. J Oral Surg 34:901, 1976.
5. Keller EE: The maxillary interpositional composite graft (LeFort I osteotomy with interpositional autogenous iliac bone graft, and titanium endosseous implants). In Worthington P, Brånemark P-I (eds): Advanced Osseointegration Surgery: Applications in the Maxillofacial Region. Carol Stream, IL, Quintessence Publishing, 1991.
6. Keller EE: Quadrangular LeFort I and II osteotomy. In Bell WH (ed): Modern Practice in Orthognathic and Reconstructive Surgery. Philadelphia, WB Saunders, 1991, pp 1797–1837.

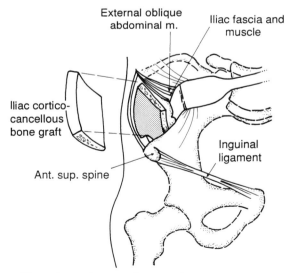

Figure 21–8. Iliac crest donor site drawing. A single block corticocancellous bone graft is harvested from the anterior-medial ilium. The superior lateral cortex and associated muscle attachments are preserved as anatomy permits. Cancellous particulate bone is also removed with chisel and curet. The one-piece corticocancellous graft contains cortex on one side (faces nasal mucosa and open antrum) and cancellous bone on the other side (faces floor of nose and floor of antrum).

7. Keller EE, Jackson IT: Treatment of skeletal deformities in the cleft patient. *In* Bardach J, Morris H (eds): Multidisciplinary Management of Cleft Lip and Palate. Philadelphia, WB Saunders, 1989, pp 515–529.

8. Keller EE, Sather AH: Quadrangular LeFort I osteotomy: Surgical technique and review of 54 patients. J Oral Maxillofac Surg 48:2–11, 1990.

9. Keller EE, Van Roekel NB, Desjardins RP, Tolman DE: Prosthetic-surgical reconstruction of the severely re-sorbed maxilla with iliac bone grafting and tissue integrated prostheses. Int J Oral Maxillofac Impl 2:155–165, 1987.

10. Obwegeser HL: Surgical correction of small or retrodisplaced maxillae. The "dish-face" deformity. Plast Reconstr Surg 43:351–365, 1969.

11. Sailer HF: A new method of inserting endosseous implants in totally atrophic maxillae. J Craniomaxillofac Surg 17:299–305, 1989.

Study Questions

1. What are the surgical options for a patient with an extremely atrophic maxilla?

2. What are the surgical options for a patient whose maxilla is severely vertically deficient and horizontally deficient, resulting in a Class III ridge relationship to the mandible?

CHAPTER 22

Maxillofacial Reconstruction in the Compromised Patient

Dale J. Misiek
John N. Kent
Revised by Michael S. Block and John N. Kent

Bone Grafting Principles
    Two-Phase Theory of Osteogenesis
    Types of Bone Grafts
    Effects of Radiation
        Case History 1: Secondary
            Reconstruction of the Mandibular
            Body in an Irradiated Field
Bone Grafting Techniques
    Case History 2: Secondary
        Reconstruction of the Mandibular
        Body, Ramus, and Condyle in a
        Nonirradiated Field
    Case History 3: Primary Reconstruction
        of the Mandibular Body and
        Symphysis in a Nonirradiated Field

Vascularized Graft Harvest Techniques
    Case History 4: Secondary
        Reconstruction of the Anterior Maxilla
        in a Nonirradiated Field with a Free
        Osteocutaneous Graft
    Case History 5: Secondary
        Reconstruction of Angle-to-Angle
        Mandibular Body Defect in a
        Radiated Field with a Free
        Osteocutaneous Graft
References

For the purpose of maxillofacial reconstruction, a compromised patient may be defined as one who has lost, or never had, a portion of facial hard or soft tissue, which prevents him or her from enjoying full function within society. Thus the goal of reconstruction should be to restore or create form to facilitate return to function.

BONE GRAFTING PRINCIPLES

The one factor common in all reconstructive efforts is the need for a bone graft.[15, 24]

The ideal bone graft should be structurally similar to the defect it is replacing, should contain all the elements necessary to promote full integration of the graft with minimal loss of shape and volume during the remodeling phase of healing, should restore function to the reconstructed region, and should not result in residual deformity or disability related to the donor site. Presently no single graft type fulfills all these requirements. Nonvascularized grafts, which rely on the host tissues for healing, undergo significant remodeling with often unpredictable volume and shape alterations, which compromise later prosthetic rehabilitation. Vascularized grafts, although they maintain their volume and shape, are usually limited in these parameters by their inherent dimensions and always result in some donor site deformity and disability.[10]

Two-Phase Theory of Osteogenesis

When bone is transplanted from one site to another within the same individual, immunologic complications for the most part do not occur. Nonvascularized grafts, involving large blocks of cortical bone, undergo resorption and remodeling resulting in form alteration. Grafting of live cells from cancellous marrow is required to induce local tissue to produce bone bulk. This initial process of bone healing, or incorporation of grafted bone, begins with osteoconduction. This involves the ingrowth of capillaries and mesenchymal cells from the recipient bed into, around, and through all forms of grafted bone. Next, osteoinduction occurs, which involves the differentiation of mesenchymal cells into bone-forming cells.[18] The process is thought to be regulated by bone morphogenic proteins (BMPs), specific enzymes, and enzyme inhibitors.[3, 19, 20–23]

There is evidence to support a two-phase theory of osteogenesis, originally advanced by Axhausen.[2, 5, 6, 8, 13] The first phase begins when transplanted cells proliferate and form osteoid. This occurs within the first few weeks, and the amount of bone regeneration depends on the amount of transplanted bone cells that survive. This first stage is responsible for the formation of most of the new bone.

The second phase of bone regeneration begins in the second week and becomes crucial 4 or 5 weeks following transplantation. Angiogenesis and proliferation of fibroblasts from the graft bed begin at the time of grafting, and osteogenesis from the host tissues soon follows. Fibroblasts and other mesenchymal cells differentiate into osteoblasts (possibly stimulated by bone morphogenic proteins) and begin to lay down new bone.[16, 17] This second phase continues indefinitely with resorption, remodeling, and replacement.

Types of Bone Grafts

AUTOGENOUS BONE GRAFTS

Autogenous grafts are composed of tissues procured from the patient and are usually considered the ideal bone graft material. These are the only types of grafts that supply living, immunocompatible bone cells essential to the initial phase of osteogenesis. Autogenous bone has advantages of providing osteogenic cells for healing, and these cells do not trigger an immunologic response. The main disadvantage may be the requirement of an additional donor site.

Nonvascularized grafts are obtained and transferred independent of a blood supply. These grafts rely on the recipient site for nutrition and revascularization. Composite grafts involve the transfer of both soft tissue and bone elements. The blood supply from the donor site is maintained during the procedure, and thus composite grafts are independent of the requirement of the well-vascularized recipient site. Because the bone is not stripped of its soft tissue pedicle, the potential for surviving osteogenic cells is much greater than for a nonvascularized graft. The free composite graft is totally removed from the body and immediately replaced, restoring its blood supply by reconnection of blood vessels with microsurgical techniques. Ilium, scapula, fibula, radius, or other suitable bone is removed along with the overlying soft tissues, including the nutrient artery and vein that supply these tissues. Once this graft is secured in place, the artery and veins are reconnected with microvascular anastomoses, thus preserving the blood supply.

Effects of Radiation

Several approaches to jaw reconstruction exist when radiation is part of the overall treatment plan. Immediate reconstruction is often not advisable because early radiotherapy may be essential in achieving a cure to the neoplastic disease.

Attempts to reconstruct bone defects in the maxillofacial region in the presence of a compromised graft bed owing to radiation are fraught with complications and failures.[1, 14] Hyperbaric oxygen therapy (HBO) was originally used postsurgically to enhance graft survival in nonvascularized grafts.[11, 25] Evidence has shown that HBO promotes osteogenesis in the grafted bone.[11] Marx and Ames[12] began using HBO presurgically to take advantage of the notable improvement in host tissue vascularity and cellularity. Their studies have shown that after 18 exposures (dives to 2.4 atm), oxygen tension in irradiated tissue plateaus at 80% to 85% of normal nonirradiated tissue. They hypothesized that this permanent increase in tissue oxygenation is due to HBO-induced angiogenesis.[4] This neovascularity promotes early revascularization of the nonvascularized bone graft as well as enhancing the survival of viable osteoprogenitor cells.[9]

As one might expect, integration of implant

fixtures is also adversely affected in irradiated bone. Success rates as low as 42% have been seen with maxillary and orbital fixtures placed in bone previously irradiated.[7]

Case History 1

SECONDARY RECONSTRUCTION OF THE MANDIBULAR BODY IN AN IRRADIATED FIELD

This 54-year-old man complained of drooling and difficulty chewing. Five years before, squamous carcinoma was diagnosed, and he underwent right mandibular body resection, hemiglossectomy, and a radical neck dissection. A deltopectoral flap was used to close the soft tissue defect, but mandibular continuity was lacking. Postoperative treatment included 6500 rads of radiation (Fig. 22–1).

Following Marx's protocol, 20 HBO dives preceded reconstruction. A low neck incision exposed the right ramus, which was properly positioned following a coronoidectomy. A large reconstruction plate then bridged the gap between the bone ends of the right ramus and the left mandibular symphysis. The medial cortex of the anterior hip was used to form the lateral border of the reconstruction with a split demineralized rib forming the superior and medial borders. Particulate cancellous marrow was compacted and placed into the defect (Fig. 21–1C). The skin flap was then closed in layers, and postoperatively the patient received 10 HBO dives.

Six months later, following an additional 10 HBO dives, a split-thickness dissection was performed over the newly formed mandible, and the reconstruction plate was removed. The deltopectoral flap was debulked and the residual tongue advanced to the symphysis. Eight hydroxylapatite (HA)–coated implants were placed, five in the graft and three in the irradiated mandible (Fig. 21–1D). The implants were countersunk 2 mm, vestibules were created, and a dermis graft was placed over the bone ridge (Fig. 22–1E).

At 4 months, the implants were exposed (Fig. 22–1F). Shouldered abutments were placed, and a hybrid, full-arch, fixed prosthesis was fabricated with a metal superstructure and acrylic teeth (Fig. 22–1G). Screw retention of the prosthesis allows for retrievability (Fig. 22–1H). At 2 years follow-up (Fig. 22–1I, J) the implants have done well both in the reconstructed and in the irradiated mandible.

BONE GRAFTING TECHNIQUES

Case History 2

SECONDARY RECONSTRUCTION OF THE MANDIBULAR BODY, RAMUS, AND CONDYLE IN A NONIRRADIATED FIELD

This 60-year-old man complained of difficulty with mastication and inability to retain a denture (Fig. 22–2). Four years before, squamous cell carcinoma was diagnosed, and he underwent a left mandibular body, ramus, and condyle resection with a suprahyoid neck dissection. A deltopectoral flap was used to close the soft tissue defect, but mandibular continuity was not reestablished. Neither radiation nor chemotherapy was included in the postoperative treatment.

On examination, the deltopectoral flap was noted to include only the retromolar, pharyngeal, and posterior soft palate mucosa. The tongue had full freedom of motion, and the residual ridge on the right side was in good position, not atrophic, but jaw movement was not reproducible. Radiographically, the right mandibular condyle, ramus, body, and symphysis were all intact and of good vertical height and width for implant reconstruction (Fig. 22–2B). The maxillary ridge as well was adequate for denture construction.

Of primary importance was reestablishment of mandibular continuity and left temporomandibular joint function. A low neck incision exposed the defect along with the stump of the symphysis and the residual glenoid fossa. A reconstruction plate with a condylar prosthesis was applied to the symphysis and positioned appropriately in the temporomandibular joint, and the glenoid fossa was reconstructed with a VK-II glenoid fossa prosthesis (Fig. 22–2C). Additionally, corticocancellous block grafts were lagged to the reconstruction plate in an effort to position the bone adequately for later implant reconstruction. Postoperatively, normal jaw function resumed after a short period of physical therapy, and good jaw contour was established.

Nine months following the reconstruction with the bone plate and corticocancellous block grafts, implants were placed in the mandible. Dissection over the reconstructed mandible revealed a significant amount of resorp-

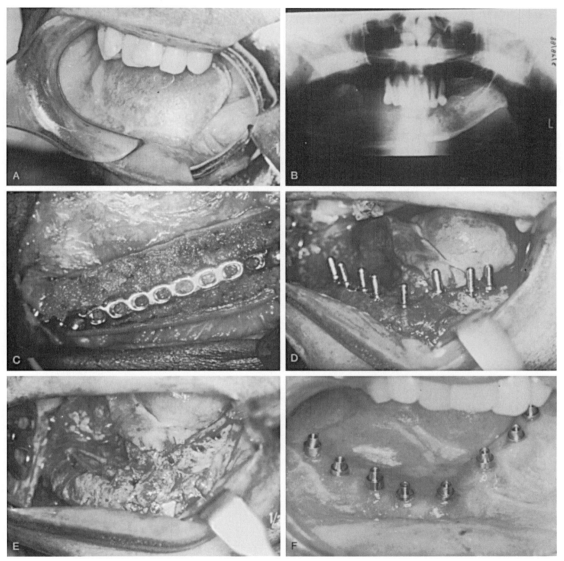

Figure 22–1. *A*, Intraoral examination indicates loss of vestibular definition and tongue displacement. *B*, Panoramic x-ray film showing right mandibular resection. *C*, Right mandibular reconstruction following 20 HBO dives. *D*, Parallel pins illustrating implant location. *E*, Ridge before placement of dermis graft. *F*, Implant exposure.

Illustration continued on following page

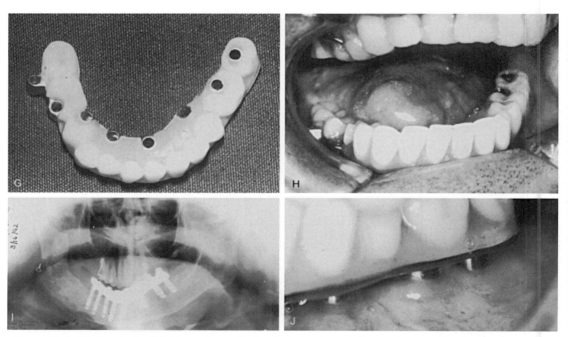

Figure 22–1 *Continued. G,* Hybrid prosthesis. *H,* Prosthesis in place. *I,* Panoramic x-ray film 2 years postoperatively. *J,* Two-year postoperative oral appearance.

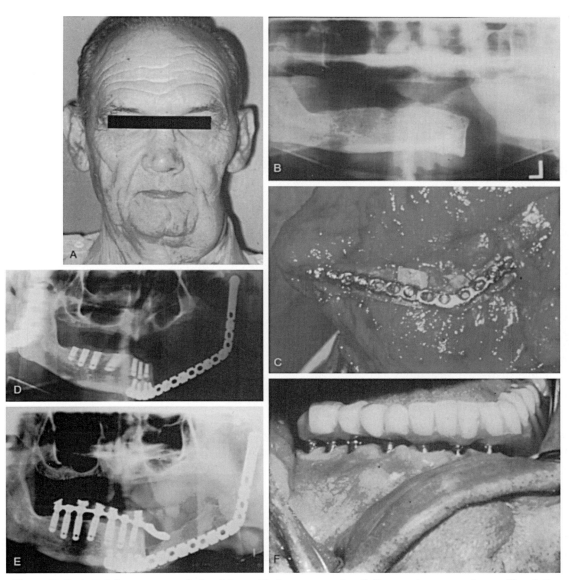

Figure 22–2. *A*, Full-face appearance before left mandibular reconstruction. *B*, Preoperative panoramic x-ray film. *C*, Bone graft to left mandible. *D*, Panoramic x-ray film of implant placement. *E*, Panoramic x-ray film 7 years postimplantation. *F*, Seven-year postoperative condition of oral tissues.

tion, primarily in a mediolateral dimension. This resulted in inability to place implants in this grafted section, and therefore only seven HA-coated implants were placed between the symphysis and the right mandibular body region (Fig. 22–2D). After 3 months, these implants were exposed, and reconstruction was completed with a hybrid, fixed prosthesis cantilevered over the left mandible using the implants in the symphysis and right mandible.

The patient has returned annually, and it is now 10 years since the implant reconstruction. There has been minimal bone loss involving the implants despite the fact that the prosthesis was cantilevered along one-third of its length (Fig. 22–2E). The patient has maintained excellent oral hygiene around the existing implants, and function with the prosthesis and alloplastic temporomandibular joint articulation has been excellent (Fig. 22–2F).

Case History 3
PRIMARY RECONSTRUCTION OF THE MANDIBULAR BODY AND SYMPHYSIS IN A NONIRRADIATED FIELD

This 53-year-old man complained of difficulty with mastication and inability to wear a removable prosthesis (Fig. 22–3A). Thirteen months before, a central mucoepidermoid carcinoma of the left mandible had been diagnosed. Following preoperative extraction and mucosal closure, the left mandibular body and symphysis were resected via an extraoral approach. Immediate reconstruction consisted of adaptation of a three-dimensional stainless steel mesh tray, which was packed with particulate cortical and cancellous bone from the posterior iliac crest, combined with demineralized bone in a 2:1 ratio of autogenous bone to allogeneic bone (Fig. 22–3B). Primary closure was achieved extraorally, and excellent mandibular contour was maintained by the three-dimensional reconstruction tray (Fig. 22–3C).

After 13 months, jaw relation records and a diagnostic wax-up were obtained to determine the ideal placement of endosseous implants (Fig. 22–3D). At the time of implant placement, excellent bone contour was found, and six HA-coated implants were placed in the graft (Fig. 22–3E). At the same time a portion of the reconstruction tray flange that had been interfering with the placement of a removable prosthesis was removed from the buccal vesti-

bule. Only 8- and 10-mm implants were used because radiographic evaluation revealed there was no mineralization indicating bone formation in the base of the reconstruction tray (Fig. 22–3F). It was hypothesized that a combination of stress shielding and hypovascularity contributed to this lack of new bone formation.

At 1 month postimplantation, persistent chronic drainage was noted around the third implant from the right. Curettage did not resolve the problem, and at 2 months, this implant was removed. Of note, the removal required trephination because of early osseointegration in the apical half of the implant. At 6 months postimplantation, the remaining implants were exposed, and no bone loss was noted (Fig. 22–3G).

Prosthetic rehabilitation included a hybrid, fixed prosthesis that was screw retained (Fig. 22–3H). Palatoversion of teeth in the anterior maxilla occurred because of the patient's prolonged period of mandibular edentulism resulting in a labial position of the anterior implants and a slightly compromised occlusion. The patient has returned annually for 8 years and has exhibited negligible bone loss around the implants and no demonstrable peri-implant mucosal disease (Fig. 22–3I). It has been decided to keep the three-dimensional reconstruction tray in place because no further bone loss has been demonstrated, and external facial contour would be compromised on its removal (Fig. 22–3J).

Vascularized Graft Harvest Techniques

Case History 4
Secondary Reconstruction of the Anterior Maxilla in a Nonirradiated Field with a Free Osteocutaneous Graft

This 25-year-old man had a rapidly enlarging mass in the anterior maxilla (Fig. 22–5A). Biopsy revealed the lesion to be an osteosarcoma. Surgery was undertaken to resect the lesion, which extended from premolar to premolar involving the floor of the nose and the maxillary alveolus. With an incision that began labially just inside the vermilion border, the tumor was resected (Fig. 22–5B). Exposed bone and denuded submucosal tissues were

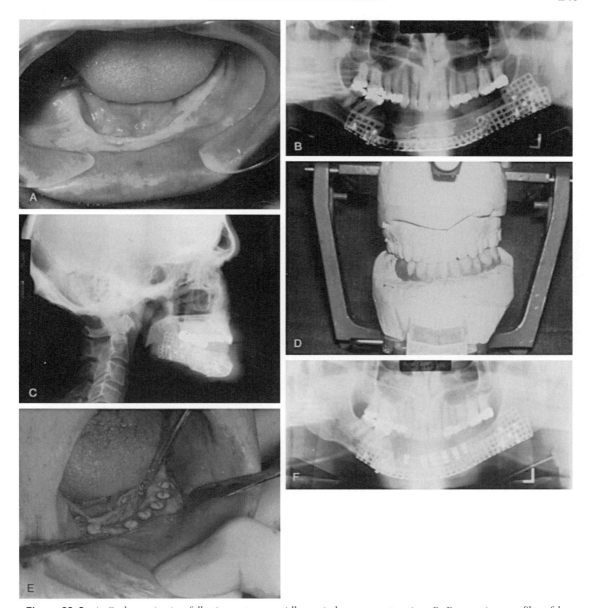

Figure 22–3. *A*, Oral examination following autogenous/allogeneic bone reconstruction. *B*, Panoramic x-ray film of bone graft reconstructed mandible. *C*, Lateral cephalogram showing good mandibular/maxillary relationships. *D*, Diagnostic wax-up. *E*, Implants at placement into consolidated bone graft. *F*, Panoramic x-ray film following implant placement.

Illustration continued on following page

covered with a skin graft (Fig. 22–5*C*) and held in place with an obturator that was sutured into position (Fig. 22–5*D*).

The surgery was followed by 6 months of chemotherapy after which planning of the reconstruction began. The area to be reconstructed would require both hard and soft tissue elements to be brought to the region because local tissues were insufficient to close the resultant defect (Fig. 22–5*E*). Three-dimensional reformatted computed tomography

(CT) identified the bone margins of the defect, which included the infraorbital rims, malar buttresses, posterior maxillae, and posterior hard palate (Fig. 22–5*F*). A scapular osteocutaneous free graft was chosen because of the length of the vascular pedicle necessary to extend from the anterior maxilla to the facial artery, where the caliber was large enough for microsurgical anastomosis (Fig. 22–4).

The lateral scapular border, based on the circumflex scapular artery, was harvested and

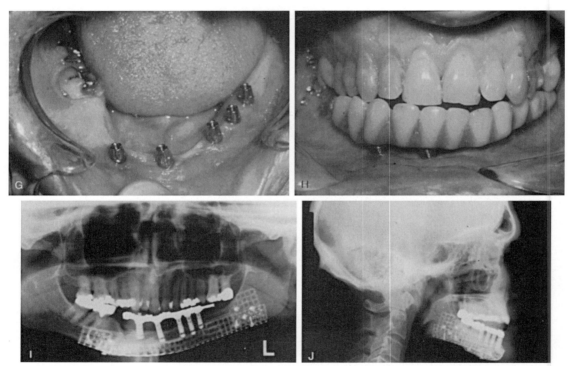

Figure 22–3 *Continued.* G, Implant exposure. H, Occlusion with hybrid prosthesis. I, Panoramic x-ray film 8 years postimplantation. J, Cephalometric x-ray film 8 years postimplantation.

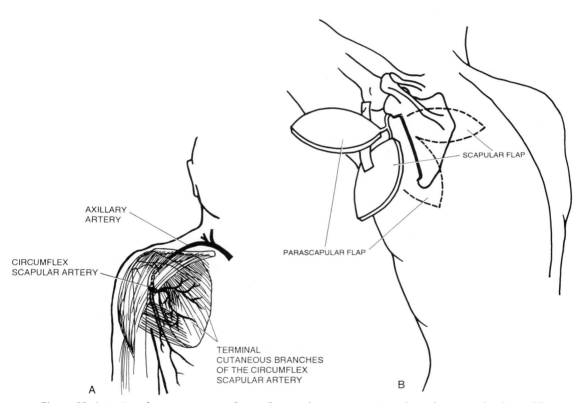

AXILLARY
ARTERY

CIRCUMFLEX
SCAPULAR ARTERY

TERMINAL
CUTANEOUS BRANCHES
OF THE CIRCUMFLEX
SCAPULAR ARTERY

A

SCAPULAR FLAP

PARASCAPULAR FLAP

B

Figure 22–4. *A*, Scapular osteocutaneous free graft—vascular anatomy. *B*, Scapular and parascapular skin paddles.

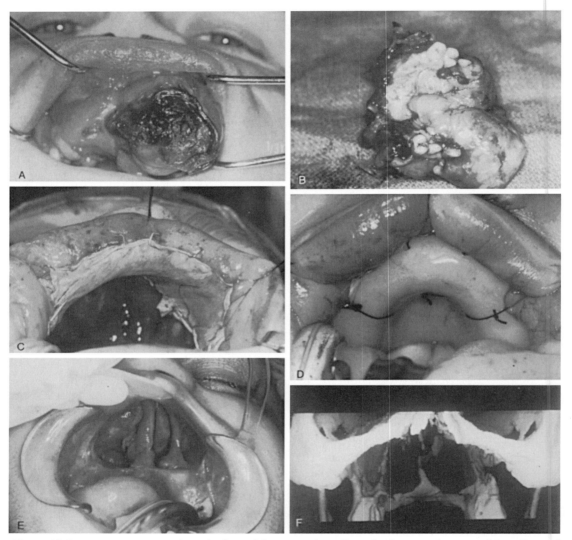

Figure 22–5. *A,* Osteosarcoma involving the floor of the nose and maxilla to the first premolar region, bilaterally. *B,* The resected anterior maxilla, intraoperatively. *C,* Postoperative resection. The defect was lined with a skin graft. *D,* A splint was placed over the defect and skin graft. (Tumor resection and reconstruction done by Dr. Elliot Black and Dr. Michael Block.) *E,* Postoperative maxillary defect. *F,* Three-dimensional reformatted CT of maxillary defect.

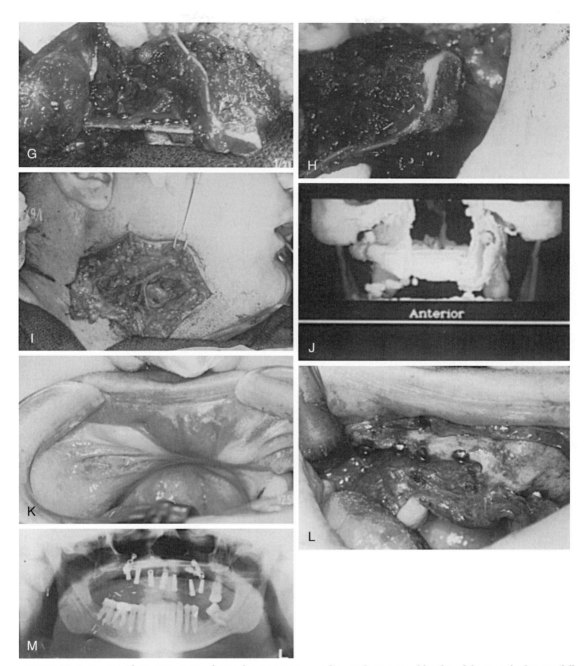

Figure 22–5 *Continued. G,* Osteotomized scapular osteocutaneous free graft. *H,* Lateral border of the scapula showing full-thickness dimensions. *I,* Facial/circumflex scapular artery and vein anastomosis site. *J,* Three-dimensional, reformatted CT following reconstruction. *K,* Intraoral view before implant placement. *L,* Intraoperative view of implants in scapula. *M,* Postimplantation panoramic x-ray film.

osteotomized to approximate the horseshoe shape of the maxillary alveolar ridge extending superiorly to the infraorbital rims (Fig. 22–5G). More than 12 mm of ridge height was provided by the full thickness of the scapular bone (Fig. 22–5H). The muscles remaining attached to the scapula were allowed to re-epithelialize without secondary skin graft coverage. The microsurgical anastomosis took place at the facial artery after creating a sub-mucosal tunnel through which the scapular vascular pedicle was passed (Fig. 22–5I).

Postoperatively reformatted three-dimensional CT reveals the form of the reconstruction (Fig. 22–5J). In addition to placement of implants, labial and buccal vestibuloplasties would be necessary (Fig. 22–5K). Ten months later, HA-coated, screw-type implants were placed in the reconstructed maxilla (Fig. 22–5L). A 4-month integration period elapsed (Fig. 22–5M). The implants were then exposed, and a metal superstructure was designed. A removable prosthesis with retention from clips onto the implant superstructure completed the rehabilitation.

Case History 5
SECONDARY RECONSTRUCTION OF ANGLE-TO-ANGLE MANDIBULAR BODY DEFECT IN A RADIATED FIELD WITH A FREE OSTEOCUTANEOUS GRAFT

This 54-year-old man complained of limited opening of and a severely retrognathic mandible (Fig. 22–6A). The history indicated that osteosarcoma of the mandible was diagnosed 4 years previously for which he received radiation therapy. Three months after this, he underwent a subtotal mandibulectomy leaving only the posterior ramus and condyles bilaterally. Six months later, an iliac osteocutaneous free graft was attempted, which subsequently failed owing to occlusion of its vascular pedicle. After 1 more year, he had successful partial mandibular reconstruction with a pedicled scapular osteocutaneous graft. After an additional 1½ years the mandibular reconstruction was completed with a free scapular osteocutaneous graft and microvascular anastomosis of the opposite scapula supported by a three-dimensional stainless steel mesh tray.

Initial oral examination revealed an intact maxilla with natural dentition (Figs. 22–6B,C). The mandible was severely retrognathic, and

the posterior maxillary teeth occluded on the mandibular ridge with only 5 mm of freeway space created during maximum opening (Fig. 22–6D). The patient still had a functional tongue. Because he lacked a labial vestibule, however, salivary control was compromised. The surgical plan was to perform a LeFort I osteotomy impacting the posterior maxilla 1 cm. At the same time, HA-coated implants would be placed in the mandible combined with overlying tissue debulking and a split-thickness graft vestibuloplasty to create a vestibule and increase flexibility.

Intraoperatively, following the performance of the standard LeFort I osteotomy, a labial incision and subsequent submucosal and subperiosteal dissection exposed the scapular graft. Debulking of the overlying flap was done at this time because primary closure and coverage of the implants were not affected by the tissue thinning. Implants were placed in the scapula, which was quite unlike drilling in an intact mandible (Fig. 22–6E). The scapular marrow retained its lamella configuration, and the density was significantly less, raising the question whether osseointegration within the graft would yield stable implants. Satisfactory closure was obtained, and a simultaneous split-thickness skin graft vestibuloplasty was performed. Alignment of the implants was satisfactory, and healing was uneventful (Fig. 22–6F).

After 7 months, all seven implants were exposed via a mucosal punch technique so as not to disturb the newly created vestibule. Bone loss of 1 to 2 mm was noted on five of seven implants; however, all were fully integrated (Fig. 22–6G). A sectional, fixed metal superstructure was fabricated to support a mandibular overdenture prosthesis (Fig. 22–6H). Six-year follow-up has revealed no restriction of masticatory function, markedly improved speech, and salivary control (Fig. 22–6I). Recurrent hyperplasia of peri-implant tissues despite excellent oral hygiene practices is treated every 18 to 24 months with debridement and tissue reduction with electrocautery. No radiographic or clinical evidence of bone loss is noted during routine follow-up examinations (Fig. 22–6J). The three-dimensional stainless steel mesh tray has been left in for the benefit of facial form (Fig. 22–6K). Extremely high patient satisfaction has resulted (Fig. 22–6L).

In summary, significant advances have been made in surgical techniques for bone harvest

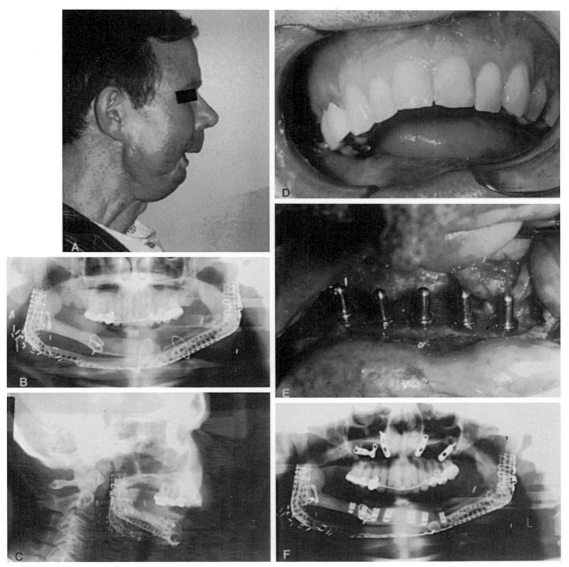

Figure 22–6. *A*, Facial appearance after multiple pedicled and free osteocutaneous flaps to complete mandibular reconstruction. *B*, Panoramic x-ray film following mandibular bone reconstruction. *C*, Cephalometric x-ray film demonstrating unfavorable mandibular position related to the maxilla. *D*, Intraoral examination showing occlusal compromise and lack of labial vestibule. *E*, Intraoperative view of implant placement in scapula. *F*, Postimplantation panoramic x-ray film.

Illustration continued on following page

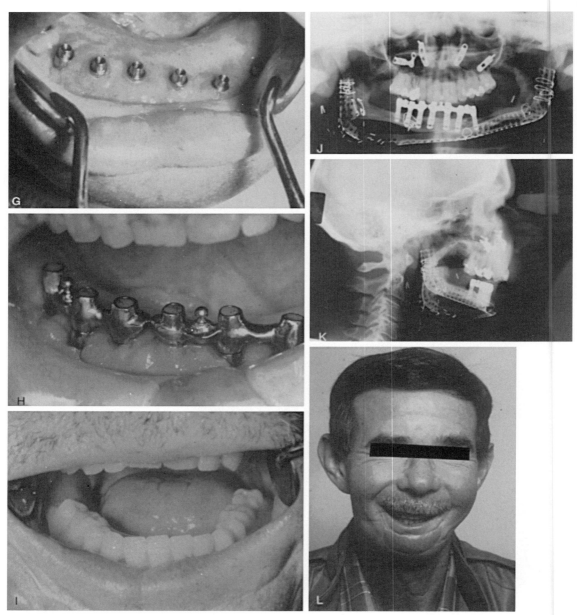

Figure 22–6 *Continued. G,* Implants exposed through skin of scapula; newly created labial vestibule. *H,* Sectional, screw-retained superstructure for overdenture prosthesis. *I,* Postrehabilitation mouth opening. *J,* Six-year follow-up panoramic x-ray film. *K,* Six-year follow-up cephalometric x-ray film. *L,* Postrehabilitation facial appearance.

over the last 20 years. There are certainly pros and cons involving each, whether it be a vascularized or nonvascularized technique; however, no one type of bone graft is so versatile that all others are obsolete. Today's reconstructive surgeon must evaluate the skeletal defect, determine the health or presence of the recipient-site soft tissue, and plan for ultimate implant prosthetic rehabilitation. It is clear that a combination of bone graft types and techniques may be necessary for a single reconstructive effect, and, if so, planning of surgical entries and re-entries must be efficient and kept to a minimum. Interdisciplinary cooperation at the outset of treatment benefits all involved from planning through execution. The goal of treatment must be maximum functional and aesthetic jaw relationships, and the ultimate beneficiary must be the patient.

Acknowledgments

We would like to thank the following for their contribution in surgical and prosthetic management of the cases illustrated in this chapter. Through their clinical excellence and their desire to work together for the benefit of our patients, successful outcomes were achieved.

Plastic and reconstructive surgeons: Elliot B. Black III, MD (Case 4) and William R. Swartz, MD (Case 5).

Oral and maxillofacial surgeons: Michael S. Block, DMD (Cases 1 and 4); Ronald B. Marks, DDS (Case 2); David M. Carlton, Jr., DDS (Case 2); C. Grady Hornsby, DDS (Case 3).

Maxillofacial prosthodontists: Israel M. Finger, DDS (Cases 1–4); Luis R. Guerra, DDS (Case 5).

We would also like to thank Kathy Martello for the preparation of illustrations, Robert Raben for photographic assistance, and Maureen Raymond for her unending patience in the preparation of this manuscript.

References

1. Adamo AR, Szal RL: Timing, results and complications of mandibular surgery. J Oral Surg 37:755, 1979.
2. Axhausen W: The osteogenetic phases of regeneration of bone, a historical and experimental study. J Bone Joint Surg 38A:593, 1956.
3. Barth A: Ueber histologische Befunde nach Knochenimplantationen. Arch Klin Chir 46:409, 1893.
4. Buhner MR, Marx RE: Hyperbaric oxygen–induced angiogenesis and fibroplasia in human irradiated tissues. Proceedings of the 65th Meeting of the American Association of Oral and Maxillofacial Surgeons, Las Vegas, 1983.
5. Burwell RG: Studies in the transplantation of bone: VII. The fresh composite homograft-autograft of cancellous bone. J Bone Joint Surg 46B:110–154, 1964.
6. Elves MW: Newer knowledge of immunology of bone and cartilage. Clin Orthop 120:232, 1976.
7. Granström G, Tjelström A, Brånemark P-I, Fornander J: Bone-anchored reconstruction of the irradiated head and neck cancer patient. Otolaryngol Head Neck Surg 108:334, 1993.
8. Gray JC, Elves M: Early osteogenesis in compact bone. Tiss Int 29:225, 1979.
9. Greenspan G: The side effects of radiation therapy and chemotherapy on the oral structures. Oral Maxillofac Clin North Am 5:347, 1993.
10. Kuriloff DB, Sullivan MJ: Mandibular reconstruction using vascularized bone grafts. Otolaryngol Clin North Am 24:1391, 1991.
11. Mainous EG, Boyne PJ, Hart DB, Terry BC: Restoration of resected mandible by grafting with combination of mandibular homograft and autogenous iliac mural, and postoperative treatment with hyperbaric oxygenation. Oral Surg 35:13, 1973.
12. Marx RE, Ames JR: The use of hyperbaric oxygen therapy in bony reconstruction of irradiated and tissue deficient patient. J Oral Maxillofac Surg 40:412, 1982.
13. Marx RE, Saunders TR: Reconstruction and rehabilitation of cancer patients. In: Fonseca RJ, Davis WH (eds): Reconstructive Preprosthetic Oral and Maxillofacial Surgery. Philadelphia, WB Saunders, 1986, p 347.
14. Obwegeser HB, Sailer HF: Experience with intraoral resection and immediate reconstruction in cases of radio-osteomyelitis. J Maxillofac Surg 6:257, 1978.
15. Shockley WW, Weissler MC: Reconstructive alternatives following segmental mandibulectomy. Am J Otolaryngol 13:156, 1992.
16. Urist MR: The substratum for bone morphogenesis. Dev Biol 4 (suppl):125, 1970.
17. Urist MR: Osteoinduction in undemineralized bone implants modified by chemical inhibitors of endogenous matrix enzymes. Clin Orthop 87:132, 1972.
18. Urist MR: Practical applications of basic research on bone graft physiology. In Evans EB, Cooper RR, et al (eds): Instructional Course Lectures, The American Academy of Orthopedic Surgery, vol 25. St Louis, CV Mosby, 1976.
19. Urist MR, Earnest F, Kimball KM, et al: Bone morphogenesis in implants of residues of radioisotope labelled bone matrix. Calcif Tis Res 15:236, 1974.
20. Urist MR, Hernandez A: Excitation transfer in bone: Deleterious effects of cobalt 60 radiation-sterilization of bank bone. Arch Surg 109:486, 1974.
21. Urist MR, Lietz A, Mizutani H, et al: A bovine low molecular weight bone morphogenetic protein (BMP) fraction. Clin Orthop 162:219, 1982.
22. Urist MR, McLean FG: Osteogenetic potency and new-bone formation by induction in transplants to the anterior chamber of the eye. J Bone Joint Sung 34:443, 1952.
23. Urist MR, Mikulski AJ, Boyd SD: A chemosterilized antigen extracted bone morphogenetic alloimplant. Arch Surg 110:416, 1975.
24. Urken ML, Buchbinder D, Weinberg H, et al: Functional evaluation following microvascular oromandibular reconstruction of the oral cancer patient: A comparative study of reconstructed and non-reconstructed patients. Laryngoscope 101:935, 1991.
25. Wilcox JW, Kolodny FC: Acceleration of healing of maxillary and mandibular osteotomies by use of hyperbaric oxygen. Oral Surg 41:423, 1976.

Study Questions

1. A patient has had a mandibular body resection, a radical neck dissection, and radiation therapy to treat cancer. Describe two surgical methods for mandibular reconstruction with implants.

2. Why use a composite bone graft, with its vasculature reattached to the carotids, in a radiated patient?

SECTION 4

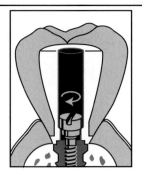

Soft Tissue and Microbiological Considerations

CHAPTER 23

Periodontal Considerations for Dental Implants

Raymond A. Yukna

The development of osseointegrated dental implants has had a major effect on periodontal education and periodontal practice. Once the implants have integrated and have been uncovered, clinical evaluation of implant health is necessary on a continuing basis and includes many soft tissue considerations. Peri-implant health should appear as noninflamed surface tissues; minimal, stable probing depths without bleeding on probing; and stable bone levels.[4, 7]

Determination of the condition of the peri-implant soft tissues includes surface evaluation for the presence and severity of inflammation. Color, contour, and consistency of the circumferential gingival tissues can be judged in descriptive terms or can be objectively scored by means of the Gingival Index or similar scoring systems. Persistent presence of inflammation suggests ongoing irritation of the tissues from plaque accumulation, rough component parts, or mobility of component parts.

Probing depth is another measure of implant health, and, as with natural teeth, minimal probing depth (<4 mm) is preferable. It is recommended that measurements of probing depths be made with calibrated plastic or nylon probes rather than metal probes to minimize scratching of the metal titanium surface of the implant abutment components. Often the suprabone/supraimplant probing depth can be determined based on the known length of the abutment head, which provides a clinical reference (Fig. 23–1).

More important than the actual millimeter probing measurement is the stability of the measurement. Increasing probing depth measurements at recall evaluations are worrisome and suggest progressive disease and possible failure of the implant. This is especially true if the probing depth increases to the point at which the

body of the implant is "probeable." Such a situation reflects crestal bone loss around the neck of the dental implant and, if progressive, suggests loss of integration of the dental implant (Figs. 23–2 through 23–4). An indicator of relative health of the peri-implant pocket is the presence or absence of bleeding on probing. Bleeding on gentle probing suggests irritation and ulceration of the soft tissue wall facing the abutment heads. Although isolated instances of bleeding on probing in a particular site may not be of consequence, continued bleeding on probing on sequential examinations strongly suggests increased potential for continued attachment and bone loss.[13, 14, 20, 21]

There is continued argument about the requirement for keratinized gingiva rather than alveolar mucosa next to the dental implant abutment head (as there continues to be concerning the type of soft tissues next to natural teeth). Although reports evaluating the health of the soft tissues adjacent to dental implants supporting

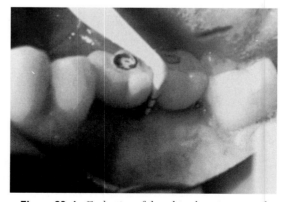

Figure 23–1. Evaluation of dental implant site using plastic periodontal probe. Stability of probing depth and presence or absence of bleeding on probing are noted.

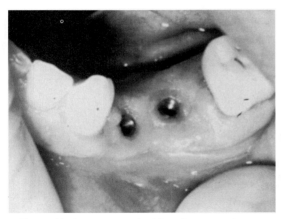

Figure 23–2. Long-term health and apparent keratinization of peri-implant tissues seen after removal of abutment heads during recall appointment.

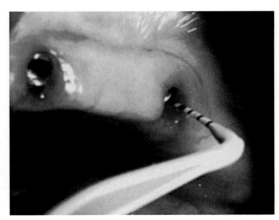

Figure 23–4. Probe verifies lack of attachment/bone loss adjacent to dental implant body at recall after removal of abutment heads.

complete denture-type restorations suggest no detrimental effects if the marginal tissues are composed of alveolar mucosa,[1, 4, 18] subjective evaluation and patient responses suggest that an adequate zone of dense, thick keratinized gingiva is preferable.[20, 21] Nonkeratinized mucosa is too readily abraded and tends to be tender to the patient during mastication and oral hygiene procedures. Additionally, it can be an aesthetic problem because the metal components can be seen through the thin mucosal tissues, and it is more subject to recession (Fig. 23–5). A good band of keratinized tissue is less movable, is more resistant to physical trauma, and provides better and more aesthetic contours.

Bone loss around dental implants can occur owing to a multitude of factors. Although ongoing research strives to elucidate the role of sev-

eral factors, current findings suggest that plaque accumulation and excessive occlusal forces are the primary causes of implant failure after integration has occurred and restorations have been placed into function.[8, 11, 15, 19, 26, 27] There are also several preloading causes of bone loss, primarily improper surgical technique that overheats the bone.[9]

Crestal and peri-implant bone levels are best determined by regular accurate radiographic evaluation. Although panoramic radiographs are commonly used for dental implant evaluation, periapical and vertical bite-wing dental radiographs used with a grid generally provide more definitive information. Again, stability of bone levels, especially following loading and restoration attachment, is critical. Progressive bone loss suggests a failing dental implant. Although a

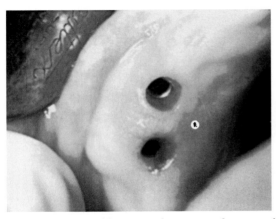

Figure 23–3. Healthy peri-implant tissues after removal of abutment heads at recall appointment.

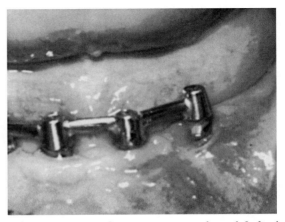

Figure 23–5. Local tissue irritation on lower left distal implant owing to loose mucosal margin and lack of dense keratinized gingival tissue.

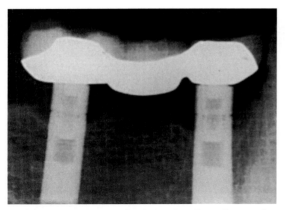

Figure 23–6. Periapical radiograph with overlying grid to verify bone levels. This 3-year radiograph shows stability of bone levels, including the saucerization at crest that became apparent in the first 3 months after loading.

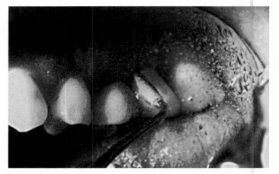

Figure 23–8. Mirror view of in-office maintenance procedure illustrating use of nylon sheath for sonic/ultrasonic unit that allows cleaning of implant parts without scratching the titanium.

well-known criteria list for dental implant success suggests that less than or equal to 0.2 mm of crestal bone loss annually is acceptable,[2] it must be realized that that same rate of bone loss reflects progressive advancing periodontal disease around natural teeth (Fig. 23–6).

The mechanism and nature of bacterial accumulation around dental implants and on dental implant parts is under investigation. Current knowledge suggests that although bacterial attachment to titanium occurs at a less rapid rate than on natural teeth, once the initial bacterial colonies have been established, the sequence of bacterial accumulation and change in flora to a more pathogenic complex occurs in the same manner. Such plaque accumulation accounts for much of the peri-implantitis that is seen. This is especially true in a "mixed dentition" situation in which both natural teeth and dental implants are present in the same mouth. It appears that the bacterial flora of the natural tooth pockets may seed the interface area of the soft tissue/dental

implant.[8, 11, 15, 17, 19, 24–27] This circumstance makes obtaining periodontal health around natural teeth imperative before exposing dental implants for restoration.

Excessive occlusal forces are another major cause of peri-implant bone loss.[26] Lateral forces, such as are present in excursive interferences or in bruxism, appear to be an important initiating factor of bone loss that then may allow pocket formation and progression into peri-implantitis with eventual implant loss. Care must be taken to establish the least amount of lateral forces possible. For patients who are suspected or known to have parafunctional habits, a soft bite-guard for protection against these forces is highly recommended (Fig. 23–7).[9, 16, 22]

The follow-up care and periodontal requirements for success are similar for dental implants as for natural teeth. In general, the follow-up and maintenance frequency for patients with dental implants would be similar to those for periodon-

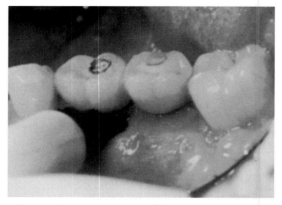

Figure 23–9. Rotary-powered brush useful for patient home care. Both InterPlak (Bausch and Lomb) and Rotadent (Pro Dentec) brushes are beneficial and may be dipped in an antibacterial rinse during use.

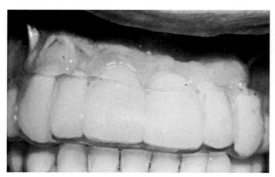

Figure 23–7. Soft bite-guard overlay to protect against damage from parafunctional forces.

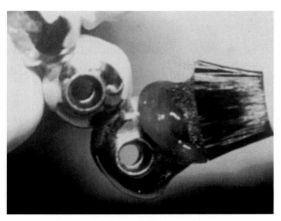

Figure 23–10. Polishing of dental implant superstructure at recall. Retrievability of implant prostheses provides many advantages for the clinician.

tal patients. It is recommended that for the first year after implant uncovering, the patient be seen every 3 months for evaluation of oral hygiene practices, tissue health, radiographic bone levels, appropriate occlusal forces, stability of the restorations, and general comfort. On a 6-month or annual basis, the superstructure (when retrievable) should be removed and the individual implant parts and peri-implant tissues evaluated more critically. This retrievable situation allows for polishing and modification of the superstructure as well as more specific hygiene instruction for the patients for any problem areas. As with patients with natural teeth, the patient's ability to perform effective oral hygiene, the condition of the soft tissues and bone levels, the type of restorations, and the need for frequent evaluation determine the actual recall intervals (Figs. 23–8 through 23–10). The more that patients can do on their own, the less they may need the dental office to help ensure long-term implant health.[12, 23, 28]

References

1. Adell R, et el: Marginal tissue reactions at osseointegrated titanium fixtures: I. A 3 year longitudinal prospective study. Int J Oral Maxillofac Surg 15:39–52, 1988.
2. Albrektsson T, Zarb G, Worthington P, Eriksson AR: The long-term efficacy of currently used dental implants: A review and proposed criteria of success. Int J Oral Maxillofac Impl 1:11–25, 1986.
3. Aspe P, Ellen RP, Overal CM, Zarb GA: Microbiota and gingival fluid collagenase activity in osseointegrated dental implant sulcus: A comparison of sites in edentulous and partially edentulous patients. J Periodontal Res 24:96–105, 1989.
4. Apse P, Zarb GA, Schmitt A, Lewis DW: The longitudinal effectiveness of osseointegrated dental implants. The Toronto study: Peri-implant mucosal response. Int J Periodont Restor Dent 11:95–111, 1991.
5. Becker W, Becker BE, Newman MG, Nyman S: Clinical and microbiologic findings that may contribute to dental implant failure. Int J Oral Maxillofac Impl 5:31–38, 1990.
6. Bergendal T, Forsgen L, Kvint S, Lowstest E: The effect of an airbrasive instrument on soft and hard tissues around osseointegrated implants. A case report. Scand Dent J 14:219–223, 1990.
7. Chaytor DV, Zarb GA, Schmitt A, Lewis DW: The longitudinal effectiveness of osseointegrated dental implants. The Toronto study: Bone level changes. Int J Periodont Restor Dent 11:113–125, 1991.
8. Ericsson I, Berglundh T, Marinello C, Liljenberg B, Lindhe J: Long-standing plaque and gingivitis at implants and teeth in the dog. Clin Oral Impl Res 3:99–103, 1992.
9. Ericsson I, et al: A clinical evaluation of fixed bridge restorations supported by the combination of teeth and osseointegrated implants. J Clin Periodontol 13:307–312, 1986.
10. Eriksson RA, Albrektsson T: The effect of heat on bone regeneration. J Oral Maxillofac Surg 42:705–711, 1984.
11. Hickey JS, O'Neal RB, Scheidt MJ, Strong S, Turgeon D, Van Dyke E: Microbiologic characterization of ligature-induced peri-implantitis in the microswine model. J Periodontol 62:548–553, 1991.
12. Jaffin R: Biological and clinical rationale for second-stage surgery and maintenance. Dent Clin North Am 33:683, 1989.
13. James RA: Peri-implant considerations. Dent Clin North Am 24:415–420, 1980.
14. Keene DM: Periodontal considerations for implant dentistry. Dent Clin North Am 20:155–179, 1976.
15. Lang NP, Brägger U, Walther D, Beamer B, Kornman KS: Ligature-induced peri-implant infection in cynomolgus monkeys: I. Clinical and radiographic findings. Clin Oral Impl Res 4:2–11, 1993.
16. Langer B, Sullivan DY: Osseointegration: Its impact on the interrelationship of periodontics and restorative dentistry: I. Int J Periodont Restor Dent 9:85–105, 1989.
17. Lekholm U, et al: The condition of soft tissues at tooth and fixture abutments supporting fixed bridges. A microbiological and histological study. J Clin Periodontol 13:558–562, 1986.
18. Lekholm U, et al: Marginal tissue reactions at osseointegrated titanium fixtures: II. A cross-sectional retrospective study. Int J Oral Maxillofac Surg 15:53–61, 1986.
19. Leonhardt Å, Berglundh T, Ericsson I, Dahlén G: Putative periodontal pathogens on titanium implants and teeth in experimental gingivitis and periodontitis in beagle dogs. Clin Oral Impl Res 3:112–119, 1992.
20. Meffert RM: Endosseous dental implantology from the periodontist's viewpoint. J Periodontol 57:531–536, 1986.
21. Meffert RM: The soft tissue interface in dental implantology. J Dent Ed 52:810–811, 1988.
22. Misch CE: Density of bone effect on treatment plans, surgical approach, healing and progressive bone loading. Int J Oral Implant 6:23–31, 1990.
23. Orton GS, Steele DL, Wolinsky LE: The dental professional's role in monitoring and maintenance of tissue-integrated prostheses. Int J Oral Maxillofac Impl 4:303–310, 1989.
24. Palmisano D, Mayo J, Block M, Lancaster D: Subgingival bacteria associated with hydroxylapatite-coated dental implants: Morphotypes and trypsin-like enzyme activity. Int J Oral Maxillofac Impl 6:313–317, 1991.
25. Quirynen M, Listgarten MA: The distribution of bacterial morphotypes around natural teeth and titanium implant ad modum Brånemark. Clin Impl Res 1:8–12, 1990.

26. Quirynen M, Naert I, van Steenberghe D: Fixture design and overload influence marginal bone loss and fixture success in the Brånemark system. Clin Oral Impl Res 3:104–111, 1992.

27. Schou S, Holmstrup P, Hjøøting-Hansen E, Lang NP: Plaque-induced marginal tissue reactions of osseointe-grated oral implants: A review of the literature. Clin Oral Impl Res 3:149–161, 1992.

28. Thompson-Neal D, Evans GH, Meffert RM: Effects of various prophylactic treatments on titanium, sapphire, and hydroxylapatite-coated implants: A SEM study. Int J Periodont Restor Dent 9:301–311, 1989.

Study Questions

1. What soft tissue indices are useful in following implant patients?

2. How would you "maintain" the dental implant patient?

3. What clinical findings are indicative of problems with the soft tissue around a dental implant?

4. Is the dental implant different than teeth, in regard to soft and hard tissue reactions? Why?

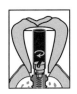

CHAPTER 24

Oral Bacteria and Dental Implants in Health and Disease

John A. Mayo
Revised by Michael S. Block

Microbiology amd Surgical Placement of
   Dental Implants
Bacterial Colonization of Intraoral Hard
   Surfaces, Including Implants
Adhesion of Bacteria to Oral Hard Surfaces:
   Teeth and Implants
Plaque Accumulation on Implant Abutment
   Cylinders

Subgingival Microbiology and Dental
   Implants
   Good Oral Health
   Edentulous versus Partially Edentulous
    Patients
   Peri-implantitis and Implant Failure
Possible Pathogenic Mechanisms in Implant
Failure
References

Even though the failure rate is low, dental clinicians and researchers are motivated to understand implant failure to improve the success rate and to reduce pain and suffering and improve quality of life for patients. The aim of this chapter is to understand the role of microorganisms in peri-implant disease and implant failure.

Implantable devices have become important in medicine as well as dentistry and have played a central role in the restoration of function and form in previously intractable cases.[3] In normal surgical practice, these devices are sterile and are placed, using aseptic surgical techniques, in microbiologically sterile body sites. Occasionally, contaminating or hematogenously disseminated bacteria ". . . win the race for the (implant) surface" and establish a biofilm on the implant surface.[18] Such biofilms act as sources of inflammation and sites for seeding of disseminated infection, thus destroying the function of the implant and even causing systemic disease. Bacteria in biofilms are notoriously resistant to antibiotics,[11] and surgical intervention and implant removal often are necessary.[14, 15, 18]

Dental implants offer a contrasting situation. Osseointegrated dental implants ultimately project from a microbiologically sterile bed of bone through the oral mucosa into the oral cavity.[10, 30] Thus, dental implants must function while exposed to an environment with a microflora that is rich both in numbers and in variety of organisms. Furthermore, this environment may contain substantial numbers of recognized periodontopathogens. Both dental implants and teeth must have a mucosal sealing mechanism to protect the microbiologically sterile root area from these oral bacteria. Finally, if that seal is breached and periodontopathogens gain access to the root area, the resulting infections may require surgical intervention and removal of the tooth or implant.

A series of studies of oral microflora in implant patients has led to four general observations. First, the microbial flora found around healthy implants is similar to that found in sulci around healthy teeth. Second, the microbial flora found around implants that are diseased or failing owing to infection is similar to that found around periodontally diseased teeth. Third, in partially edentulous patients, implant microflora is similar to that of the remaining teeth. Fourth, in edentulous patients, the microbial flora of implants is different from the implant microflora of partially edentulous patients. These observations suggest the following questions concerning dental implants and oral microorganisms:

1. Which oral bacteria will colonize dental implants?
2. What mechanisms are involved in the interaction of oral bacteria with implant materials?
3. What is the source of these bacteria?
4. Are different implant materials and surface types colonized by different groups of oral bacteria?
5. Which oral bacteria are associated with healthy implants, and which are responsible for peri-implant disease and implant failure?
6. Are nonoral bacteria ever responsible for implant failure?
7. How do these bacteria cause loss of oral soft and hard tissue leading to implant failure?
8. How can peri-implant disease and implant failure be prevented or treated?

MICROBIOLOGY AND SURGICAL PLACEMENT OF DENTAL IMPLANTS

Endosseous root-form dental implants are sterile as provided by the manufacturers and are placed using sterile instruments and aseptic surgical techniques. If good surgical technique is practiced, loss of endosseous implants to infection during healing and osseointegration should be rare, and this seems to be the case.[4, 9, 23]

After healing and osseointegration, endosseous implants are exposed and abutments attached, which project into the oral cavity. Such sites can be colonized both with normal oral flora[44] and with "classic" implant pathogens such as *Staphylococcus aureus* and *Pseudomonas aeruginosa*.[19]

BACTERIAL COLONIZATION OF INTRAORAL HARD SURFACES, INCLUDING IMPLANTS

Osseointegrated implants and their associated abutments in the oral cavity can be regarded as analogous to natural teeth.[10, 30] Studies have indicated that teeth and implants are colonized by similar groups of oral bacteria, that the principles and mechanisms of colonization are similar, and that similar groups of periodontopathogens are involved in both periodontal diseases and *peri-implantitis*.

ADHESION OF BACTERIA TO ORAL HARD SURFACES: TEETH AND IMPLANTS

Bacterial adhesion to surfaces is driven by short-range weak bonds, primarily hydrophobic interactions.[20, 59] In the human oral cavity, bacterial adhesion is influenced by other factors as well.

All oral surfaces are bathed in saliva, and oral hard surfaces, such as teeth, implants, restorations, and prostheses, are coated by an acquired pellicle derived from saliva.[57, 60] Receptors in acquired pellicle can serve as specific binding sites for adhesins on bacterial cell surfaces; adhesins are specific adhesion-mediating bacterial proteins.[65] This type of interaction has been invoked as a mechanism to explain the specific distribution of different groups of oral bacteria on different oral tissues.[57, 60] For example, *Streptococcus sanguis* is a pioneer species in the colonization of tooth surfaces[32] and forms complexes in vitro with pellicle.[5] Colonization is mediated by an adhesin and can be blocked or inhibited by protease treatment of bacterial cell surfaces or by incubation of bacterial cells with antibody directed against the adhesin protein.[65] Acquired pellicle is a ubiquitous feature of the oral environment, and all intraoral structures, including implants, are coated with pellicle. This is consistent with the generalization that solid surface interfaces with liquids are coated with a *conditioning film* derived from the liquid phase and with which bacteria interact.[11] Nonspecific factors that influence bacterial adhesion to oral hard surfaces include hydrophobicity,[59] surface zeta potential,[46] surface roughness,[52, 53] and surface free energy.[1, 52, 53, 64]

The preferred materials for implants are titanium or hydroxylapatite (HA)-coated titanium, for reasons of biocompatibility and osseointegration.[10] These materials provide high-energy surfaces, and high-energy surfaces are regarded as important for successful osseointegration.[8] Regardless of composition of the root-form portion, the exposed part of these implants is smooth-surfaced titanium. Plaque accumulation on this high-energy surface has been reported to be less than on natural teeth,[2] and this may be due to the smoothness of the surface. It follows that implant maintenance procedures should avoid roughening, scratching, or marring the exposed portion of the implant because this may have the undesirable effect of enhancing plaque accumulation.

Despite the importance attached to understanding of interactions between oral bacteria and implant materials, few such studies are found in the literature. With the use of an in vitro adherence model, it was found that *S. sanguis* bound approximately equally to saliva-treated enamel and saliva-treated titanium, whereas *Actinomyces viscosus* bound significantly less to saliva-treated titanium than to saliva-treated enamel.[66] Furthermore, three times as many *S. sanguis* cells bound to saliva-coated titanium as did *A. viscosus* cells, despite equal binding of the two organisms to saliva-coated enamel. In an in vivo study, plaque formation was studied on discs of a variety of implant materials placed in splints, which were worn intraorally for 4 or 48 hours.[43] Materials studied included single-crystal and polycrystal alumina (PA), polycrystal zirconia, HA, and titanium. PA and HA had the greatest surface roughness, with average roughness (Ra) values approximately nine and five times greater than enamel. After 4 hours, pellicle adherence and bacterial colonization were seen on all materials, with PA and HA accumulating twice as many bacterial cells as the other materials. After 48 hours, the greatest bacterial numbers still were found on PA and HA, although the relative differences with other materials were somewhat smaller than at 4 hours. Statistical analysis was not presented, and significance of the differences with respect to material and time cannot be assessed. For all materials, *Streptococcus* species were the predominant early colonizers, and anaerobes were present in significant numbers only in the 48-hour samples.

The general picture to be drawn from all of these studies is that implant materials are coated with salivary pellicle and colonized by oral bacteria essentially as is seen with natural teeth. Surface roughness of implant material is an important variable, with increased roughness promoting bacterial accumulation. For this reason, implant maintenance procedures should avoid roughening, scratching, or marring the exposed portion of the implant.[36, 37]

PLAQUE ACCUMULATION ON IMPLANT ABUTMENT CYLINDERS

Plaque accumulation is regarded as a risk factor for implant loss.[38] In an animal study, poor oral hygiene after implant placement appeared to lead to looser junctional epithelium with fewer hemidesmosomes and intercellular desmosomes.[25, 29] A study of edentulous patients with mandibular implants found that lack of oral hygiene was the most significant factor associated with bone loss around the margins of the implants. It is accepted that disruption of the mucosal seal around implants and loss of supporting bone are effects produced by oral bacteria, but definitive studies relating this pathogenesis to accumulation of plaque on exposed implant abutments have not yet been done.

Studies investigated the effect of scrupulous control of supragingival plaque on the amount and composition of subgingival bacterial accumulations in periodontal pockets.[13, 21, 35, 61] The general findings of these investigations were that scrupulous, frequent removal of supragingival plaque resulted in marked reduction of total viable counts in pockets, increase in numbers of subgingival gram-positive organisms, and decrease in numbers and proportions of presumed periodontal pathogens such as spirochetes and *Porphyromonas gingivalis*. It was concluded that saliva and supragingival plaque could serve as reservoirs for colonization of subgingival areas by periodontopathogens.

SUBGINGIVAL MICROBIOLOGY AND DENTAL IMPLANTS

A general picture has emerged that in both health and disease the subgingival microfloras of teeth and implants are essentially the same. The major observations (and references) are given in Tables 24–1 and 24–2. In addition, this topic has been discussed in several reviews.[10, 17, 24, 38, 45, 62]

Good Oral Health

It is well established[57, 60] that in good oral health, the microflora of teeth is relatively sparse, mainly gram-positive, and mainly facultative, with the genera *Streptococcus* and *Actinomyces* predominating. With established gingivitis, the plaque is more abundant and has shifted to predominantly gram-negative and anaerobic, with presence of putative periodontal pathogens such as *P. gingivalis*, *Prevotella intermedia*, and spirochetes. Colonization and plaque formation seem to follow the same pattern on implants as on teeth.

Colonization and plaque formation on implants have been investigated in humans receiving transmucosal titanium[40] or permucosal HA implants and after exposure and loading of tita-

Table 24–1. Subgingival Microbiology and Dental Implants: Major Observations

Observation	References
In good oral health, teeth and implants have similar microflora with streptococci and nonmotile rods predominating	Apse et al, 1989[6]
	Lekholm et al, 1986[26]
	Mombelli et al, 1987[41]
	Mombelli and Mericske-Stern, 1990[40]
	Newman and Flemming, 1988[45]
	Palmisano et al, 1991[48]
	Quirynen and Listgarten, 1990[51]
The same groups of recognized periodontopathogens are involved in periodontal diseases and in peri-implantitis or infectious failure of implants	Apse et al, 1989[6]
	Becker et al, 1990[7]
	Mombelli et al, 1987[41]
	Mombelli et al, 1988[39]
	Nakou et al, 1987[44]
	Newman and Flemming, 1988[45]
	Palmisano et al, 1991[48]
	Rosenberg et al, 1991[58]
In partially edentulous patients, crevices around teeth may serve as sources of bacteria, which can colonize crevices around implants	Apse et al, 1989[6]
	Quirynen and Listgarten, 1990[51]
In addition to the recognized periodontopathogens, *Staphylococcus* spp. may be important in infectious failure of dental implants	Rams et al, 1990[54]
	Rams et al, 1991[56]
	Rosenberg et al, 1991[58]

nium or HA endosseous implants[54] and in beagle dogs with exposed endosseous titanium implants.[28] The general approach in these studies was for several weeks or months to obtain samples of subgingival microflora for culturing and for microscopic assay and at the same time to take clinical measurements at the sampled sites, including gingival and plaque indices, probing depth, and bleeding on probing, and in some instances radiographs. The predominant subgingival morphotypes in healthy sites were cocci and nonmotile rods. The predominant cultivable subgingival bacteria were streptococci and actinomycetes, in terms of both percent of cultivable microflora and frequency of isolation. Putative periodontopathogens such as *Porphyromonas gingivalis*, *Prevotella intermedia*, and spirochetes were minor components of the microflora in healthy sites or were not found at all.

Edentulous versus Partially Edentulous Patients

Investigations summarized previously indicated that supragingival plaque on teeth could serve as a reservoir for periodontopathogens and other organisms that colonize subgingival habitats.[13, 21, 35, 61] These results suggest the possibility

Table 24–2. Predominant Subgingival Microflora of Healthy and Failing Dental Implants

Assay System	Healthy	Failing Noninfectious	Failing Infectious
Microscopic examination	Cocci	Cocci	Cocci
	Nonmotile rods	Nonmotile rods	Nonmotile rods
	Spirochetes		Motile rods
			Spirochetes
Culture	*Streptococcus* spp.	*Streptococcus* spp.	Gram-negative and gram-positive periodontopathogens
	Actinomyces spp.		*Staphylococcus* sp. Gram-negative enteric and facultative rods
			Yeasts

Adapted from Rosenberg ES, Torosian JP, Slots J: Microbial differences in 2 clinically distinct types of failures of osseointegrated implants. Clin Oral Impl Res 2:135–144, 1991.

that microflora of remaining teeth could serve as the source of inoculum for colonization of implants in partially edentulous patients. Comparison of implant sites in edentulous and partially edentulous patients, however, showed significant differences. Culturing studies showed significantly higher percentages of so-called black-pigmented *Bacteroides* and *Capnocytophaga* species around implants of partially edentulous patients.[6] With microscopic analysis, Quirynen and Listgarten[51] found that implant sites in partially edentulous patients have significantly fewer cocci and significantly more motile rods and spirochetes than similar sites in edentulous patients, although Apse et al[6] found such a difference for motile rods only. Overall, these studies suggest the strong possibility that subgingival microflora of teeth can influence the subgingival microflora of implants in partially edentulous mouths. This reinforces the importance of rigorous oral hygiene programs in implant patients, especially partially edentulous patients.

Peri-implantitis and Implant Failure

Despite the high success rate of well-designed, well-executed implant programs, there still are occasional failures. Early studies concluded that implant failure after primary healing and osseointegration was due to infection or extensive and excessive occlusal stress and suggested that in failure due to infection, the microflora was similar to that which produces periodontal disease.[45]

The microbial cause of periodontal diseases has been clarified greatly over the past 15 years, and strong associations of microorganisms with various classes of periodontal disease have been developed.[62] Because of the age distribution of patients receiving implants, adult periodontitis is the most realistic model for peri-implant disease or peri-implantitis. The species associated with adult periodontitis include *Actinobacillus actinomycetemcomitans*, *Bacteroides forsythus*, *Porphyromonas gingivalis*, *Prevotella intermedia*, and *Wolinella recta*. Oral spirochetes are associated with increasing severity of periodontal disease and may constitute as much as 50% of the microscopic count in active periodontal lesions.[31] They may be involved with the progression rather than the initiation of such lesions.

All failing implants are characterized by mobility and peri-implant radiolucency.[60] Implants failing as a result of infection are additionally characterized by pain, bleeding on probing, sup-

puration, increased probing depth, high gingival and plaque indices, attachment loss, and granulomatous tissue on removal. Implants failing for traumatic reasons (surgical trauma, faulty design of prostheses, or overloading) may be painful, but otherwise lack the additional characteristics associated with infectious failure. Implants showing the signs and symptoms of infectious failure but not yet mobile may be said to be "ailing."[36, 37]

Implants suffering traumatic failure have subgingival microflora resembling that of periodontal health, with cocci and nonmotile rods as the predominant morphotypes and *Streptococcus* and *Actinomyces* species as the predominant cultivable microflora (see Table 24–2). In contrast, with infectious failure, spirochetes, motile rods, nonmotile rods, and cocci were seen in approximately equal numbers by microscopic analysis. Predominant cultivable subgingival flora in infectious failure included *Porphyromonas gingivalis*, *Prevotella intermedia*, *W. recta*, *Peptostreptococcus micros*, *Fusobacterium* species, *Candida* species, *Pseudomonas aeruginosa*, and enteric gram-negative rods. Also found were lesser numbers of *A. actinomycetemcomitans*, *S. aureus*, and *S. epidermidis*.[60] A second study comparing successful and failing osseointegrated titanium implants yielded similar results.[41] Successful implant sites had subgingival microflora with cocci as predominant morphotypes, few fusiforms or motile or curved rods, and no spirochetes. Failing sites were characterized microscopically by numerous spirochetes, fusiforms, motile rods, and curved rods and by a cultivable flora with a large proportion of gram-negative anaerobic rods, including *Fusobacterium* species and so-called black-pigmented *Bacteroides*. In a third study, DNA probe technology was used for detection of three putative periodontopathogens subgingivally in implants that were failing as defined by mobility and peri-implant radiolucency.[7] DNA probe analysis was done on a total of 28 sites in 13 patients, with blade, subperiosteal, and several types of osseointegrated implants. No periodontopathogens were detected in four sites, which presumably were suffering traumatic failure. In general, moderate levels of *A. actinomycetemcomitans*, *Porphyromonas gingivalis*, or *Prevotella intermedia* were detected in the remaining sites; most sites had at least two of the three organisms.

The conclusion to be drawn from these studies and the additional investigations reviewed by others[10, 17, 24, 38, 45, 62] is that the subgingival bacteria associated with infectious implant failure are the same as those associated with adult periodontitis.

Subgingival staphylococci (*S. aureus* and *S. epidermidis*) have been isolated from about 50%

of gingivitis and periodontitis patients and from 55% of a small sample of ailing or failing implants.[54] A notable finding was that staphylococci were 15% of the cultivable subgingival flora in peri-implantitis but only 1.2% in periodontitis lesions and 0.06% in gingivitis. This was a statistically significant difference, and the authors suggested that staphylococci may play a role in at least some implant failures.

Oral spirochetes have been implicated as periodontopathogens because they can be as much as 50% of the microscopic count in active lesions, because high levels of spirochetes are associated with active disease, and because in some patients treatment with metronidazole to eliminate spirochetes also eliminates disease activity (Fig. 24–1).[31, 32] Subgingival spirochete levels in healthy implants have been reported to be low or even zero[6, 27, 40, 41, 44, 48, 51, 56] and to be elevated in ailing or failing implants.[41, 58]

POSSIBLE PATHOGENIC MECHANISMS IN IMPLANT FAILURE

The hallmarks of implant failure are disruption of the perimucosal seal and loss of peri-implant bone, analogous to the destruction of soft and hard tissue seen in periodontitis. The mechanisms leading to implant failure have not yet been defined. The subgingival microfloras associ-

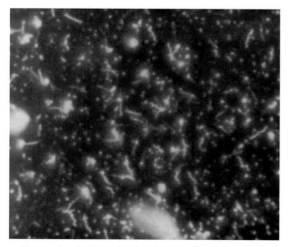

Figure 24–1. Spirochetal infection of a failing implant. Before retrieval, supragingival plaque was removed from a failing HA-coated titanium implant. Subgingival plaque then was removed and examined by darkfield microscopy, original magnification 640 ×. Numerous spirochetes are present, suggesting a massive spirochetal infection. (Clinical material courtesy of Dr. J. Kwan.)

ated with implant failure and periodontitis are similar, however, and it is reasonable to expect that the pathogenic mechanisms also would be similar. Current thinking is that destruction of periodontal tissue is a consequence of interactions involving endotoxin, cytokines, and cells of the periodontal region.[12, 22, 42, 47]

The key bacterial virulence factor for destruction of periodontal tissue is endotoxin, a ubiquitous component of the cell walls of all gram-negative bacteria. Gram-negative bacteria associated with periodontitis include A. actinomycetemcomitans, B. forsythus, Porphyromonas gingivalis, Prevotella intermedia, and W. recta. Oral spirochetes also are gram-negative. In periodontal tissue, the primary target of endotoxin is the macrophage. Endotoxin-activated macrophages produce proteases that can degrade collagen and proteoglycans, ultimately producing degradation of extracellular matrix. Furthermore, activated macrophages produce the cytokines interleukin-1 (IL-1) and prostaglandin E_2 (PGE_2).

IL-1 has two targets: macrophages and fibroblasts. In an autocatalytic feedback loop, IL-1 stimulates macrophages to produce more IL-1. Fibroblasts are activated in two ways by IL-1. First, they are activated to produce additional proteases, which can degrade collagen and proteoglycans. Second, they are activated to produce PGE_2.

The PGE_2 produced by endotoxin-activated macrophages and IL-1–activated fibroblasts has as its target the osteoclast. PGE_2 activates osteoclasts, leading to resorption of alveolar bone and loss of support. This completes the circuits leading to destruction of soft and hard periodontal tissue. The likelihood is that these mechanisms are active in implant failure. If ailing implants are to be treated analogously to the way in which periodontally involved teeth are managed, it is important to detoxify the surface of the ailing implant to remove all traces of endotoxin.[67]

This picture is complicated by the finding that in in vitro systems implant materials are not physiologically inert and can activate pathways that possibly could lead to loss of alveolar bone. Activation of complement was studied after exposure of human serum to samples of 10 different implant systems, including titanium, plasma-sprayed titanium, and HA-coated titanium implants.[49] Exposure of serum to implants generated a sixfold increase in level of C3a and a twofold increase in C5a. Both are inflammatory peptides, and C5a stimulation of macrophages causes release of IL-1. In a second study,[50] human peripheral blood monocytes were collected from donors with good medical and periodontal health. These cells were suspended in culture medium and incubated with samples of five different types of titanium and HA-coated implants. Implants were used as received after sterilization by the manufacturers. Levels of IL-1 and tumor necrosis factor (another cytokine) were measured in the culture fluid, and four of five implant types produced significant increases in levels of both cytokines. The authors of these two studies suggested that under some circumstances implants themselves could elicit cytokine responses, leading to bone loss and implant failure. They also pointed out that endotoxin is a potent activator of complement and of IL-1 production and that the implants used in these experiments may have received endotoxin contamination during manufacture and sterilization. The relevance of these in vitro studies to peri-implantitis and implant failure in vivo is not clear. It is obvious, however, that further studies are required to determine whether implants are contaminated with endotoxin during the manufacturing/sterilizing process and to determine the exact mechanisms causing loss of soft and hard tissue supporting implants.

References

1. Absolom DR, Lamberti FV, Polocova Z, Zingg W, van Oss CJ, Neumann AW: Surface thermodynamics of bacterial adhesion. Appl Environ Microbiol 46:90–97, 1983.
2. Adell R, Lekholm U, Rockler B, Brånemark P-I: A 15-year study of osseointegrated implants in the treatment of the edentulous jaw. Int J Oral Surg 10:387–416, 1981.
3. Albrektsson T, Zarb GA (eds): The Brånemark Osseointegrated Implant. Chicago, Quintessence, 1989.
4. Albrektsson T, Zarb G, Worthington P, Eriksson AR: The long-term efficacy of currently used dental implants: A review and proposed criteria of success. Int J Oral Maxillofac Impl 1:11–25, 1986.
5. Appelbaum B, Golub E, Holt SC, Rosan B: In vitro studies of dental plaque formation: Adsorption of oral streptococci to hydroxyapatite. Infect Immunol 25:717–728, 1979.
6. Apse P, Ellen RP, Overall CM, Zarb GA: Microbiota and crevicular fluid collagenase in the osseointegrated dental implant sulcus: A comparison of sites in edentulous and partially edentulous patients. J Periodont Res 24:96–105, 1989.
7. Becker W, Becker BE, Newman MG, Nyman S: Clinical and microbiologic findings that may contribute to dental implant failure. Int J Oral Maxillofac Impl 5:31–38, 1990.
8. Block CM, Mayo JA, Evans GH: Effects of the Nd:YAG dental laser on plasma-sprayed and hydroxyapatite-coated titanium dental implants: Surface alteration and attempted sterilization. Int J Oral Maxillofac Impl 7:441–449, 1992.
9. Bosker H, Jordan RD, Sindet-Pedersen S, Koole R: The transmandibular implant: A 13-year survey of its use. J Oral Maxillofac Surg 49:482–492, 1991.
10. Carmichael RP, Aspe P, Zarb GA, McCulloch CAG: Biological, microbiological, and clinical aspects of the peri-

11. Costerton JW, Cheng K-J, Geesey GG, Ladd TI, Nickel JC, Dasgupta M, Marrie TJ: Bacterial biofilms in nature and disease. Annu Rev Microbiol 41:435–464, 1987.
12. Creamer HR: A novel hypothesis concerning the mechanisms of activation, and of control, of periodontal bone loss. Med Hypoth 35:115–121, 1991.
13. Dahlen G, Linde J, Sato K, Hanamura H, Okamoto H: The effect of supragingival plaque control on the subgingival microbiota in subjects with periodontal disease. J Clin Periodontol 19:802–809, 1992.
14. Dougherty SH: Pathobiology of infection in prosthetic devices. Rev Infect Dis 10:1102–1117, 1988.
15. Dougherty SH, Simmons RL: Endogenous factors contributing to prosthetic device infections. Infect Dis Clin North Am 3:199–209, 1989.
16. Doyle RJ, Nesbett WE, Taylor KG: On the mechanism of adherence of Streptococcus sanguis to hydroxyapatite. FEBS Microbiol Lett 15:1–5, 1982.
17. Ellen RP, Apse P: Periimplant infections of the oral cavity. In Wadstrom T, Eliasson I, Holder I, Ljundh A (eds): Pathogenesis of Wound and Biomaterial-Associated Infections. New York, Springer-Verlag, 1990, pp 245–253.
18. Gristina AG: Biomaterial-centered infection: Microbial adhesion versus tissue integration. Science 237:1588–1595, 1987.
19. Heimdahl A, Kondell PA, Nord CE, Nordenram A: Effect of insertion of osseointegrated prosthesis on the oral microflora. Swed Dent J 7:199–204, 1983.
20. Hjerten R, Wadstrom W: What types of bonds are responsible for the adhesion of bacteria and viruses to native and artificial surfaces? In Wadstrom T, Eliasson I, Holder I, Ljundh A (eds): Pathogenesis of Wound and Biomaterial-Associated Infections. New York, Springer-Verlag, 1990, pp 245–253.
21. Katsanoulas T, Renee I, Attstrom R: The effect of supragingival plaque control on the composition of the subgingival flora in periodontal pockets. J Clin Periodontol 19:760–765, 1992.
22. Katz J, Goultschin J, Benoliel R, Ben-Sasson Z: The interleukin concept and the periodontal diseases. Med Hypoth 29:251–254, 1989.
23. Kent JN, Block MS, Finger IM, Guerra L, Larsen H, Misiek DJ: Biointegrated hydroxylapatite coated implants: Five year clinical observations. J Am Dent Assoc 121:138–144, 1990.
24. Klinge B: Implants in relation to natural teeth. J Clin Periodontol 18:482–487, 1991.
25. Koth DL, Lemons JE, Braswell LD, Fritz ME: Root and plate form tissue interfaces from dogs and primates (abstract). J Dent Res 71(spec iss):637, 1992.
26. Lekholm U, Adell R, Lindhe J, Brånemark P-I, Eriksson B, Rockler B, Lindvall A-M, Yoneyama T: Marginal tissue reactions at osseointegrated titanium fixtures (II). A cross-sectional retrospective study. Int J Oral Maxillofac Surg 15:53–61, 1986.
27. Lekholm U, Ericsson I, Adell R, Slots J: The condition of the soft tissues at tooth and fixture abutments supporting fixed bridges. A microbiological and histological study. J Clin Periodontol 13:558–562, 1986.
28. Leonhardt A, Berglundh T, Ericsson I, Dahlen G: Putative periodontal pathogens on titanium implants and teeth in experimental gingivitis and periodontitis in beagle dogs. Clin Oral Impl Res 3:112–119, 1992.
29. Lindquist LW, Rockler B, Carlsson GE: Bone resorption around fixtures in edentulous patients treated with man-

dibular fixed tissue-integrated prostheses. J Prosthet Dent 59:59–63, 1988.

30. Listgarten MA, Lang NP, Schroeder HE, Schroeder A: Periodontal tissues and their counterparts around endosseous implants. Clin Oral Impl Res 2:1–19, 1991.

31. Loesche WJ, Laughon B: Role of spirochetes in periodontal disease. *In* Genco RJ, Mergenhagen SE (eds): Host-Parasite Interactions in Periodontal Disease. Washington, DC, American Society for Microbiology, 1982, pp 62–75.

32. Loesche WJ, Syed SA, Schmidt E, Morison EC: Bacterial profiles of subgingival plaques in periodontitis. J Periodontol 56:447–456, 1985.

33. Marsh PD, Martin M: Oral Microbiology, ed 2. Wokingham, UK, Van Nostrand Rheinhold, 1984.

34. Mayo JA, Oertling K, Andrieu SC: Bacterial biofilm: A source of contamination in dental air-water syringes. Clin Prev Dent 12:13–20, 1990.

35. McNabb H, Mombelli A, Lang NP: Supragingival cleaning 3 times a week. The microbiological effects in moderately deep pockets. J Clin Periodontol 19:348–356, 1992.

36. Meffert RM: Periodontal considerations in endosseous implantology. *In* Caswell CW, Clark AE Jr (eds): Dental Implant Prosthodontics. Philadelphia, JB Lippincott, 1991, pp 287–304.

37. Meffert RM: Treatment of failing dental implants. Curr Opin Dent (Periodont Restor Dent) 2:109–114, 1992.

38. Meffert RM, Langer B, Fritz ME: Dental implants: A review. J Periodontol 63:859–870, 1992.

39. Mombelli A, Buser D, Lang NP: Colonization of osseointegrated titanium implants in edentulous patients. Early results. Oral Microbiol Immunol 3:113–120, 1988.

40. Mombelli A, Mericske-Stern R: Microbiological features of stable osseointegrated implants used as abutments for overdentures. Clin Oral Impl Res 1:1–7, 1990.

41. Mombelli A, van Oosten MAC, Schurch E, Lang NP: The microbiota associated with successful or failing osseointegrated titanium implants. Oral Microbiol Immunol 2:145–151, 1987.

42. Mundy GR: Inflammatory mediators and the destruction of bone. J Periodont Res 26:213–217, 1991.

43. Nakazato G, Tsuchiya H, Sato M, Yamauchi M: In vivo plaque formation on implant materials. Int J Oral Maxillofac Impl 4:321–326, 1989.

44. Nakou M, Mikx FHM, Oosterwall PJM, Kruijsen JCWM: Early microbial colonization of permucosal implants in edentulous patients. J Dent 66:1654–1657, 1987.

45. Newman MG, Flemming TF: Periodontal considerations of implants and implant associated microbiota. J Dent Educ 52:737–744, 1988.

45a. Nilius AM, Spencer SC, Simonson LG: Stimulation of *in vitro* growth of *Treponema denticola* by extracellular growth factors produced by *Porphyromonas gingivalis*. J Dent Res 72:1027–1031, 1993.

46. Olsson J, Glantz P-O, Krasse B: Surface potential and adherence of oral streptococci to oral surfaces. Scand J Dent Res 84:240–242, 1976.

47. Page R: The role of inflammatory mediators in the pathogenesis of periodontal disease. J Periodont Res 26:230–242, 1991.

48. Palmisano DA, Mayo JA, Block MS, Lancaster DM: Subgingival bacteria associated with hydroxylapatite-coated dental implants: Morphotypes and trypsin-like enzyme activity. Int J Oral Maxillofac Impl 6:313–318, 1991.

48a. Passariello C, Berlutti F, Selan L, Amadeo C, Comodi-Ballanti MR, Serafino L, Thaller MC: Microbiological and morphological analysis of dental implants removed for incomplete osseointegration. Microbial Ecol Health Dis 6:203–207, 1993.

49. Perala D, Chapman R, Gelfand J: Complement activation by dental implants. Int J Oral Maxillofac Impl 6:136–141, 1991.

50. Perala DG, Chapman RJ, Gelgand JA, Callahan MV, Adams DF, Lie T: Relative production of IL-1β and TNFα by mononuclear cells after exposure to dental implants. J Periodontol 63:426–430, 1992.

51. Quirynen M, Listgarten MA: The distribution of bacterial morphotypes around natural teeth and titanium implants ad modem Brånemark. Clin Oral Impl Res 1:8–12, 1990.

52. Quirynen M, Marechal M, Busscher HJ, Weerkamp AH, Darius PL, van Steenberghe D: The influence of surface free energy and surface roughness on early plaque formation. An in vivo study in man. J Clin Periodontol 17:138–144, 1990.

53. Quirynen M, Marechal M, van Steenberghe D, Busscher HJ, van der Mei HC: The bacterial colonization of intraoral hard surfaces in vivo: Influences of surface free energy and surface roughness. Biofouling 4:187–198, 1991.

54. Rams TE, Feik D, Slots J: Staphylococci in human periodontal diseases. Oral Microbiol Immunol 5:29–32, 1990.

55. Rams TE, Link CC Jr: Microbiology of failing dental implants in humans: Electron microscopic observations. J Oral Implantol 11:93–100, 1983.

56. Rams TE, Roberts TW, Feik D, Molzan AK, Slots J: Clinical and microbiological findings on newly inserted hydroxylapatite-coated and pure titanium human dental implants. Clin Oral Impl Res 2:212–217, 1991.

57. Rosan B: Mechanisms of oral colonization. *In* Slots J, Taubman MA (eds): Contemporary Oral Microbiology and Immunology. St. Louis, Mosby-Year Book, 1992, pp 283–298.

58. Rosenberg ES, Torosian JP, Slots J: Microbial differences in 2 clinically distinct types of failures of osseointegrated implants. Clin Oral Impl Res 2:135–144, 1991.

59. Rosenberg M, Kjelleberg S: Hydrophobic interactions: Role in bacterial adhesions. Microb Ecol 9:353–393, 1986.

60. Schonfeld SE: Oral microbial ecology. *In* Slots J, Taubman MA (eds): Contemporary Oral Microbiology and Immunology. St. Louis, Mosby-Year Book, 1992, pp 267–274.

60a. Simonson LG, McMahon KT, Childers DW, Morton HE: Bacterial synergy of *Treponema denticola* and *Porphyromonas gingivalis* in a multinational population. Oral Microbiol Immunol 7:111–112, 1992.

61. Smulow JB, Turesky SS, Hill RG: The effect of supragingival plaque removal on anaerobic bacteria in deep periodontal pockets. J Am Dent Assoc 107:737–742, 1983.

62. Tanner A: Microbial etiology of periodontal diseases: Where are we? Where are we going? Curr Opin Dent (Periodont Restor Dent) 2:12–24, 1992.

63. Weerkamp AH, Quirynen M, Marechal M, van der Mei HC, van Steenberghe D, Busscher HJ: The role of surface free energy in the early in vivo formation of dental plaque on human enamel and polymeric substrata. Microbial Ecol Health Dis 2:11–18, 1989.

64. Weerkamp AH, van der Mei HC, Busscher HJ: The surface free energy of oral streptococci after being coated with saliva and its relation to adhesion in the mouth. J Dent Res 64:1204–1210, 1985.

65. Weerkamp AH, van der Mei HC, Engelen DPE, de Windt CEA: Adhesion receptors (adhesins) on oral streptococci. *In* ten Cate JM, Leach SA, Arends J (eds): Proceedings Bacterial Adhesion and Preventive Dentistry. Oxford, IRL Press Ltd, 1984, pp 85–97.

66. Wolinsky LE, de Carmago PM, Erard JC, Newman MG: A study of in vitro attachment of *Streptococcus sanguis*

and *Actinomyces viscosus* to saliva-treated titanium. Int J Oral Maxillofac Impl 4:27–31, 1989.

67. Zablotsky M, Diedrich D, Meffert R, Wittrig E: The ability of various chemotherapeutic agents to detoxify the endotoxin infected HA-coated implant surface. Int J Oral Impl 8:45–49, 1991.

Study Questions

1. What are the normal bacteria found on healthy dental implants?

2. What are the bacteria found on dental implants that have gingival hyperplasia and bone loss?

3. Describe the treatment of an unhealthy dental implant in regard to most likely bacteria involved with the surface, from a microbiological point of view.

4. What is the mechanism for bacterial attachment to dental implant surfaces?

5. Describe the differences in bacterial accumulation with rough and smooth surfaces.

CHAPTER 25

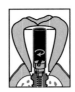

Diagnosis and Treatment of the Ailing/Failing Dental Implant

Raymond A. Yukna

Treatment of Failing Implants
References

Although osseointegrated dental implants have been shown to be successful, they are not perfect therapy. Because some dental implants encounter problems of increasing pocket depth and advancing bone loss, protocols must be established to manage these problems.

First, the cause of the adverse clinical changes should be determined, if possible. Among the reasons for dental implant failure are:

> 1. Hard tissue problems.
> 2. Soft tissue problems.
> 3. Bacterial accumulations (hygiene).
> 4. Prosthetic problems.
> 5. Occlusal excessive forces.
> 6. Host factors.
> 7. Combinations of the above reasons.

Hard tissue problems are most often initiated at the dental implant placement surgery. Overheating of the bone, improper fit of the dental implants, and lack of stability of the dental implants at placement all have the potential to create a fibrous tissue interface rather than osseointegration.[5] This histologic situation may not become clinically manifest until uncovering and loading of the dental implants.

Soft tissue problems can include tissue hyperplasia or recession. Both of these are often related to the presence of alveolar mucosa rather than keratinized gingiva adjacent to the implants and their abutment heads. Lack of firm adherent tissue adjacent to dental implants can foster food and bacterial accumulations with subsequent inflammation and patient discomfort.[14]

Bacterial accumulations are probably the most significant etiologic factor in dental implant failure (Figs. 25–1 and 25–2). Although it may take longer for oral bacteria to colonize titanium surfaces, once colonized, the sequence of bacterial succession proceeds as on natural teeth.[1–3, 7, 9, 11, 12, 15, 16, 18]

Prosthetic problems mainly involve improper contours that compromise the patient's ability to perform effective oral hygiene. Because of the slim cylindrical shape of the dental implant and abutment head, the restoration shape, especially in fixed prosthetics, often creates ridge lap areas, closed embrasures, or other plaque and food retentive areas (Fig. 25–3). All implant-borne restorations must allow for and, in fact, facilitate

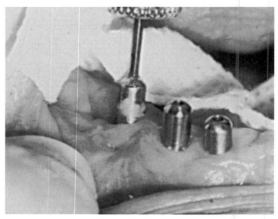

Figure 25–1. Subgingival plaque and food accumulation on transgingival healing cuff. Despite the apparent surface cleanliness, this finding suggests infrequent or incomplete regular home care procedures.

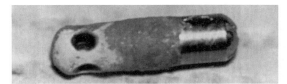

Figure 25–2. Retrieved failed implant showing dense bacterial accumulations on the surface. Patient confessed to a total lack of home care as well as ignoring restrictions on wearing the temporary denture.

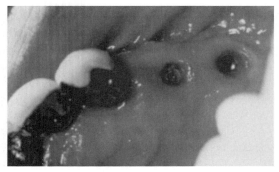

Figure 25–4. Clinical mirror image photograph showing broken abutment head screw in maxillary implant. The remaining screw part was removed with the hex driver, and a new abutment head was placed, preserving the superstructure.

effective oral hygiene. Although such proper shape may compromise the aesthetic goals of the patient, long-term peri-implant health and, therefore, long-term retention of dental implants and their restorations must be the overriding consideration.[4, 10] A great advantage of retrievability of dental implant prostheses is that they can be readily removed, inspected, and modified to facilitate oral hygiene and tissue health.

Prosthesis fabrication and fit are another potential source of implant failure. Superstructures on dental implants require a greater level of exactness and a better passive fit on the abutment heads than restorations on natural teeth because there is no periodontal ligament cushion to give or accommodate an inexact fit.[20] If the superstructure framework does not fit exactly and passively at try-in, its use is detrimental to the dental implants because of the torquing stresses it will deliver.

Occlusal forces are also influenced by prosthetic design. Oversized occlusal tables and cuspal designs that create excessive lateral forces may transmit forces to the bone-implant interface that may cause *disintegration* (Fig. 25–4). In addition, other mechanical parts of the implant system[6, 17] may be overstressed by improper and heavy forces leading to bending or fracture of the parts, such as abutment head posts or retaining screws[8, 19] (Fig. 25–5).

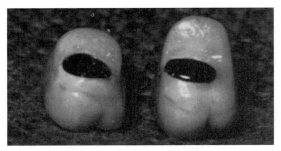

Figure 25–3. Example of modification of crown superstructure owing to retrievability of prosthesis. Premodification status is at right, showing extensive ridge lap that precludes patient access for oral hygiene. Postmodification status on left allows better access.

Parafunctional habits have great potential for producing occlusal force overload for dental implants. Because most patients exhibit signs of parafunction even in the absence of knowledge or outright denial of same, it must be taken into consideration in prosthesis design and treatment planning.[17] At least some sort of protection for the prosthesis, implant parts, and bone must be provided. This may take the form of selection of certain types of "softer" restorative materials, use of removable appliances with some cushioning effect, or fabrication of a soft biteguard for fixed restorative and "mixed dentition" (implant plus natural teeth) cases.

Host factors are a great unknown in dental implant failure. All patients have a multitude of systemic and social factors that may play a role in implant success. Medical conditions, such as osteoporosis, diabetes, and others, may affect bone repair and the solidity of the integration. Such medical conditions may also affect the sensitivity of the bone-implant interface to adverse postrestorative influences. Medications, such as oral contraceptives, corticosteroids, or antineoplastic drugs, can also alter tissue metabolism, the repair response, and the resistance to irritants.

Patients' social habits may play a role as well. There is abundant evidence from the orthopedic, oral surgery, and periodontal literature that smoking, stress, and alcohol intake have an adverse effect on wound healing and tissue integrity. The presence of one or more of these factors in a patient's background should give the clinician pause and lead to a lower prognosis for long-term success unless those factors can be discontinued.

Perhaps more than with other forms of dental treatment, a thorough, accurate medical and

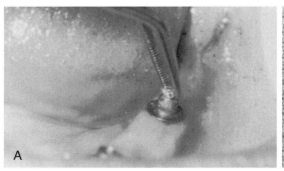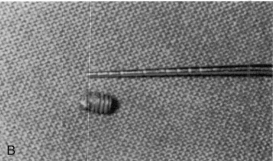

Figure 25–5. *A,* Broken solid coping retaining-screw being grasped with cotton pliers. *B,* Retrieved screw portion, allowing replacement with new retaining-screw.

dental history may indicate that other types of dental treatment may be preferable to the use of dental implants for a particular patient.

Pinpointing a single cause of dental implant failure is difficult. Most often, combinations of these various factors come into play. A marginal medical history, improper surgical technique, inadequate zone of keratinized gingiva, poor prosthesis design, inadequate oral hygiene, heavy occlusal forces, and lack of follow-up care by the patient create a negative environment and compromise the short-term and long-term prognosis for dental implants.

TREATMENT OF FAILING IMPLANTS

Clinical and radiographic evidence that peri-implant conditions are not stable and that continuing advancing bone loss is occurring indicates the need for intervention. Clinical testing of the individual implants must show immobility of the implant despite the clinical bone loss. Mobility is tested manually as is done for natural teeth or with an instrument such as the PerioTest mobility device. Before any corrective treatment, the cause(s) should be identified and reduced or eliminated.

If the problems are mainly of the suprabony type (horizontal regular bone loss without vertical defects), management can focus on correction of the soft tissue portion of the peri-implant "pocket." Standard techniques, such as gingivectomy or apically positioned flaps, are used in these situations to reduce the pocket and improve access for oral hygiene. Regeneration of bone is not a goal of corrective treatment in these situations, and care must be taken not to reduce or eliminate surgically the zone of keratinized gingiva (Fig. 25–6).

When the bone loss around the dental implants is irregular with localized dehiscences and vertical defects, regenerative therapy may be indicated. Protocols for these types of "rescue" treatments are still under development,[13] but one that has been effective for me, at least in the short-term, is described as follows.

Patients with failing dental implants should be placed on a regimen of systemic antibiotics. Antibiotics of choice include doxycycline, 100 mg twice a day; clindamycin, 150 mg three times a day; or amoxicillin/augmentin, 500 mg four times a day—all started 2 days before surgical treatment and continued for 10 days afterward.

Whenever possible, the superstructures should be removed and a healing cover screw/cap placed on the head of the implants. Access to the problem area is achieved by means of a full-thickness flap to expose the dental implant and the adjacent bone. Flap reflection must be extensive enough to gain clear appraisal of the exposed pathologically involved implant surface. As part of flap development, the granulomatous tissue next to the implant and in the adjacent bone defects must be removed with hand curets, files, or hoes. Neither ultrasonic instruments nor lasers should be used during these procedures.

Once the dental implant has been uncovered, the clinically exposed surfaces must be cleansed and decontaminated. The Cavi-jet/Prophy-jet provides mechanical cleansing of the implant surface by means of a baking soda "sandblasting" effect. Care should be used not to damage, ditch, or remove too much of the implant surface but rather simply to clean the surface mechanically. If the implant has a hydroxylapatite (HA) coating, the sodium bicarbonate sandblasting action removes some or all of the HA coating in areas where excess time of application and high pressure from the air/powder spray are directed onto a small area of the implant.

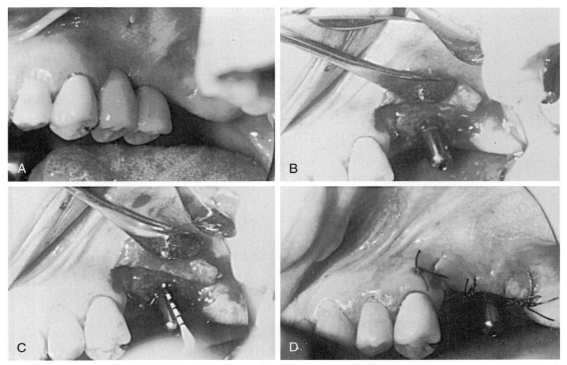

Figure 25–6. *A,* Failing dental implant on patient's upper left. Clinical probing depth increased on two successive recalls, suggesting the need for intervention. *B,* Clinical photograph at surgical entry demonstrating slight horizontal bone loss around the implant. *C,* Plastic periodontal probe verifies slight horizontal nature of bone loss. Healing post has replaced abutment head. *D,* Treatment consisted of decontamination of the exposed implant surface and apical positioning of flap. Healing was uneventful, and the original superstructure was replaced after 1 month of healing.

Chemical detoxification is then carried out by applying hydrogen peroxide intermittently with sequential soaked pellets for 5 minutes. This is followed by a similar application of tetracycline paste (250 mg capsule of tetracycline dissolved in 5 ml of sterile water or sterile saline) for 5 minutes with similar sequential 1-minute applications. The use of tetracycline in this manner is particularly effective when an HA coating is present because tetracycline binds and is slowly released in active form from HA, thereby providing a reservoir of antibacterial activity. Citric acid, pH 1, may also be used in this capacity.

If a dehiscence on only one surface or a true infrabony defect is present, placement of a grafting material seems to be beneficial. Bioactive material such as demineralized freeze-dried bone allograft particles or filler materials such as HA, HTR polymer, or BIOCORAL particles can be used.

Research has shown the advantage in certain applications of using guided tissue regeneration barrier materials to "seal" the surgical site. Use of substances such as GoreTex Augmentation Material, allogeneic freeze-dried dura mater, col-

lagen barriers, Vicryl and other polymer-based materials, and others can handicap the race between bone formation and gingival tissue closure of the defect in favor of selecting for bone regeneration (Fig. 25–7). Nonresorbable guided tissue regeneration barriers must be removed, generally at 4 to 6 weeks after placement. Rarely they remain comfortably and asymptomatically in place until uncovering of the "rescued" dental implant. Resorbable barriers, of course, can remain in place until dissolved or incorporated as part of wound repair.

If at all possible, the flaps should be coronally positioned or laterally positioned to cover the dental implant and the repair area. This often requires submucosal releasing dissections to gain enough release of the tissues for primary coverage of the surgical area. Such total coverage is also possible only if the prosthesis and abutment heads are retrievable, so a healing screw can be placed as at the time of original dental implant placement. Because of the tension present in the flaps, the shallowing of the vestibule, and the need for long-term closure, atraumatic, nonirritating, nonresorbable sutures should be used.

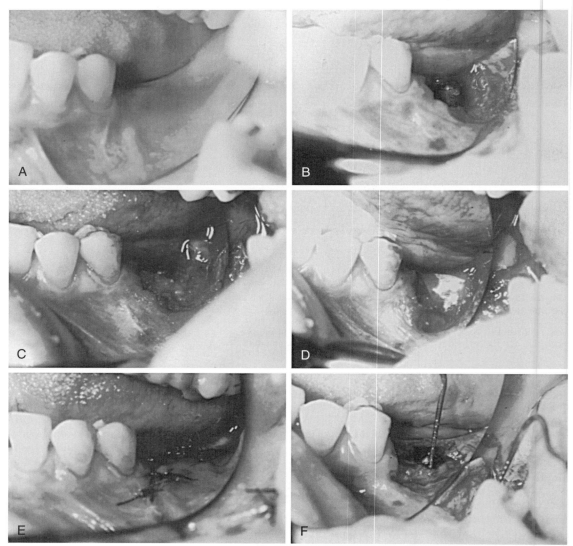

Figure 25–7. *A,* Dental implant site on lower left that had experienced problems, including multiple infections during the early postsurgical period. Soft tissue healing at the 6-month phase II uncovering surgery appears within normal limits. *B,* Clinical appearance of implant site at uncovering. Extensive horizontal and vertical bone loss was present, and most of the HA coating had dissolved from the exposed portion owing to the acidic pH associated with the infection. Root decontamination with air/powder abrasive, tetracycline paste, and hydrogen peroxide was performed. *C,* Defect around and adjacent to the implant grafted with demineralized freeze-dried bone allograft. *D,* Resorbable guided tissue barrier (lyophilized allogeneic dura mater) placed over treatment site. *E,* Surgical area closed to rebury the implant. This required decreasing the vestibular depth temporarily until the later uncovering surgery would be performed. *F,* Six months later, uncovering of the implant demonstrated substantial repair of the area with inability to probe around the implant. (*Note:* Metal probe was used in this instance because the implant surface had already been altered.)

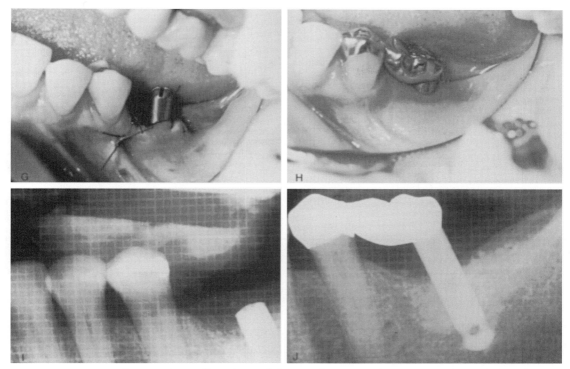

Figure 25–7 *Continued. G,* Healing cuff in place and flap apically positioned to recapture the vestibule and create a satisfactory zone of keratinized gingiva. *H,* Restoration placed after 6 weeks of healing. Crown on the implant is connected with a stress breaker to the crown on the natural tooth. Note access for hygiene around the implant abutment head. *I,* Radiograph taken at time of original uncovering illustrating bone loss that was seen clinically in part *B. J,* Twelve-month post-treatment radiograph illustrating stability of bone fill area around implant.

Follow-up care, including nonloaded healing, proceeds as with the initial implant placement. Repair and reintegration are allowed to proceed for 4 to 6 months, at which time re-uncovering and reattachment of the prosthesis can occur. The uncovering is usually performed with a flap approach to reclaim the vestibular depth and secure a good zone of keratinized gingiva. Before prosthesis replacement, however, any etiologic factors contributing to the treated problems around the implants must be corrected.

The combination of recognition of problems as they arise, appropriate intervention, correction of etiologic factors, and good follow-up care can "rescue" ailing/failing dental implants and preserve the patient's investment in the implants themselves and the attached prosthesis.

References

1. Aspe P, Ellen RP, Overal CM, Zarb GA: Microbiota and gingival fluid collagenase activity in osseointegrated dental implant sulcus: A comparison of sites in edentulous and partially edentulous patients. J Periodont Res 24:96–105, 1989.

2. Becker W, Becker BE, Newman MG, Nyman S: Clinical and microbiologic findings that may contribute to dental implant failure. Int J Oral Maxillofac Impl 5:31–38, 1990.

3. Ericsson I, Berglundh T, Marinello C, Liljenberg B, Lindhe J: Long-standing plaque and gingivitis at implants and teeth in the dog. Clin Oral Impl Res 3:99–103, 1992.

4. Ericsson I, et al: A clinical evaluation of fixed bridge restorations supported by the combination of teeth and osseointegrated implants. J Clin Periodontol 13:307–312, 1986.

5. Eriksson RA, Albrektsson T: The effect of heat on bone regeneration. J Oral Maxillofac Surg 42:705–711, 1984.

6. French A, Bowles C, Arham P, et al: Comparison of peri-implant stresses transmitted by four commercially available osseointegrated implants. Int J Periodont Restor Dent 9:221–229, 1989.

7. Hickey JS, O'Neal RB, Scheidt MJ, Strong S, Turgeon D, Van Dyke E: Microbiologic characterization of ligature-induced peri-implantitis in the microswine model. J Periodontol 62:548–553, 1991.

8. Jemt T: Failures and complications in 391 consecutively inserted fixed prostheses supported by Brånemark implants in edentulous jaws: A study of treatment from the time of prosthesis placement to the first annual check-up. Int J Oral Maxillofac Impl 6:272–275, 1991.

9. Lang NP, Brägger U, Walther D, Beamer B, Kornman KS: Ligature-induced peri-implant infection in cynomolgus monkeys: I. Clinical and radiographic findings. Clin Oral Impl Res 4:2–11, 1993.

10. Langer B, Sullivan DY: Osseointegration: Its impact on

the interrelationship of periodontics and restorative dentistry: I. Int J Periodont Restor Dent 9:85–105, 1989.

11. Lekholm U, et al: The condition of soft tissues at tooth and fixture abutments supporting fixed bridges: A microbiological and histological study. J Clin Periodontol 13:558–562, 1986.

12. Leonhardt Å, Berglundh T, Ericsson I, Dahlén G: Putative periodontal pathogens on titanium implants and teeth in experimental gingivitis and periodontitis in beagle dogs. Clin Oral Impl Res 3:112–119, 1992.

13. Meffert RM: Treatment of failing dental implants. Curr Opin Dent 2:109–114, 1992.

14. Meffert RM: Endosseous dental implantology from the periodontist's viewpoint. J Periodontol 57:531–536, 1986.

15. Palmisano D, Mayo J, Block M, Lancaster D: Subgingival bacteria associated with hydroxylapatite-coated dental implants: Morphotypes and trypsin-like enzyme activity. Int J Oral Maxillofac Impl 6:313–317, 1991.

16. Quirynen M, Listgarten MA: The distribution of bacterial morphotypes around natural teeth and titanium implant ad modum Brånemark. Clin Impl Res 1:8–12, 1990.

17. Quirynen M, Naert I, van Steenberghe D: Fixture design and overload influence marginal bone loss and fixture success in the Brånemark system. Clin Oral Impl Res 3:104–111, 1992.

18. Schou S, Holmstrup P, Hjorting-Hansen E, Lang NP: Plaque-induced marginal tissue reactions of osseointegrated oral implants: A review of the literature. Clin Oral Impl Res 3:149–161, 1992.

19. Worthington P, et al: The Swedish system of osseointegrated implants: Problems and complications encountered during a 4-year period. Int J Oral Maxillofac Impl 2:77–84, 1987.

20. Zarb GA: Osseointegration: A requiem for the periodontal ligament? Int J Periodont Restor Dent 11:88–91, 1991.

Study Questions

1. What are the criteria for a diagnosis of the "failing" implant?

2. Why do implants "fail?"

3. Based on the answer to question 2, what are the solutions?

4. You place an implant and two years after restoration, the patient presents with 4 mm of bone loss with purulent drainage. What do you do?

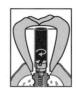

CHAPTER 26

Medical-Legal Ramifications of Dental Implants

Arthur W. Curley
Ronald Marks

Implants and the Public
Dental Implant Community
Legal System
Malpractice Defined
Plaintiff's Proof
Statute of Limitations
Abandonment
Comparative Negligence
Respondeat Superior
Patient Confidentiality
Duty to Refer
Informed Consent
    Consent Documentation
Charting and Record Keeping
    Records Defined
    Ownership/Maintenance
    Contents/Style
    Alterations
    Implant Records
Legal Issues for Implants
    Patient Candidacy
    Planning Issues
    Restorative/Occlusal Issues
American Dental Association Approval
Experience
Failure Recognition
Continuing Education/Politics of Implants

Dental implants offer new, exciting opportunities for today's dental patient and practitioner. Unfortunately, they also pose significant exposure to claims of malpractice. American juries have awarded patients verdicts in excess of $1.5 million in cases in which the plaintiff alleged negligent and unnecessary placement of dental implants, causing physical and emotional injuries.

To avoid such claims, today's practitioner must have a basic understanding of the legal environment, risk-management tools, and office practice techniques. This chapter is intended to offer primary insight to the medical-legal ramifications of dental implants. The prudent practitioner should seek out risk-management courses covering all areas of the dental practice and apply those guidelines to the principles set forth herein to maximize the benefits and protection that may be obtained.

IMPLANTS AND THE PUBLIC

As a result of the significant advances in technology and health care as well as the effects of advertising and the promotion of dentistry, the public today sees the dental practitioner as delivering a product with all the attendant expectations associated with most consumer goods.

Today's dental patient, particularly in the field of implants, expects the process to be pain and failure free. If problems develop, the public first thinks of a product defect or operator error. People are resistant to the concept of poor patient cooperation or accommodation as a cause or contributing factor to implant failure.

Consequently, patient education and the documentation of such efforts are as important to risk management as careful operative technique.

DENTAL IMPLANT COMMUNITY

Unfortunately the early years of implants were mired in the politics associated with divergent philosophies of implant placement and integration as well as competing brands of implants.

There are several methods and brands available to implant patients, and the careful practitioner can make a significant contribution to risk management by avoiding negative comments regarding the care of other health care practitioners unless and until all the facts are known.

Most dental malpractice cases are initiated by a dissatisfied patient who obtains opinions from another health care provider disparaging the treating dentist or surgeon. The law does not require a health care provider except for quality or peer review committees to investigate or criticize another practitioner. Rather the prudent practitioner must diagnose pathology or its potential and recommend treatment without speculating about the treatment of another dentist.

LEGAL SYSTEM

Actions against dentists involving claims associated with the placement of dental implants most often involve two fundamental areas of American law. *Civil, or tort, litigation* involves suits or claims filed by individual patients against dentists and seeks monetary awards. The plaintiff must prove the case by a preponderance of the evidence (greater than 50%). In a case of *criminal litigation*, an action is brought by the district attorney, who must prove guilt by a much higher standard, "beyond a reasonable doubt," and is seeking the levy of a fine, incarceration of the defendant, or both.

Torts include claims of negligence, such as failure to diagnose periodontal disease, lack of informed consent, or prescription of the wrong medication. Criminal cases involve allegations, such as fraudulent insurance billing, sexual molestation, and assault and battery.

MALPRACTICE DEFINED

In most states, dental malpractice is defined as negligence on behalf of the dental practitioner who failed to meet the *standard of care*. The standard of care is defined as *that level of care provided by a reasonable practitioner, of similar skill and learning, practicing under the same or similar circumstances and in the same or similar location and time*.

In the field of dental implants, the *location* rule is a national standard, and expert witnesses need not be licensed in the state where the suit is filed.

Except in areas of health care in which specialists or medical/dental societies have promulgated guidelines or standards of practice (American Society of Anesthesiologists and the American Association of Oral and Maxillofacial Surgeons), the standard of care is determined by the testimony of expert witnesses and not set forth in statutes or textbooks. It is the role of the American jury to judge the credibility of expert witnesses as well as the parties in determining whether or not the standard was violated.

The standard of care may be violated by providing the wrong treatment (extracting the wrong tooth), failing to provide the correct treatment (failing to diagnose periodontal disease), abandoning care (refusal to continue treatment), or failing to obtain informed consent.

PLAINTIFF'S PROOF

To prevail in a malpractice case, a patient must prove the following: substandard care that probably (greater than 50% of the evidence) caused physical or emotional injuries. The patient may then recover monetary damages to compensate for special damages (lost wages, medical and dental bills) and general damages (pain and suffering). Sometimes, in cases involving gross or intentional conduct (sexual molestation, altered records, unnecessary treatment) the jury may award punitive damages. These damages are designed to punish the doctor rather than compensate the patient, are generally not covered by insurance, and are usually a portion of the defendant's net worth (3% to 10%).

STATUTE OF LIMITATIONS

The statute of limitations is that period after a negligent act or the occurrence of an injury within which a lawsuit must be filed with the court. The statutory limit is usually extended in the case of minors until they reach the age of majority.

The time in which a patient must file a suit for malpractice varies with each state and generally ranges from 1 to 3 years. Most states, however, provide that the time does not begin to run until that patient "knew or should have known" of the negligent conduct and the associated injury. The time is also tolled until the patient discovers a retained nontherapeutic device, such as a sponge or broken root canal file.

The statute of limitations may also be extended until the discovery of a fraud. Examples of such cases include cases in which the patient was told that a nerve injury was "normal" and would heal, the patient paid for gold and received semi-precious metal, or treatment was unnecessary.

ABANDONMENT

A patient may terminate care or change doctors at any time and does not need the permission of the health care provider. Abandonment is defined as the health care provider's withdrawal from or refusal of further care without the consent or knowledge of the patient. For there to be a claim for abandonment, there must be a previously established doctor-patient relationship and a resulting injury to the patient.

The health care provider may not terminate care without reasonable notice to the patient. Failure to give such notice is abandonment and substandard care, and the patient may claim damages for problems incurred until another health care provider is obtained. The health care provider is required to complete treatment of the patient so as to stabilize the dental condition; however, this may not require completion of the entire treatment plan. The doctor must continue to provide care and seek legal remedies to recover monies owed (collection action or filing a law suit).

It is also abandonment to withhold treatment unless a patient pays monies owed (refusal to cement permanent crown, place implant attachment, or deliver final bridge) or refuse treatment to disabled persons (federal law defines disabled to include persons with acquired immunodeficiency syndrome [AIDS]).

Withdrawal from care, where not otherwise prohibited, should be by way of written notice to the patient and stating that the office will be available for emergencies only for a reasonable period (usually 30 days).

Claims for abandonment are often associated with the sale of a practice, treatment of human immunodeficiency virus (HIV) patients, orthodontics, and patients who were unable to locate or reach the doctor for an emergency.

COMPARATIVE NEGLIGENCE

The health care provider will not be responsible for injuries sustained as a result of the patient's failure to follow instructions. To be afforded this protection, however, the dental practitioner must carefully document problems with patient compliance: missed appointments, poor home care, failure to wear appliance, failure to take medications, or failure to act on a referral to another doctor or therapist.

Most states provide a defense of comparative negligence. The negligence of the patient, however, is merely a partial offset of the negligence of the defendant unless the plaintiff's injuries were exclusively due to patient negligence. In these cases, the jury award to the patient is reduced by that portion of the patient's negligence (usually less than 50%).

RESPONDEAT SUPERIOR

Respondeat superior is the legal principle that holds the owner of the dental practice responsible for the negligent acts of all the employees acting within the scope and course of their employment even if they fail to follow instructions or guidelines. This principle is also known as *vicarious liability*.

If a receptionist incorrectly marks a referral slip for the extraction of teeth or placement of implants, gives the patient the wrong prescription, or refuses to appoint an AIDS patient, the owner of the practice is liable and subject to malpractice claims.

To avoid such claims, it is recommended that the staff have duties that are carefully delineated, be subject to periodic assessment of performance, be encouraged to attend continuing education courses (particularly risk management), regularly check and have equipment serviced, and have clear lines of authority and supervision.

PATIENT CONFIDENTIALITY

Before the AIDS epidemic, breach of patient confidentiality was not a significant source of claims of malpractice. This new environment, however, creates a potential exposure for negligent failure to maintain confidentiality about a patient's health care status. The law provides that a patient may sue for emotional injury owing to humiliation as a result of a breach of this duty.

The most frequent source of the breach of confidentiality occurs when a staff member, usually a receptionist, discusses a patient's case on the telephone or at the reception desk in hearing distance of other patients or in a loud voice. Confidentiality issues should be clearly outlined to all employees. Conduct and communication issues must also be applied to social as well as professional settings.

Many states prohibit the communication of a patient's HIV status to other health care providers without the patient's written permission and then only to persons *directly* involved in the care of the patient. Thus, care should be exercised before disclosing an AIDS patient's status to a bookkeeper, billing clerk, or receptionist not directly involved in patient care.

DUTY TO REFER

A treating dentist must refer to or consult with a specialist where a prudent dentist in similar circumstances would do so or where the dentist does not have a specialist's knowledge or skill sufficient to perform adequately the treatment indicated or at the standard of a specialist.

Referral is indicated where the diagnosis remains unclear, the usual treatment has proved ineffectual, the required treatment is best handled by a specialist, and another treatment not ordinarily provided by the dentist might be more beneficial for the patient.

Referrals should be in writing and specific information included: reasons for the referral, any special dental or medical history of importance, medication requirements, the nature of the consultation, and a request for a follow-up report.

The careful practitioner documents the patient's lack of compliance with the referral as well as the response from the specialist. Further, the referring dentist should have a basic understanding as to the experience and skills of the health care provider to whom the patient was referred. This is particularly true when communicating with a dentist who had not previously seen implant patients.

A dentist may be liable for negligent referral if a patient is injured as a result of substandard care rendered by someone the defendant knew or should have known was inexperienced or poorly trained.

INFORMED CONSENT

The doctrine of informed consent is a critical risk-management issue for dentistry and particularly for implant patients.

In cases involving alternative forms of treatment, informed consent is defined as the consent to provide or withhold care after a patient has been informed in lay terms of the nature of the treatment, tests, or care; the known risks of serious bodily injury or death associated with the treatment or refusal of treatment; the alternatives to treatment or care; all facts deemed to be material (not commonly appreciated by laypersons); any information necessary for the patient to make a decision; and those facts that other practitioners of good standing (standard of care) would advise a patient under similar circumstances.

Obtaining informed consent, before the placement of implants, has several benefits. The consent process keeps patient expectations reasonable. A well-informed patient is less likely to sue in the event of a bad result. Finally the patient-doctor relationship is strengthened as a result of the dialogue.

The law does not list or delineate the risks that must be disclosed. The prudent practitioner should never offer a warranty or guarantee of the results. The patient may not consent to substandard care.

Consent Documentation

Implants should never be planned or placed without first obtaining a signed, dated, and witnessed written acknowledgment of informed consent. The consent form should state the nature, placement, type, and number of implants; the requirements for patient cooperation; and the risks of permanent nerve damage (lip, chin, tongue), sinus communication, bone or jaw fracture (requiring further treatment), serious infections (and the need for treatment and medication), or temporomandibular dysfunction or limited jaw openings. Finally, the patient must be advised of the risks and complications associated with implant failure and the fact that additional treatment might be indicated following implant removal.

It is recommended that a copy of the consent form be given to the patient at the early stages of the implant consultation and that the signed form be copied for the restorative dentist to enhance team support in the event of a poor result or complication.

CHARTING AND RECORD KEEPING

Inadequate, lost, or altered records are the primary problems in the defense of most claims involving dental implants. Thorough, well-maintained records are the primary defense in cases involving surgical complications, infections, and implant failures. Counsel for a dissatisfied patient most often reviews a copy of the treating doctor's records before deciding to file a suit.

Records Defined

Dental records are defined in the law as all tangible items created in the process of providing care for a patient. Such items include updated and current health history, dental history, tooth charting, treatment records, x-rays, models, wax bites, laboratory slips, photographs, letters, insurance forms, prescriptions, phone logs, tracings, drawings, mountings, and ledger and billing records.

Ownership/Maintenance

The original dental records are the exclusive property of the dentist and should not be released without first consulting with an attorney or insurance carrier. The patient is entitled to copies of all of the records on request regardless of any monies owed or the progress of treatment. The practitioner may charge only a nominal fee for the copying process and may not charge for professional time or services to make the copies. In most cases, the copies must be provided within 5 days. If the request from the patient is that the records be sent to an attorney or another health care provider, the copies should be delivered only on receipt of a written request.

Owing to the tolling provisions associated with the statutes of limitation and the crowded condition of the courts, cases seldom go to trial less than 2 years after suit is filed. It is recommended that original records be maintained for at least 10 years from the last patient contact and ideally indefinitely or until retirement or the sale of the practice.

Contents/Style

Because of the changes in the profile of today's dental patient as well as the more complex forms of treatment, a detailed, frequently updated health history is essential. Further, communication with the family physician is encouraged any time there is a question regarding the patient's health status.

A good charting system requires that four basic subjects be noted *at every chart entry:* SOAP—(1) the patient's *symptoms* or the lack thereof, (2) clinical *observations*, (3) *assessment*/advice given, and (4) recommended *plan* or procedure. The practitioner should also consider and note the what, where, why, and how of each assessment, including a written plan and problem list.

Alterations

Many claims against dentists are lost because of altered records rather than substandard care. The pages of dental charts should be maintained in numbered sequence, each entry properly dated and signed by the maker. Some states require by statute that all chart entries be signed or initialed.

Altered or forged records seriously challenge the defendant's credibility and subject the defense to a claim for spoilation of evidence and punitive damages. There are many technical ways to detect alterations. Today, most of the inks used in pens are registered and dated with the federal government such that the date of the entry may be compared with the age of the ink on the paper. Some experts state they can determine authenticity by handwriting style.

Necessary changes should be made by putting a line through the error and writing in the correct information followed by the author's initials. Unless the correction is made at the same time as the original entry, the date of the correction should also be noted.

The preferred technique is careful and complete recording from the beginning.

Implant Records

Dental implants require special record keeping. The complete chart should include the following: periodontal probing, full mouth x-ray, hygiene assessment, health history, occlusal analysis, temporomandibular joint (TMJ) examination, and patient candidacy assessment. A written treatment plan should be approved by the patient.

After choosing to place implants and obtaining written informed consent, the records should reflect an analysis of the bone quality and size with special consideration given to the location of nerves and the sinus cavities.

The brand, type, and size of the implants, the attachments, and the restorations should be noted. Postimplantation charting must include an assessment of the healing and periodontal status, including the lack of any problems. Immediate postoperative x-rays are recommended so that potential problems of angulation, sinus communication, or nerve contact may be assessed early and at a time when the implant can be easily removed or repositioned. Photographs are perhaps the best risk-management tool, particularly in cases of poor patient compliance.

LEGAL ISSUES FOR IMPLANTS

Claims and suits involving dental implants most often involve poor patient candidacy, poor planning, lack of informed consent, failure to assess periodontal status, surgical complications, restorative and occlusal problems, periodontal tissue follow-up and maintenance, and failure to refer.

Patient Candidacy

Not all patients, despite their dental needs or condition, are candidates for implants. The practitioner must carefully evaluate and record the patient's medical condition, soft and hard tissue quality, and the patient's physiologic profile to achieve a successful and long-term result.

The most common cause of implant failure is chronic infection. Claims against dentists have alleged failure to appreciate the patient's reduced health status, poor home care, or systemic conditions that reduce healing. The practitioner should note the lack of problems in these areas to verify and record that these areas were considered in determining patient candidacy.

Planning Issues

Claims involving planning for implants primarily focus on imaging issues. Today's practitioner must be cognizant of the status of the debate as to the minimal imaging required for treatment planning: panoramic computed tomography versus magnetic resonance imaging. The practitioner must consider the need for more defined imaging during the evaluation of the area into which the implants are to be placed.

Planning cases frequently involves injuries and complications such as nerve damage, bone fracture, and sinus communication. Obtaining informed consent for these risks will not protect the doctor if it is shown that inadequate imaging was used and that the injury could have been avoided with better studies.

Claims of substandard planning also involve inadequate assessment of the patient's home care skills. This is particularly important in cases in which implants are being used to replace teeth lost because of periodontal disease. Continued patient motivation is essential to success in such cases and must be assessed and documented, including periodic periodontal charting.

Restorative/Occlusal Issues

TMJ/TMD is a subject frequently presented in the media, and accordingly the public is keenly aware of the condition and its association with dental care and treatment. The status of the occlusion and its effect on the TMJ must be considered, particularly as the restorative phase of treatment becomes more extensive.

Claims of TMD associated with implants most often allege inadequate assessment of the TMJ, a change of the bite without first considering splint treatment, and failure to refer to a specialist at the first signs of a problem. The careful practitioner must record the lack of TMD signs or symptoms as well as any problems with occlusion or the bite.

AMERICAN DENTAL ASSOCIATION APPROVAL

Several suits against dentists have alleged failure to inform the patient of the use of a non-American Dental Association approved implant or the unique risks associated with a particular system of implants. Currently, there are several brands and types of dental implants on the market that may be used to treat the same dental condition. The ADA has approved several implants as dental devices. The law requires that the practitioner have a basic understanding of the implant system to be used as well as an appreciation for the risks/benefits offered by other systems.

The law does not require ADA approval for the placement of an implant system. The practitioner must be familiar with the system and obtain the patient's consent to use a nonapproved device.

EXPERIENCE

The patient is entitled to know the basic experience level of the dental practitioner before consenting to implant placement. Failure to inform the patient is the same as failing to obtain informed consent. This doctrine does not mean the dentist must list the number of cases treated. A patient is entitled to know, however, if the dentist is placing implants for the first time following a brief instructional course.

Advising the patient of the practitioner's experience level often serves to keep the patient's expectations reasonable, and if a practitioner obtains a good result with the first few cases placed, the informed patient is often impressed and the patient-doctor bond strengthened.

FAILURE RECOGNITION

Many claims of malpractice are related to late recognition of the failing implant, abutment, or restoration. Close follow-up minimizes or eliminates these cases as potential claims. The practitioner must carefully communicate and be sure that someone in the implant team is monitoring the patient and the soft tissue status in addition to implant stability.

Patients, often after years of using a removable device, are reluctant to acknowledge a failing implant yet cannot be motivated to improve hygiene. The careful practitioner must be firm in the decision to remove or treat a failing implant and not be swayed by the patient's promises to improve home care.

The problems that can be created by an infected implant (heart valve infection, brain abscess, osteomyelitis) greatly exceed the disappointment associated with the failure.

CONTINUING EDUCATION/ POLITICS OF IMPLANTS

The state of the art of dentistry and implants is rapidly changing. Imaging is more accurate and more available. New techniques such as lasers offer new opportunities, potential problems, and the need for risk management. The prudent implant dentist needs to be current on these and other changing issues, such as the use of keratinized tissue grafts for mandibular implants.

The standard of care requires that dentists stay informed of the developments addressed in readily available publications or presented in national meetings on the subject of implants. The information obtained should be considered in selecting an implant system and in determining the information to be given to a patient to obtain informed consent.

In summary, dental implants have all the risks associated with the extraction of teeth and the restoration of crowns except the dentist can plan where to put the implant to minimize complications. Careful planning, execution, and follow-up with a fundamental appreciation of the legal principles applied to thorough documentation will minimize the risks of litigation. The careful practitioner can then fully enjoy the rewards and satisfaction of placing dental implants.

Study Questions

1. Why do dentists get sued over dental implants?

2. What can you do to prevent a malpractice claim against you?

3. Your consent form is 6 pages long and the patient refuses to read it, but agrees to sign it. Is this "informed consent?" What must you do?

INDEX

Note: Page numbers in *italics* refer to illustrations; page numbers followed by t refer to tables.

Abandonment, 283
Abutment(s), analogs for, in hybrid denture impressions, 115, *116*
  angled, for fixed prosthodontics, 130–131, *131*
  cemented, after placement of prosthesis, 87
    disadvantages of, 87, *88*
  customized, 131
  for fixed prosthodontics, preparation of, 130
    selection of, 130–131, *131*
    transfer of, 129, *129*
  for hybrid dentures, oral hygiene instructions for, 119–120
    verifying fit of, 119, *119*
  physical misfit of prosthesis and, *70,* 70–71
  plaque accumulation on, 267
  provided on attachments, 101, *102*
  replacements for, in single-tooth restorations, 135
  selection of, for implant-supported overdentures, 102
  shouldered, in overdenture fabrication, 106, *106*
  stiffness of, 69
  tensile forces on, 69–70
  transfer of implants instead of, in overdenture fabrication, 108, *108*
Acquired immunodeficiency syndrome (AIDS), abandonment concept related to, 283
  patient confidentiality issues and, 283–284
Acrylic resin(s), as occlusal surface material, 80–81
  for temporary restorations, 144, *144*
  reduction of stress by, 139
Acrylic template(s). See *Stent(s), clear acrylic.*
Actinobacillus actinomycetemcomitans, 269
Actinomyces species, 269
Actinomyces viscosus, 267, 268, 268t
Adams' dental implant, 4
Adhesion, bacterial, 266–267
Aesthetic restorations, abnormally long teeth in, 114
  exposure techniques for, 155–156, *155–156*
  for fixed prosthetics, 123, *123,* 132, *132*
  for hybrid dentures, 113, *114,* 119
  in single-tooth restorations, 134, 135
  malpositioned implants in, solutions for, 80
  prosthetic options for, 79–80
  removable acrylic facade for, 114, *114*
Aging, wound healing and, 50–51
AIDS. See *Acquired immunodeficiency syndrome (AIDS).*
Ailing implant(s), 269. See also *Implant failure.*
Alcohol abuse, preoperative assessment of, 19–20
Allogeneic bone graft(s), for composite bone grafts, 233, 238–239
  mineralized, creeping substitution of, 208
  of alveolar crest defect, 159, *160–163*
  of maxillary sinus, 208
Alloplast graft(s), for composite bone grafts, 233
  of alveolar crest defect, 158–159, *159*
  of maxillary sinus, 209
Alveolar bone. See also *Alveolar ridge.*
  grafting of. See *Bone grafting.*
  height of, panoramic radiographs for determining, 36
  loss of, around implant, acceptable amount of, 262

Alveolar bone *(Continued)*
    as indication of implant failure, 260
    causes of, 261–262
    occlusal forces in, 139, 261, 262, *262*
    radiographic evaluation of, 261, *262*
    treatment of, 276–279
    with overdentures, 94
  due to poor oral hygiene, 267
  occlusal planning and, 143–144, *143–144*
  progressive loading of, occlusion and, 143
  quality of, classification of, 122
    determining, for fixed prosthetics, 122–123
    for single-tooth restorations, 133, 133t
    in advanced maxillary resorption, 232
    number of implants determined by, 78
    pre-prosthetic evaluation of, 76–77
    records of analysis of, 285
    wound healing related to, 50
Alveolar mucosal tissue. See *Mucosal tissue.*
Alveolar nerve, inferior, 175–181
  anatomic and structural arrangement of, *178*
  anatomic location of, 21, *22–24,* 24
  anesthetic block of, 150
  injuries to, after implant placement, 180, *181*
    after nerve lateralization, 180–181, *181*
    classification of, 178
    during instrumentation and implant placement, 179–180, *180*
    following implant placement, 178–179
    primary repair of, 178
    radiographic evaluation of, 179, *179*
    secondary repair of, 178–179
    treatment algorithms for, 179–180, *180–181*
  repositioning of, 175–178
    advantages and disadvantages of, 176
    anterior approach to, 176, *176–177*
    indications for, 175–176
    paresthesias after, 177
    posterior approach to, 177, *177–178*
    surgical procedures for, 176–177, *176–178*
Alveolar ridge, defects of, after implant placement, alloplast grafting of, 158–159, *159*
  dehiscence, *189*
    case history of, *196,* 197, *198*
    guided tissue regeneration for, *192,* 193
    mandibular, case history of, 197, *200–202*
  fenestration, *189*
    case history of, *202–204,* 205
    guided tissue regeneration for, *193,* 193–194
  large, autogenous and allogeneic grafting for, 159, *160–163*
    guided tissue regeneration for, 159, *164–165*
  residual intraosseous, case history of, 197, *199–200*
    guided tissue regeneration for, *192–193,* 193
  small, alloplast grafting of, 158–159, *159*
  maxillomandibular relationship of. See *Jaw relation.*
  resorption of, 10–15
    as indication for inferior alveolar nerve repositioning, 175

Alveolar ridge *(Continued)*
   bone grafting for. See *Bone grafting.*
   categories of, 10
   classification of, 207t
   factors in, 10, *11*
   general changes in, 10–12, *11–12*
   in women, 10, *11*
   intermaxillary relationship changes in, 12–13, *13*
   jaw relation changes due to, 113
   labial bone loss in, 28, *28*
   maxillary changes in, 12, *12*
   patterns of, 10
   prosthetic considerations in, 13, 15, *15*
   pyramidal architecture in, 13, *13*
   soft tissue changes in, 13, *14*
   stages of, 11, *11*
   treatment implications of, 13, 15
   with denture use, 10
  width of, diagnostic cast for determining, 82
American Dental Association, implant approval by, 286
Amino acids, wound healing and, 50
Amoxicillin/Augmentin, for implant failure, 276
Anatomy, mandibular, 21–25
  maxillary, 27–31
Ancient dental implants, 4
Anesthesia, for implant exposure, 153
  intravenous sedation as, 150
  local, 150
   in hypertensive patients, 18–19
   types of, 150
Angina, preoperative assessment of, 19
  unstable, 19
Angiogenesis, in bone healing, 243
Antibiotic therapy, for implant failure, 276, 277
Antivibrational thread compound(s), 88
Anxiety, increased oxygen demand in, 19
Arch. See *Dental arch.*
Attachment(s). See also *Fixation technique(s).*
  ASC-52, 98t, 101, *102*
  ball-type, 98t, *103*
  bar and clip, for implant-borne overdentures, 100, 101,
   101t
   for tissue-borne overdentures, 96–97, *97*, 98t
  Ceka attachment, 79
  combination bar, for implant-borne overdentures, 101t
   for tissue-borne overdentures, 98t
  Dalla Bona, 98t, *103*
  Dolder bar, 98t, 101, 101t
  ERA, *97*, 98t, 102, *103*
  for implant-borne overdentures, *100*, 100–102, 101t, *103–104*
  for tissue-borne overdentures, 96–97, 98t
  O-ring, *79*, 98t, 101, *102–103*
  plunger-type, 98t, 101
  selection of, factors in, 100
   interocclusal space considerations in, 100
   requirements for implant-borne overdentures in, 101–102
  slant-lock type, *99*, 101t
  spark-erosion type, *100*, 101t
  special designs for, 101t
  stress-breaking, for tissue-borne overdentures, 97, 98t, *100*
  stud-type, 98t, 101, *102*
   placement of, during overdenture fabrication, 107
  supporting partial removable dentures, 78, *78*
  Swiss anchor, 98t, 101, *102*
  without splinting bar, *79*, 79
Austenal (corporation), 4
Autogenous bone graft(s), for atrophic edentulism. See
  Bone grafting, for atrophic edentulism.

Autogenous bone graft(s) *(Continued)*
  for composite bone grafts, allogeneic bone preparations
   . with, 238–239
  of advanced maxillary resorption, 233
   in full-arch onlay graft, 234, *235*
   in interpositional graft with LeFort I osteotomy, 234,
    238–240, *239–240*
   in sinus inlay graft, 234, *235–238*
  in maxillofacial reconstruction, 243
  of alveolar crest defect, 159, *160–163*
  of maxillary sinus, 208, *212–215*

Bacteria, oral, 265–271. See also *Plaque accumulation.*
  accumulation of, around implants, 262
  adhesion of, to hard surfaces, 266–267
  attachment of, to titanium, 262
  biofilm of, 265
  colonization of implants by, after exposure of implants,
   266
   implant failure due to, 274, *274–275*
   natural teeth *vs.,* 266
  endotoxins from, implant failure and, 270, 271
  plaque accumulation and, 267
  subgingival, 267–270
   edentulousness and, 268–269
   good oral hygiene and, 267–268
   implant failure and, 269–270, *270*
    possible pathogenic mechanisms in, 270–271
   major observations about, 268t
   predominant types of, 268, 268t
Bacteroides forsythus, 269
Bacteroides species, black-pigmented, 269
Ball-type attachments, 98t, *103*
Bar and clip attachment(s), for implant-borne overdentures,
  100, 101, 101t
  for tissue-borne overdentures, 96–97, *97*, 98t
Bar assembly, implant-supported, for partial removable
  dentures, 78
Bar attachment(s). See also *Attachment(s).*
  combination, for implant-borne overdentures, 101t
  for tissue-borne overdentures, 98t
Barrier(s), in guided tissue regeneration. See also specific
  types, e.g., *Expanded polytetrafluoroethylene
  membrane (e-PFTE).*
  result of, *184*
  types of, *184–185*, 184–186
Basal lamina–hemidesmosomal complex, in implant healing,
  48
Bioactive materials, 48t, 54
Biocompatible materials, 55–61. See also implants of
  specific materials, e.g., *Titanium implant(s).*
  classifications of, 48t, 54
  compatibility with bony tissue, 48t
  fixation techniques for, 56–60
   calcium phosphate ceramic coatings in, 58, *58*, 59t, 60,
    60
   direct bone apposition in, 56, *57*
   motion at bone-implant interface and, 61
   optimizing, 60–61
   porous ingrowth attachment in, 56–58, *57*
   surgical fit and, 61
   testing results for hydroxylapatite-coated implants in,
    59t
  surface and interface properties of, 47t
  surface-active ceramics, 55t, 55–56, *56*
  titanium and titanium-based alloys, 55
Biofilm, bacterial, 265
Bioglass ceramics, 55, 55t

Bioinert materials, 48t, 54

Biologic factors, in residual ridge resorption, 10, *11*

Biomechanics of dental implants, 61–71. See also *Screw mechanics.*

  biting forces in, 63–64, *63–64*

  edentulous mandible and, 65, *66–67*, 67

  forces on implants supporting bridgework in, 64–65, *65*

  implant angulation effects in, 67–68, *68*

  partial edentulousness and, 67

  stiffness in, analysis of tooth connected to implant and, 69

    definition of, 68–69

    prosthesis supported by abutments and, 69

Biotolerant materials, 48t, 54

Bite guard, for protection against occlusal forces, 262, *262*

Biting force, 63–64, *63–64*, 139

Blade implant, Linkow's designs for, *5, 6*

Bleeding. See also *Hemorrhage.*

  on probing, as sign of implant failure, 260

Blood clot, in guided tissue regeneration, 194

Body region, of mandible, 21, *22*

Bone(s), alveolar. See *Alveolar bone.*

  healing of, 45–46, *46*, 47t

  increased mass of, in response to stress, 167

  loss of. See *Alveolar bone, loss of; Alveolar ridge, resorption of.*

  skeletal, guided tissue regeneration of, 186

  surgical trauma to, poor wound healing related to, 48, 274

Bone grafting. See also *Guided tissue regeneration.*

  composite, for advanced maxillary resorption, 232–240

    bone graft considerations in, 233

    bone quality in, 232

    cosmetic considerations in, 233

    full-arch onlay grafts in, *233*, 234, *235*

    interpositional, with LeFort I osteotomy, 234, 238–240, *239–240*

    one-stage *vs.* two-stage procedure in, 233, *233*

    preoperative considerations in, 232–233

    sinus inlay graft in, 234, *235–238*

    surgical technique of, 233–240

  in maxillofacial reconstruction, 243

  for alveolar crest defect, large, autogenous and allogeneic grafts for, 159, *160–163*

  with hydroxylapatite, 158–159, *159*

  for atrophic edentulism, 223–231

    alignment stents for, 224, *224*

    anatomic replacement of bone in, 224

    case histories in, for denture retention and function, 228–231, *229–230*

      for severe maxillofacial injuries, 226–228, *227–229*

    closure of, without tension, 225

    coverage of implant by graft in, 225

    implant anchorage in native bone and, 225

    implants anchored in graft alone, failure of, 225

    interface between natural bone and graft in, 224

    patient selection in, 225–226

    provisional denture requirements in, 225, *226*

    requirements for, 224–226

    rigid fixation with screws in, 224–225

    types of grafts in, 223

  for implant failure, 277

  in maxillofacial reconstruction, 242–257

    for primary mandibular reconstruction, case history of, 248, *249–250*

    for secondary mandibular reconstruction, case histories of, 248–249, *251–253*, 254

      angle-to-angle defect, in irradiated field, 254, *255–256*

      in irradiated field, 244, *245–246*

Bone grafting *(Continued)*

    in nonirradiated field, 244, *247*, 248

    principles of, 242–244

  of maxillary sinus, 206–221

    choice and behavior of materials for, 208–209, 211, *212–220*

    classification of alveolar bone in, 207t

    clinical results of, 207t, 211, 220–221

    complications of, 221, *221*

    surgical procedures for, *209–211*, 211

    treatment planning for, 206–208, 207t

  resorption of graft, during healing, 225

Bone morphogenetic proteins (BMPs), in bone healing, 243

Bone-implant interface. See also *Fixation technique(s); Osseointegration.*

  direct bone apposition at, 56, *57*

  motion at, 61

  occlusal forces at, implant failure due to, 275

  stress transfer capabilities at, 54

  surgical fit and, 50, 61

  wound healing and, 46–47, 47t–48t

Brånemark, P.I., 2, 6

Bridge(s), implant as substitute for, in orthopedic treatment, 168

  implant-supported, forces on, 64–65, *65*

  number of implants required for, 79

Brush(es), for oral hygiene around abutments, 120

Calcium homeostasis, wound healing related to, 50–51

Calcium phosphate ceramics. See also *Hydroxylapatite.*

  biocompatibility of, 55

  bone-bonding capability of, 56

  coating of implants with, 58, *58*, 59t, 60, *60*

Cancellous bone graft(s), for composite bone grafts, 233

  in interpositional graft with LeFort I osteotomy, 234

  in sinus inlay graft, 234, *235–236*

  of maxillary sinus, 208, *216–220*

Candida species, implant failure due to, 269

Cantilever(s), avoiding, on maxillary arch, 99

  for hybrid dentures, 117, *117,* 119

  occlusal planning and, 145, *145*

Capnocytophaga species, 269

Carbocaine (Mepivacaine), 18

Cardiac Risk Index, 17–18

  categories in, 18t

  risk variables in, 17, 18t

Cardiovascular assessment, 17–18, 18t

Cast(s). See *Diagnostic cast(s).*

Cavi-jet, 276

Ceka attachment, 79

Cephalometric radiographs, lateral, 36, *37, 38*

Ceramics. See *Glass ceramics.*

Cervital ceramics, 55, 55t

Charting. See *Dental records.*

Chief complaint, in clinical evaluation, 75

Chin, as source of bone, for maxillary sinus bone graft, *212*

  avoiding laxity of, 151

Chlorhexidine rinse, 187, 195

Cigarette smoking, wound healing and, 19

Citric acid, for implant failure, 277

Civil litigation, 282

Clamping force(s), definition of, 88

  development of, 89

  for prevention of screw loosening, 89

Clear acrylic template(s). See *Stent(s), clear acrylic.*

Clindamycin, for implant failure, 276

Clip attachment(s). See *Bar and clip attachment(s).*

Clot, in guided tissue regeneration, 194

Coagulopathy, wound healing related to, 51
Coating(s) for implants, for porous ingrowth attachment, 56–58
  hydroxylapatite as. See also *Hydroxylapatite-coated implants.*
    grit-blasted titanium *vs.*, 58, *58*, 60, *60*
    mechanical testing results for, 59t
    types of, 57, *57*
Cobalt-chromium-molybdenum (Co-Cr-Mo) alloy, 55
Collagen membrane(s), in guided tissue regeneration, 185–186
Combination syndrome, in residual ridge resorption, 12, *14*
  maxillary sinus bone graft in, *219–220*
Comparative negligence, 283
Complement activation, implant failure and, 270, 271
Composite bone grafting. See *Bone grafting, composite.*
Compressive force, exposure of implants to, 63
Computed tomography (CT), 38–43
  bone height determination by, 38, *40*
  clear acrylic template in, 38, *41*
    for implant placement in extraction sites, 159, 163, *165*
  dental processing software in, 38, *42–43*, 43
  of maxillary sinuses, 36, *37*
  panographic views in, 38, *39*
Conditioning film, on oral surfaces, 266
Condylar angle(s), occlusal planning and, 142
Connective tissue, grafting of, for aesthetic restorations, 155, *155*
Continuing education, for risk management, 287
Copings. See *Transfer copings.*
Core-Vent implants, 7
Coronary artery bypass grafting, 19
Coronary artery disease, preoperative assessment of, 19–20
Cortical cancellous bone graft(s). See *Cancellous bone graft(s).*
Corticosteroid therapy, wound healing and, 51
Creep, definition of, 68
Creeping substitution, of mineralized allogeneic bone, 208
Crestal bone defect. See *Alveolar ridge, defects of.*
Crestal incision, for maxillary sinus bone graft, *211*
  of anterior mandible, 151, *151*
  of posterior mandible, 152, *152*
Criminal litigation, 282
Crossbite occlusion, 140, *140*
Crown-to-root ratio, in fixed prosthetics, 124, 125t, *126*
CT. See *Computed tomography (CT).*
Curve of Wilson, 27
Cuspid disclusion, 144, *144*, 145
Cytokine(s), implant failure and, 270, 271

Dalla Bona attachment(s), 98t, *103*
3D/Dental software, for computed tomography, 38
Dehiscence defect(s), case history of, *196*, 197, *198*
  cause of, *189*
  guided tissue regeneration for, *192*, 193
  mandibular, case history of, 197, *200–202*
Demineralized bone graft(s), of maxillary sinus, 208–209
Dental arch, diagnostic casts of, arch length determination by, 82
  arch width determination by, 81, *81*
  interarch space determination by, 82, 113
  maxillomandibular relationship determination by, 82
  ridge width determination by, 82
  form of, occlusal planning and, 139–140, *140*
  interarch distance in, occlusal planning and, 140–141, *140–141*
Dental evaluation, pre-prosthetic, 76
Dental Implant Consensus Conference, 2

Dental records, 284–286
  alterations to, 285
  content and style of, 285
  definition of, 285
  of implant procedures, 285–286
  ownership/maintenance of, 285
Dent/a/Scan software, for computed tomography, 38
Dentist(s), continuing education for, as risk management strategy, 287
  experience level of, legal issues related to, 286–287
  responsibilities of, in team approach to prosthodontics, 75
Denture(s), diagnostic, in hybrid denture construction, 114
  hybrid. See *Hybrid denture(s).*
  overdenture-type. See *Overdenture(s).*
  partial removable, implants for improving, 78, *78*
  provisional, after bone grafting, in case history, 229–230, *230*
    of atrophic edentulous jaw, 225, *226*
  residual ridge resorption due to, 10
Design of implants. See *Implant design.*
Diabetes mellitus, wound healing and, 51
Diagnostic cast(s), 81–82
  arch length determination by, 82
  arch width determination by, 81, *81*
  for hybrid dentures, 113, 118
  interarch space determination by, 82
  maxillomandibular relationship determination by, 82
  ridge width determination by, 82
Diagnostic denture(s), in hybrid denture construction, 114
Diagnostic wax-up, 82–84, *83*
  for fixed prosthetics, 123–124
  for hybrid dentures, 116, *116*
  for phonetic problems, 80
  index for, 83–84, *83–84*
  uses for, 83
Digastric fossa, anatomy of, 21, *22*, 25
Disabled persons, abandonment of care of, 283
Displacement, definition of, 68
Dolder bar attachment(s), 98t, 101, 101t
Doxycycline, for implant failure, 276
Drug(s). See also specific drug or drug group.
  implant failure and, 275
Duty to refer, 284

Early dental implants, 4, *4*
Edentulous jaw, atrophic, bone grafting of, 223–231
    case histories of, 226–231, *227–230*
    requirements for, 224–226, *224*, *226*
  bacterial colonization and, 268–269
  biomechanical forces on implants in, 65, *66–67*, 67
  bite force and, 64
  exposure of implants in, 153–154
  incidence of, 94, 112
  maxillary, composite bone grafting of, 232–240
    full-arch onlay grafts in, 233, 234, 235
    interpositional, with LeFort I osteotomy, 234, 238–240, *239–240*
    preoperative considerations in, 232–233
    sinus inlay graft in, 234, 235–238
    surgical technique of, 233–240
  occlusal plane of, 141–142
  occlusal planning and, 145–146
  partial, bacterial colonization and, 268–269
    biomechanical forces on implants in, 67
    exposure of implants in, 155
    occlusal plane of, 141
    occlusal planning and, 144–145, *144–145*
  weakening of, after implant placement in opposite arch, 142

Education, continuing, for risk management, 287
    of patient, pre-prosthetic, 76
Encapsulation of implant, fibrous, 48, 49, 56
Endotoxin, bacterial, in implant failure, 270, 271
Epinephrine, in local anesthesia, 150
    in hypertensive patients, 18–19
e-PTFE. See *Expanded polytetrafluoroethylene membrane
        (e-PTFE)*.
ERA attachment(s), 97, 98t, 102, *103*
Excursive contacts, as joint-separating forces, 90
Expanded polytetrafluoroethylene membrane (e-PTFE),
        background of, 186–187, *187*
    considerations for use of, 194–195, *194–196*
    maintenance of space beneath, 194–195, *194–195*
    natural space-making defect and, 194, *194*
    non-space-making defect and, 194, *195*
    potential bone regeneration using, *189*
    premature exposure of, 196
    removal procedure for, 196–197
    stabilization of, 195, *195*
Expert witness(es), standard of care determined by, 282
Exposure of implants, 153–156
    anesthesia for, 153
    for aesthestic restorations, *155*, 155–156
    for hybrid denture placement, 115
    technique of, 153, *154*, 155
    timing of, 153
Extraction site(s), alveolar bone resorption and, 10
    defects in, guided tissue regeneration for, *192–193*, 194
    placement of implants in, 157–166, *190*
        bone grafting for crestal defects in, 158–159, *159–163*
        clear acrylic template for, 159, 163, *165*
        common locations for, 158
        contraindications to, 157–158
        delayed, 158
        guided tissue regeneration in, 159, *164–165*, 166
        immediate, 157–158
        in anterior maxilla, 159, 163, *163–165*, 166
        indications for, 157
        palatal location and, 166
        simultaneous, 158–159, *158–163*, 163, 166
        soft tissue grafting for, 163, 166
        treatment planning for, 157–158

Fabrication of overdentures. See *Impression technique(s),
        for overdentures*.
Facial structures, support of, by prosthetics, 113, 123
Failure of implants. See *Implant failure*.
Fenestration defect(s), *189*
    case history of, *202–204*, 205
    guided tissue regeneration for, *193*, 193–194
Fibroblast(s), IL-1 activated, implant failure and, 270
    in bone healing, 243
Fibrous encapsulation of implant, due to premature loading,
        49
    due to surgical trauma, 48
    stress distribution affected by, 56
Film, conditioning, on oral surfaces, 266
Fixation technique(s). See also *Attachment(s)*.
    for implants, 56–60. See also *Bone-implant interface;
            Osseointegration*.
        calcium phosphate ceramic coatings in, 58, *58*, 59t, 60,
                60
        direct bone apposition in, 56, *57*
        motion at bone-implant interface and, 61
        optimizing, 60–61
        porous ingrowth attachment in, 56–58, *57*
        surgical fit and, 61

Fixation technique(s) *(Continued)*
        testing results for hydroxylapatite-coated implants in,
                59t
    for rigid bone grafts, 224–225
Fixed prosthodontics. See *Prosthodontics, fixed*.
Fixtures (titanium screws), development by Brånemark, 6, 7
Flap development, for implant failure, 276, 277
    in inferior alveolar nerve repositioning, 176, 177
    of lip mucosa, during incision procedure, 151, *151*
    palatal, for aesthetic restorations, 155, *156*
Force(s). See also *Biomechanics of dental implants; Screw
        mechanics*.
    biting, 63–64, *63–64*
    compressive, 63
    direction along long axis of implant, in fixed prosthodon-
            tics, 125–126
    Newton as unit of, 64
    occlusal, implant failure due to, 261, 262, *262*, 275
        parafunctional habits and, 275
    on implants supporting bridgework, 64–65, *65*
    stress, acrylic resin for reducing, 139
        implant angulation and, 68
        increased bone mass in response to, 167
    tensile, 63
        on abutments, preload and, 69–70
Framework(s). See also *Superstructure*.
    for fixed prosthodontics, 131–132, *132*
    for hybrid dentures, characteristics of, 118t
        fabrication of, 116, *117*
        fitting of, 117–119
        metals for casting of, 118
        verification of, 118, *118*
    for overdentures, fabrication of, 105–106
    forceful seating of, bone damage due to, 118
        implant failure due to, 105, 131
    non-passive, implant loosening due to, 91, *91*
Freeze-dried bone graft(s), of maxillary sinus, 208
Full-arch only composite graft, *233*, 234, *235*
Furcations, Gore-Tex periodontal material for, 184–185, *185*
Fusobacterium species, implant failure due to, 269

Genial tubercles, anatomy of, 21, *22*, 25
Genioglossus muscle, 25
Geniohyoid muscle, 25
Gershkoff subperiosteal implant, 4, *5*
Gingiva, grafting of, before exposure of implants, 153
        before implant placement, 77
        from palate, 155–156
    keratinized, as preferred tissue around implants, 77, 260–
            261, *261*
        creation of, with split-thickness free palatal graft, 155–
                156
        for fixed prosthetics, 123
        preservation of, during exposure of implants, 153, *154*
            during posterior mandible incision, 151–152, *152*
Glass ceramics, 55–56
    biocompatibility of, 55–56
    chemical composition of, 55t
    surface and interface properties of, 47t
Gold implants, 4
Goldberg subperiosteal implant, 4, *5*
Gore-Tex augmentation material, in guided tissue
        regeneration, 187, *188*
Gore-Tex periodontal material, for furcations, 184–185, *185*
    regrowth of attachment using, 184
Grafting, of bone. See *Bone grafting*.
    of connective tissue, for aesthetic restorations, 155, *155*
    of gingiva, before implant exposure, 153

Grafting (Continued)
    before implant placement, 77
    from palate, 155–156
    soft tissue, for implant placement in extraction sites, 163, 166
Greenfield two-piece basket implant, 4, 4
Group function type of occlusion, 143, 144, 144
Guided tissue regeneration, 183–205
    around endosseous implants, 186–187, 187
    around natural teeth, 183–186, 184–185
    background of, 183–186
    barriers (membranes) in, for implant failure, 277, 278–279
        prerequisites for successful use of, 187, 190
        results of use of, 184
        types of, 184–185, 184–186
    case reports of, for cortical dehiscence defect, 196, 197, 198
        of mandible, 197, 200–202
        for fenestration defect, 202–204, 205
        for intraosseous defect, 197, 199–200
    expanded polytetrafluoroethylene membranes in, background of, 186–187, 187
        considerations for use of, 194–195, 194–196
        maintenance of space beneath, 194–195, 194–195
        potential bone regeneration using, 189
        premature exposure of, 196
        removal procedure for, 196–197
    follow-up care in, 195–196
    for alveolar crest defect, 159, 164–165, 166
    for dehiscence defect, 189, 192, 193
    for fenestration defect, 189, 193, 193–194
    for residual intraosseous defect, 193, 193
    Gore-Tex augmentation material for, 187, 188–190
    in skeletal bones, 186
    indications for, 192–193, 192–194
    postoperative considerations in, 195–196
    principles of, 183–184

Hard palate. See Palate.
Healing. See Wound healing.
Heat, from rotary instruments, implant failure due to, 274
    wound healing and, 48
Hematologic disorder(s), wound healing and, 51
Hemidesmosome(s), in implant healing, 48
Hemorrhage. See also Bleeding.
    due to lingual artery injury, 25
    during inferior alveolar nerve repositioning, 179
Hex system(s), antirotational, 88
History of implants, ancient implants in, 4
    blade implants in, 6, 6
    early implants in, 4
    endosteal root-form implants in, 6, 6–7, 8
    one-stage devices in, 6
    osseointegration in, 2
    sequence of development in, 2, 3
    subperiosteal implants in, 4, 5
    transosteal implants in, 6
Hollow-basket implants, examples of, 7
    Greenfield's two-piece design for, 4, 4
Host factor(s), in implant failure, 275
Howmedica Corporation, 4
Hybrid denture(s), 112–120. See also Overdenture(s).
    aesthetic considerations in, 113, 114
    diagnostic casts for, 112
    diagnostic dentures for, 114
    factors affecting construction of, 112–114
    healing period for, before implant exposure, 115

Hybrid denture(s) (Continued)
    impression technique for, 115–116, 115–116
    jaw relationship and, 113
    number of implants required for, 79, 113, 114
    patient selection for, 112–113
    prosthesis placement for, 119–120, 119–120
    stent fabrication for, 114–115
    structure of, 112, 113
    superstructure design for, 116–119, 117–119
        aesthetic considerations in, 119
        cantilever dimensions in, 117, 117, 119
        framework considerations in, 117–119, 118, 118t
        metals for frameworks in, 118
Hydrogen peroxide, for implant failure, 277
Hydroxylapatite. See also Calcium phosphate ceramics.
    bone bonding capability of, 56, 56
    bone grafting with, for small alveolar crest defects, 158–159, 159
        in maxillary sinus, 209, 211
            resorbable HA and, 209
            sintered HA particles and, 209
    composition of, 55
Hydroxylapatite-coated implants, bacterial attachment to, predominant types of bacteria in, 268, 268t
        surface roughness and, 267
    biomechanical properties of, 58, 58, 60, 60
        mechanical testing results for, 59t
    in primary mandibular reconstruction, case history of, 248
    in secondary mandibular reconstruction, case histories of, angle-to-angle defect, with free osteocutaneous graft, 254
        in irradiated field, 244, 245
    in secondary maxillary reconstruction, case history of, 253, 254
    removal of coating in, by Cavi-jet/Prophy-jet treatment, 276
Hyperbaric oxygen therapy (HBO), after radiation therapy, bone graft survival and, 243
        case history of, 244
    improved implant integration with, 51
Hypertension, preoperative assessment of, 18–19

Iliac crest, as bone graft source, for composite bone graft, 233
        in full-arch onlay graft, 233, 234
        in interpositional graft, 238, 239–240
        in sinus inlay graft, 234, 235–236
    for maxillary sinus, 211, 215–216, 219–220
    for maxillofacial reconstruction, case history of, 248
Implant(s), ailing, 269
    as substitute for bridges, 168
    biomechanics of, 61–71. See also Biomechanics of dental implants.
    coatings for, 56–58, 58, 59t, 60, 60. See also Hydroxylapatite-coated implants.
    colonization by and accumulation of bacteria on. See under Bacteria, oral.
    early, 4, 4
    exposure of, 153–156. See also Exposure of implants.
    gold, 4
    health of, probing depth as measure of, 260, 260
    history of, 2–7. See also History of implants.
    IMZ, 2, 7, 8
    ITI, 7, 8
    legal aspects associated with, 281–287. See also Legal aspects of implants.
    loading of. See also Loading of implants.
        premature, 49

Implant(s) (Continued)
    malpositioned, solutions for, 79
    periodontal status of, 260–263. See also Periodontal status
        of implants.
    placement of, in extraction sites. See Extraction site(s),
        placement of implants in.
    preloading of, failure due to, 261
    screw-retained, 87–92. See also Screw-retained
        implants.
    titanium. See Titanium implant(s).
Implant design. See also Biocompatible materials.
    antirotational screw design in, 88, 88
    calcium phosphate ceramic coatings in, 58, 58, 59t, 60, 60
    direct bone apposition and, 56, 57
    hollow-basket design in, 7
        Greenfield's two-piece, 4, 4
    legal aspects of, 286
    Linkow blade implant designs in, 5, 6
    one-stage endosteal pins, screws, and cylinders, 6
    oral hygiene considerations in, implant failure and, 274,
        274–275
    porous ingrowth attachment and, 56–58, 57
    root-form, as dominant design, 2
        endosteal, 6, 6–7, 8
    subperiosteal, 4, 5
    transosteal, 6
Implant failure, bacterial role in, 265, 274, 274–275. See
        also Bacteria, oral.
    possible mechanisms of, 270–271
    types of bacteria in, 269–270
    bone loss in, as sign of integration loss, 260, 261
        horizontal, therapy of, 276
        irregular and vertical, therapy of, 276–279, 278–279
    causes of, 274
    hard tissue problems in, 274
    host factors in, 275
    legal aspects of, 287
    motion at bone-implant interface and, 61
    of implants anchored in bone graft alone, 225
    oral hygiene and, 76, 274–275
    parafunctional habits in, 275
    plaque accumulation and, 261, 274, 274
    prosthesis fabrication and fit in, 275
    prosthetic problems in, 274–275
    social habits and, 275
    soft tissue problems in, 274
    traumatic, 274
        vs. infectious, 269
    treatment of, 276–279
        antibiotic therapy in, 276, 277
        follow-up care in, 279
        for soft tissue problems, 276, 277
        regenerative therapy in, 276–279, 278–279
Implant fixation techniques. See Fixation technique(s).
Impression post(s), impression tray required for, 105, 106
    in overdenture fabrication, 105, 105
    in transfer of fixed prosthodontics, 129, 129–130
Impression technique(s), for fixed prosthodontics, 128
    transfer system for, 128–130, 128–130
    for hybrid dentures, 115–116, 115–116
    for overdentures, 102–103
        double-impression type of, 103–106, 104–106
        single-impression type of, 106–109, 106–109
IMZ implant, examples of, 7
    plasma-spray press-fit, 2, 8
Incisal guide angle(s), occlusal planning and, 142
Incision(s), 150–153
    anterior mandibular, 150–151, 151
    breakdown of, after maxillary sinus bone grafting, 221
        prevention of, 152

Incision(s) (Continued)
    for maxillary sinus bone graft, 210–211
    maxillary, 152–153, 153
    posterior mandibular, 151–152, 152
Infection(s). See also Bacteria, oral.
    as contraindication to implant placement in extraction
        site, 157–158
    control of, for fixed prosthodontic preparation, 130
Inferior alveolar nerve. See Alveolar nerve, inferior.
Inflammation, around implant. See Peri-implantitis.
Inflammatory phase, of wound healing, 45, 46t
Informed consent, documentation of, 284
    for bone grafting of atrophic edentulism, 226
    legal aspects of, 284
Inlay composite graft, of maxillary sinus, 234, 235–238
Interarch space, determination of, 82
    for hybrid dentures, 113
    occlusal planning and, 140–141, 140–141
Interleukin-1 (IL-1), implant failure and, 270, 271
Interlock system, antirotational, 88, 88
Interpositional composite graft, with LeFort I osteotomy,
    234, 238–240, 239–240
Intramobile element, in implant connected to tooth, 69,
    124, 139
ITI implants, 7, 8

Jaw. See also Mandible; Maxilla.
    as class 3 lever, 63, 63
    edentulous. See Edentulous jaw.
Jaw relation, diagnostic cast for determining, 82
    hybrid denture construction and, 113
    occlusal planning and, 140–141, 140–141
    pre-prosthetic evaluation of, 77
    prognathic (Cl III), 113
    record of, in overdenture fabrication, 108
    retrognathic (Cl II), 113
Joint-separating force(s), clamping force vs., 89, 89
    definition of, 88
    excursive contacts in, 90
    implant attachment to natural teeth and, 91
    lateral excursions in, 90, 90
    maximizing resistance to, 91–92, 92
    minimizing, 90–91, 90–91
    non-passive frameworks and, 91, 91
    off-axis centric contacts in, 90, 91
Junctional epithelium, in implant healing, 48

Keratinized gingiva. See Gingiva, keratinized.

Labial plate, alveolar maxillary, 27, 28, 28–29
Lateral cephalometric radiographs, 36, 37, 38
LeFort I osteotomy, with interpositional composite graft,
    234, 238–240, 239–240
Legal aspects of implants, 281–287
    abandonment and, 283
    approved implant types and, 286
    charting and record-keeping requirements and, 284–286
    comparative negligence and, 283
    continuing education and, 287
    duty to refer and, 284
    implant failure recognition and, 287
    informed consent and, 284
    malpractice, defined, 282
    patient confidentiality and, 283–284

Legal aspects of implants (*Continued*)
   patient selection and, 286
   plaintiff's proof and, 282
   planning issues and, 286
   practitioners' experience and, 286–287
   professional relations and, 281–282
   public expectations and, 281
   punitive damages and, 282
   respondeat superior principle and, 283
   restorative/occlusal issues and, 286
   statute of limitations in, 282–283
   types of litigation in, 282
Lidocaine, for local anesthesia, 150
Lingual artery, sharp injury to, life-threatening hemorrhage
   from, 25
   sublingual branch of, 25
Lingual foramen, 25
Lingual nerve, anatomy of, 21
Linkow blade implant design, 5, 6
Lip, flap development in, during incision, 151, *151*
   prosthetic support of, 113, 123
Loading of implants. See also *Preload.*
   in fixed prosthodontics, considerations in, 132
      transitional and provisional, 128
   in single-tooth restorations, 133, 134
   overloading in, bone loss due to, 139
   preloading in, implant failure due to, 261
   premature, wound healing and, 49
   progressive concept of, 143
Loosening of screw-retained implants. See *Screw-retained*
   implants, loosening of.

Macrophage(s), endotoxin-activated, in implant failure, 270
Magnetic resonance imaging, 43
Malpositioned implants, solutions for, 79
Malpractice. See also *Legal aspects of implants.*
   definition of, 282
   statute of limitations and, 282–283
Mandible. See also *Jaw.*
   abnormal movement of, occlusal planning and, 142
   anatomy of, 21–25
   anterior, implant placement into extraction sites in, 158
   body region of, 21, *22*
   bone quality of, wound healing related to, 50
   dehiscence defect of, case history of guided tissue regen-
      eration for, 197, *200–202*
   incisions of, crestal, 151, *151*
      in anterior mandible, 150–151, *151*
      in posterior mandible, 151–152, *152*
      vestibular, 151, *151*
   inclination of teeth in, 28
   inferior alveolar nerve location in, 21, 22–24, *24*
   number of implants required in, for hybrid dentures, 79,
      113, *114*
      for overdentures, 99
   primary reconstruction of, case history of bone grafting
      in, 248, *249–250*
   relationship of, to maxilla, diagnostic cast for determining,
      82
      hybrid denture construction and, 113
   residual ridge resorption of. See *Alveolar ridge, resorp-*
      tion of.
   saddle deformity of, alveolar nerve and, 175
   secondary reconstruction of, for angle-to-angle defect, in
      irradiated field, case history of, 254, *255–256*
      in irradiated field, case history of, 244, *245–246*
      in nonirradiated field, case history of, 244, *247*, 248
   symphysis region of, 24–25, *24–25*

Mandibular canal, anatomy of, 21–22, *22–23*, 24
Mandibular foramen, anatomy of, 21–22, *22*
Maturation phase, of wound healing, 45, 46t
Maxilla. See also *Jaw.*
   alveolar arch morphology of, 27–29, *28–29*
      labial plate in, 27, 28, *28–29*
      palatal plate in, 27, 28, *28–29*
   anatomy of, 27–31
   anterior, implant placement into extraction sites in, 158,
      159, 163, *163–165*, 166
   bone quality of, wound healing and, 50
   bone volume determination in, by panoramic radiographs,
      36, *37*
   expansion of maxillary sinus into, 29–30, *30*
   implant-supported overdentures in, 95
   incision of, 152–153, *153*
   inclination of teeth in, 27, *28*
   location of implants in, for hybrid dentures, 113, *114*
   mucosal tissues of, 30–31, *31*
   number of implants required in, 79
   osseous foundation of, 27, *27*
   phonetic problems and, 80, 142
   reconstruction of, case history of bone grafting in, 248–
      249, *251–253*, 254
   relationship of, to mandible, diagnostic cast for determin-
      ing, 82
      hybrid denture construction and, 113
   residual ridge resorption in, changes in, 12, *12*
      combination syndrome in, 12, *14*
      intermaxillary relationship changes in, 12–13, *13*
      prosthetic considerations in, 13, 15
      soft tissue changes in, 13
   transfer of masticatory forces in, 27, *27*
Maxillary sinus, anatomy of, 29–30, *30*
   bone grafting of, 206–221
      allogeneic grafts in, 208
      alloplastic materials in, 209
      autogenous bone in, 208, *212–215*
      choice and behavior of materials for, 208–209, 211,
         212–220
      classification of alveolar bone in, 207t
      clinical results of, 207t, 211, 220–221
      complications of, 221, *221*
      cortical-cancellous bone in, 208, *216–220*
      demineralized bone in, 208–209
      freeze-dried bone in, 208
      history of, 206
      hydroxylapatite in, 209, 211
      incision design for, *210–211*
      inlay composite graft in, 234, *235–238*
      onlay grafts in, 208
      perforation of sinus membrane in, *211*
      surgical procedures for, 209–211, *211*
      treatment planning for, 206–208, 207t
   CT imaging of, 36, *37*, 209
   expansion of, into alveolus, 29–30, *30*
   ostium of, 30, *30*
Maxillofacial reconstruction, 242–257
   bone grafting in, 242–244
      after trauma, case history of, 226–228, *227–229*
      nonvascularized grafts in, 242, 243
      radiation effects and, 243–244
      two-phase theory of osteogenesis in, 243
      types of grafts in, 243
      vascularized grafts in, 242–243
         case history of, 248–249, *251–253*, 254
   primary mandibular, in nonirradiated field, case history
      of, 248, *249–250*
   secondary mandibular, for angle-to-angle defect, in irradi-
      ated field, case history of, 254, *255–256*

Maxillofacial reconstruction *(Continued)*
in irradiated field, case history of, 244, *245–246*
in nonirradiated field, case history of, 244, *247*, 248
secondary maxillary, in nonirradiated field, case history of, 248–249, *251–253*, 254
Mechanical factors, in residual ridge resorption, 10, *11*
Medical evaluation, 17–20
cardiovascular assessment in, 17–18, 18t
elements of, 17
of coronary artery disease, 19–20
of healthy patient, 20
of hypertension, 18–19
Medical-legal aspects of implants. See *Legal aspects of implants.*
Medication(s). See also specific medication.
implant failure and, 275
Mental foramen, panoramic radiographs for locating, 33, 36
Mental fossa, 24, *24*
Mental protuberance, 24, *24*
Mental tubercle, 24, *24*
Mentalis muscle, chin laxity and, 151
Mepivacaine (Carbocaine), 18
Metal biomaterial(s), 47t, 80
Metronidazole, for spirochete infection, 270
Millipore filter(s), in guided tissue regeneration, 184, *184*
Minerals, wound healing and, 50
Mobility, definition of, 68
of implant, factors in, 138–139
testing for, 276
stiffness and, 68
Moment, exposure of implants to, 64, *64*
Mucoepidermoid carcinoma, primary mandibular reconstruction after, case history of, 248, *249–250*
Mucogingival junction, 31
Mucoperiosteal-implant interface, wound healing and, 47–48, *49*
Mucoperiostium, 31
Mucosal tissue, 30–31
alveolar, around implants, implant failure related to, 274
keratinized gingiva *vs.*, 260–261, *261*
masticatory, 31
keratinized, 30
non-keratinized, 30
of hard palate, 31, *31*
Mylohyoid ridge, anatomy of, 21, *22*
Myocardial infarction, preoperative assessment of, 19

Nasopalatine nerve and vessel, in alveolar bone loss, 28
Natural teeth. See *Tooth (teeth).*
Negligence, duty to refer and, 284
respondeat superior principle and, 283
Newton, as unit of force, 64
Nicotine, wound healing and, 19
Nonrotational implant system, for retrievable prostheses, 79
for single implants, 79
Nutritional status, wound healing and, 50

Occlusal force(s), implant failure due to, 261, *262*, 262, 275
in natural teeth *vs.* implants, 139
overloading of implants by, bone loss due to, 139
Occlusal surface materials, 80–81
Occlusion, 138–146
abnormal mandibular movements and, 142
arch form and, 139–140, *140*
balanced, bilateral, 145, 146
full-balance, 109

Occlusion *(Continued)*
bone support and, 143–144, *143–144*
centric, 143
choice of schemes for, 143
condylar guide angle and, 142
cuspid disclusion in, 144, *144*, 145
disclusion of posterior teeth in, 143
flat plane type of, 109
for overdentures, implant-borne, 109
tissue-borne, 108–109
group function type of, 143, 144, *144*
impact load in, 138–139
incisal guide angle and, 142
interarch distance and jaw relationship in, 140–141, *140–141*
legal issues related to, 286
lingualized, 109
of implants, in edentulous patient, 145–146
in partially edentulous patient, 144–145, *144–145*
lack of proprioception with, 138, 139
orientation of occlusal plane and, 141–142
phonetic considerations in, 142, *142–143*
pre-prosthetic considerations in, 81
requirements for, 138, 139
soft tissue attachments and, 141, *141*
stress load transfer in, 138–139
Off-axis centric contact, as joint-separating force, 90, *91*
OmniVac machine, 84
Onlay graft(s), full-arch composite, *233, 234*, 235
of maxillary sinus, 208
types of, for atrophic edentulism, 223
Onplant(s), in orthodontic treatment, 171–173, *171–173*
Oral bacteria. See *Bacteria, oral.*
Oral hygiene, bacterial colonization and, 267–268, 268t
for hybrid dentures, 113, 115
around abutments, 119–120
lack of, bone loss due to, 267
patient commitment to, in pre-prosthetic evaluation, 76
prosthesis design and, implant failure related to, *274*, 274–275
O-ring attachment(s), 79, 98t, 101, *102–103*
Orthodontic treatment, implant(s) in, 167–173
advantages and disadvantages of, 167–169
animal studies of, 167
as anchor, 169, *169–170*
as onplant, 171–173, *171–173*
for orthopedic development, 169, 171, *171*
movement of, with vertical elongation of alveolus, *168*, 168–169
submergence of, 169
patient compliance in, 167
Osseointegration. See also *Bone-implant interface; Fixation technique(s).*
biology of, *46*
discovery of, 2
hydroxylapatite-coated implants and, 58, *58*, 59t, 60, *60*
importance of, in history of dental implants, 6
life-table analysis of, *3*
surgical fit of bone to implant in, 49–50, 61
with bioinert materials, 54
Osteoclast(s), PGE_2-activated, implant failure and, 270
Osteoconduction, in bone healing, 243
Osteogenesis, two-phase theory of, 243
Osteoinduction, in bone healing, 243
Osteoporosis, wound healing related to, 50–51
Osteosarcoma, secondary mandibular reconstruction after, case histories of, 248–249, *251–253*, 254, *255–256*
Osteotomy, for maxillary sinus bone graft, *210*
LeFort I, with interpositional composite graft, 234, 238–240, *239–240*

Ostium, of maxillary sinus, 30, *30*
Overdenture(s), 94–109. See also *Hybrid denture(s).*
  advantages of, 94
  double impression techniques for, 103–106, *104–106*
  implant systems for support of, 95–96, *95–96*
    criteria for selecting, 96
  implant-borne, *99–100,* 99–103
    advantages of, 94
    attachments for, *100,* 100–102, 101t, *103–104*
    cementable-type superstructure in, 100
    disadvantages of, 95
    fabrication of, 102–103
    impression techniques for, 102–103
  jaw relation records for, 108
  number of implants for support of, 79, 99, *99*
  occlusion for, 108–109
  single impression techniques for, 106–109, *106–109*
  success rate with, 94, 95
  tissue-borne, 96–99
    attachments for, 97, *97,* 98t
    multiple implants in, 97–99
    splinting of, 99
  types of, 95

Palatal plate, alveolar maxillary, 27, 28, *28–29*
Palate, flap development in, for aesthetic restorations, 155, *156*
  grafting of, for creation of keratinized gingiva, 155–156
  hard, median raphe of, 31, *31*
    mucosal tissue of, 31, *31*
    implant location in, 166
Palatine bone(s), transfer of masticatory forces by, 27, *27*
Panoramic radiographs, 33, 36, *36–37*
Papilla(e), preservation of, during implant exposure, 155
Parafunctional habits, occlusal force generated by, 275
Partial edentulousness. See *Edentulous jaw, partial.*
Patient confidentiality, 283–284
Patient education, pre-prosthetic, 76
Patient selection, for bone grafting, of atrophic edentulism, 225–226
  for hybrid dentures, 112–113
  legal aspects of, 286
Pellicle, acquired, in bacterial adhesion, 266
Peptostreptococcus micros, implant failure due to, 269
Periapical radiographs, 33
Peri-implant sulcus, 48
Peri-implantitis, as indication of periodontal status, 260
  bacterial colonization and, 266
  due to plaque accumulation, 262
  implant failure due to, bacterial colonization and, 269–270
Periodontal status of implants, 260–263
  bacterial accumulation in, 262. See also *Bacteria, oral.*
  bone loss in, 261–262, *262*
    loss of integration due to, 260, *261*
    occlusal forces and, 262, *262*
    radiographic evaluation of, 261, *262*
  follow-up care and, 262–263, *262–263*
  inflammation in, 260
  plaque accumulation in, 262
  probing depth in, 260, *260*
  soft tissues in, 260–261, *261*
Periodontitis, bacteria associated with, 269
  guided tissue regeneration for, barrier materials for, 185–186
    Gore-Tex periodontal material in, 184, *185*
PerioTest mobility device, 276
Personnel, dental. See *Staff, dental.*

Phonetics, occlusal planning and, 142, *142–143*
  pre-prosthetic planning for, 80
  with hybrid dentures, 117
Physical evaluation, pre-prosthetic, 75
Placement of implants, in extraction sites. See *Extraction site(s), placement of implants in.*
Plaintiff's proof, in malpractice cases, 282
Planning. See *Radiologic planning; Treatment planning.*
Plaque accumulation, as cause of implant failure, 261, 274, *274*
  on high-energy titanium implant surface, 266
  on implant abutment cylinders, 267
  peri-implantitis due to, 262
Platinum/palladium alloy, for frameworks, 118
Plunger-type attachment(s), 98t, 101
Polycrystal alumina (PA), surface roughness of, bacterial colonization and, 267
Polylactic acid membranes, in guided tissue regeneration, 185
Polymeric biomaterials, surface and interface properties of, 47t
Polysiloxane impression material, 104
Porcelain, as occlusal surface material, 80
Porous ingrowth attachment mechanisms, 56–58, *57*
Porphyromonas gingivalis, implant failure due to, 269
  in periodontitis, 269
  in plaque, 267, 268
Postoperative care, for guided tissue regeneration, 195–196
Practitioner(s). See *Dentist(s).*
Preload, biomechanics of, 69–71, *70*
  development of, torque in, 89, *90*
Preloading of implants. See also *Loading of implants.*
  failure due to, 261
Premature loading of implants, 49. See also *Loading of implants.*
Prevotella intermedia, implant failure due to, 269
  in periodontitis, 269
  in plaque, 267, 268
Probing depth, as measure of implant health, 260, *260*
Prognathic jaw relation (Cl III), 113
Proliferative phase, of wound healing, 45, 46t
Prophy-jet, 276
Prostaglandin E$_2$ (PGE$_2$), implant failure and, 270
Prosthesis retrievability, advantages of, 87
  cemented abutments and, 87
  nonrotational implant system for, 79
Prosthodontics, 74–85
  aesthetics of, 79–80
  arch length and, 82
  arch width and, 81, *81*
  clinical evaluation in, 75–77
    dental, 76
    for chief complaint, 75
    general physical, 75–76
    of bone, 76–77
    of ridge relationships, 77
    of soft tissue, 77
    psychological, 76
  diagnostic casts in, 81–82
  diagnostic wax-up in, 82–84, *83*
  fixed, 122–135
    abutment head selection for, 130–131, *131*
    aesthetic considerations in, 132, *132*
    clinical and biomechanical considerations in, 122–126
    connection to teeth in, 124–125, *124–125*
    crown-to-root ratio in, 125, 125t, *126*
    direct connection of restoration to implant in, 132, *132*
    direction of forces along implants and, 125–126
    fabrication of restorations for, 128–130
    hard tissue factors in, 122–123

Prosthodontics (*Continued*)
    implant orientation in, 125–126
    impression technique for, 128
    infection control for, 130
    laboratory considerations for, 130–132
    loading forces on, 132
    metal framework for, 131–132, *132*
    number of implants for, 124
    provisional or temporary restorations in, 127–128, *127–128*
    retrievable *vs.* cementable restorations in, 126–127, *126–127*
    single-tooth restoration considerations in, *123*, 132–135
        anterior, *134*, 134–135
        posterior, *133*, 133–134
        retention issues in, *134–136*, 135
        treatment planning for, 132–133, *132*, 133t
    soft tissue factors in, 123, *123*
    spacing of implants for, 123–124, *124*
    transfer systems for, 128–130, *128–130*
    transitional and provisional loading of, 128
    types of restorations required in, 122
    interarch space and, 82, *82*
    maxillomandibular relationships in, 82
    number of implants required and, 78–79, *79*
    occlusal requirements in, 81. See also *Occlusion.*
    occlusal surface materials in, 80–81
    phonetic considerations in, 80
    prosthetic requirements and, 77–78, *78–79*
    radiographic evaluation in, 77, *77*
    surgical stent in, 84–85, *83–85*
    team approach *vs.* individual practitioner and, 75
Proxy brush, for oral hygiene around abutments, 120
Pseudomonas aeruginosa, implant failure due to, 269
Psychological evaluation, pre-prosthetic, 76
Punitive damages, in malpractice cases, 282

Radiation therapy, bone grafting after, 243–244
        in secondary mandibular reconstruction, 244, *245–246*
        of angle-to-angle defect, with free osteocutaneous graft, 254, *255–256*
    wound healing related to, 51
Radiography, for inferior alveolar nerve injury, 179, *179*
    for placement of implants in extraction sites, 159
    in evaluation of implant health, 261, *262*
    lateral cephalometric, 36, *37*, 38
    panoramic, 33, 36, *36–37*
    periapical, 33
Radiologic planning. See also *Treatment planning.*
    computed tomography in, 38, *39–43*, 43
    conventional tomography in, 38
    decision-making process in, for mandibular implants, *35*
    for maxillary implants, *34*
    legal aspects of, 286
    magnetic resonance imaging in, 43
    pre-prosthetic, 77, *77*
Reconstructive maxillofacial surgery. See *Maxillofacial reconstruction.*
Records. See *Dental records.*
Referral to specialists, 284
Regeneration, in wound healing, 45
Reparative healing, 45
Residual intraosseous defect. See *Alveolar ridge, defects of.*
Residual ridge resorption. See *Alveolar ridge, resorption of.*
Respondeat superior principle, 283
Retrognathic jaw relation (Cl II), 113
Ridge, alveolar. See *Alveolar ridge.*
Risk management. See also *Legal aspects of implants.*

Risk management (*Continued*)
    continuing education for, 287
Root-form implant, as dominant design, 2
    endosteal, 6, *6–7*, 8
Rotary instruments, heat and trauma from, implant failure due to, 274
    wound healing and, 48, 49

Saddle deformity, mandibular, alveolar nerve and, 175
Saliva, in bacterial adhesion and colonization, 266, 267
Scapula, implant placement in, for secondary mandibular reconstruction, 254, *255*
    osteocutaneous free graft from, in secondary maxillary reconstruction, 249, *251*, 254
Screw joint, biomechanics of, 69–70, *70*
    definition of, 88
Screw mechanics, 88–90. See also *Biomechanics of dental implants.*
    clamping force in, 88–89
    joint-separating forces in, 88–89
    preload in, 89, *90*
    torque in, 89, 89–90
Screwdriver, for torque application, 89
Screw-retained implants, 87–92
    cemented abutments and, 87, *88*
    limitations on screw size in, 90
    loosening of, 87–88
        joint-separating forces in, 90
        maximizing resistance to, 91–92, *92*
        minimizing, 90–91, *90–91*
        prevention of, 88, *88*, 92
    prosthesis retrievability and, 87
    segmented *vs.* nonsegmented, 87, *87*
    undertightening of, 92
Sedation, intravenous, 150
Sex factors, in residual ridge resorption, 10, *11*
SIM/PLANT software, for computed tomography, 38, *42–43*, 43
Single-tooth restoration(s), 132–135
    anterior, *134*, 134–135
    occlusal scheme for, 145
    posterior, *133*, 133–134
    retention methods for, *134–136*, 135
    treatment planning for, *132*, 132–133, 133t
Sinus, maxillary. See *Maxillary sinus.*
Sinusitis, after maxillary sinus bone grafting, 220, 221
Skalak model, *66–67*, 69, *70*
Slant-lock type of attachment, *99*, 101t
Smile line, fixed prosthetics and, 123, *123*
    hybrid dentures and, 113, *114*
    single-tooth restoration and, 134
Smoking, wound healing and, 19
Smoothness of implant surface, bacterial attachment related to, 266, 267
Social habit(s), implant failure and, 275
Soft tissue(s). See also *Gingiva.*
    changes of, in residual ridge resorption, 13, *14*
    grafting of, for placement of implants in extraction sites, 163, 166
    implant failure related to, 274
        treatment of, 276, 277
    occlusal planning and, 140–141, *140–141*
    preferred type of, around implant, 260–261, *261*
    quantity of, for fixed prosthetic implants, 123
Spark-erosion attachment(s), *100*, 101t
Spinous foramen, 25
Spirochetes, implant failure due to, 270, *270*
    in periodontitis, 269

Spirochetes *(Continued)*
in plaque, 267, 268, 268t
Splinting, of implant-borne overdentures, 99
Squamous cell carcinoma, secondary mandibular
reconstruction after, case histories of, 244, *245–247,*
248
Staff, dental, patient confidentiality issues and, 283–284
respondeat superior principle and, 283
Standard of care, definition of, 282
determined by expert witness testimony, 282
Staphylococcus aureus, implant failure due to, 269–270
Staphylococcus epidermidis, implant failure due to, 269–270
Statute of limitations, in malpractice cases, 282–283
Stent(s), clear acrylic, fabrication of, 84–85, *83–85*
for bone graft placement, 224, *224*
case history of, 227, *227*
for hybrid dentures, 114–115
in computed tomography (CT), 38, *41*
for implant placement in extraction sites, 159, 163,
165
Stiffness, coordinate system for, 68
creep and, 68
definition of, 68–69
displacement and, 68
mobility and, 68
of abutments, 69
of tooth connected to implant, 69
Streptococcus sanguis, 266, 267
Streptococcus species, colonization of tooth surface by, 267,
268, 268t
implant failure due to, 269
Stress, acrylic resin for reducing, 139
implant angulation and, 68
increased bone mass in response to, 167
Stress-breaking attachment(s), 97, 98t, *100*
Strock, placement of first long-term implant by, 4
Stud-type attachment(s), 98t, 101, *102*
placement of, during overdenture fabrication, 107
Subgingival bacteria. See *Bacteria, subgingival.*
Sublingual fossa, anatomy of, 21, *22*
Submandibular fossa, anatomy of, 21, *22*
Subperiosteal implants, history of, 4, *5*
Sulcus, creation of, aesthetic considerations in, 155
peri-implant, 48
Superfloss, for oral hygiene around abutments, *119,* 120
Superstructure. See also *Framework(s).*
for hybrid dentures, 116–119, *117–119*
aesthetic considerations in, 119
cantilever dimensions in, 117, *117,* 119
framework considerations in, 117–119, *118,* 118t
metals for frameworks in, 118
for implant-borne overdentures, cementable-type, 100
Surface(s), conditioning film on, 266
occlusal, materials for, 80–81
oral, bacterial adhesion to, 266–267
smoothness of, bacterial colonization and, 266–267
Surgeon, responsibilities of, in team approach to
prosthodontics, 75
Surgical stent(s). See *Stent(s).*
Surgical technique, bone-implant fit in, wound healing and,
49–50
trauma in, wound healing and, 48–49
Swiss anchor attachment(s), 98t, 101, *102*
Symphysis, mandibular, anatomy of, 24–25, *24–25*

Team approach, to prosthodontics, 75
Teeth. See *Tooth (teeth).*
Template(s), clear acrylic. See *Stent(s).*

Temporomandibular joint disease, legal issues related to,
286
Tensile force, exposure of implants to, 63
on abutments, preload and, 69–70
Tetracycline, for implant failure, 277
Thread compound(s), antivibrational, 88
Tissue-borne overdenture(s), 96–99. See also
Overdenture(s).
Titanium implant(s). See also *Biocompatible materials.*
bacterial attachment to, 262, 266–267
predominant types of bacteria in, 268, 268t
surface smoothness and, 266, 267
biocompatibility and biomechanics of, 55
chemical bonding of, to bone, 46–47
grit-blasted, *vs.* hydroxylapatite-coated implants, 58, *58,*
59t, 60, 60
protection of, against scratching, plastic or nylon probes
for, 260, *260*
screw-shaped, development of, by Brånemark, 6, *7*
tightening forces tolerated by, 92
with composite bone grafts, in full-arch onlay graft, 234,
235
in interpositional graft with LeFort I osteotomy, 238,
240, 240
in sinus inlay graft, *236–237*
Titanium-aluminum-vanadium (Ti–6A1–4V) alloy, 55
Tomography, computed. See *Computed tomography (CT).*
conventional, 38
Tooth (teeth), bacterial adhesion to, 266–267
bacterial colonization of, compared with implants, 266
congenitally missing, single-tooth restoration for, 133
connection of, to implants, biomechanics of, 69
in fixed prosthetics, 124–125, *124–125*
crown-to-root ratio in, 124, 125t, *126*
intramobile element in, 69, 124, 139
joint-separating forces and, 91
extraction of, alveolar bone resorption after, 10
guided tissue regeneration around, 183–186, *184–185*
maxillary, inclination of, 27, *28*
occlusal force of, implants *vs.,* 139
Torque, attachments for controlling, 101, *102*
countertorque mechanisms and, 92
definition of, 89
exposure of implants to, 64, *64*
factors limiting application of, 89
in clamp load, 89
maximum values for, 92
mechanisms for controlling, 88, *88*
optimum tightening, calculation of, 89–90
preload development and, 89, *90*
Torque wrench(es), 88, 89
Tort litigation, 282
Trace elements, wound healing and, 50
Transfer copings, for fixed prosthodontics, 129, *129*
for hybrid denture impressions, 115–116, *116*
for overdenture impressions, 104, *104*
Transfer system, for fixed prosthodontics, 128–130, *128–130*
for overdentures, implants transferred instead of abutments in, 108, *108*
Transosteal implants, 6
Trauma, during surgery, wound healing and, 48–49
from rotary instruments, implant failure due to, 274
to alveolar nerve. See *Alveolar nerve, inferior, injuries to.*
Treatment planning. See also *Radiologic planning.*
for bone grafting, of maxillary sinus, 206–208, 207t
for placement of implants in extraction sites, 157–158
for single-tooth restorations, *132,* 132–133, 133t
legal aspects of, 286
Tribasic calcium phosphate ceramics, 55. See also
Hydroxylapatite.

Vestibular incision, of anterior mandible, 151, *151*
Vicarious liability, 283
Vitamin C, wound healing related to, 50
Vitamin D, wound healing related to, 50
VK-II glenoid fossa prosthesis, 244, *247*
Vomer, transfer of masticatory forces by, 27, *27*

Wax-up. See *Diagnostic wax-up.*
Wilson, curve of, 27
Witch's chin, 151
Withdrawal of care, 283
Wolff's law, 167
Wolinella recta, implant failure due to, 269
  in periodontitis, 269
Women, residual ridge resorption in, 10, *11*
Wound healing, 45–51
  aging and, 50–51
  bone healing in, 45–46, *46*, 47t
  bone quality in, 50
  bone-implant contact and, 49–50
  bone-implant interface in, 46–47, 47t–48t

Wound healing *(Continued)*
  cigarette smoking and, 19
  corticosteroid therapy and, 51
  diabetes mellitus and, 51
  factors affecting, 48
  health status of patient in, 50–51
  hematologic disorders and, 51
  inflammatory phase of, 45, 46t
  maturation phase of, 45, 46t
  mucoperiosteal-implant interface in, 47–48, *49*
  nutritional status of patient and, 50
  premature loading of implants and, 49
  proliferative phase of, 45, 46t
  radiation therapy and, 51
  regeneration in, 45
  reparative, 45
  surgical trauma and, 48–49
Wrench, for torque application, 88, *89*

Zygomatic bones, transfer of masticatory forces by, 27, *27*